MECHANISMS OF VIRUS DISEASE

VOLUME
ONE

ICN ICN-UCLA SYMPOSIA
ON
MOLECULAR & CELLULAR BIOLOGY

MECHANISMS
OF
VIRUS
DISEASE

EDITED BY

WILLIAM S. ROBINSON
Stanford University

C. FRED FOX
University of California, Los Angeles

W. A. Benjamin, Inc.
Menlo Park, California. Reading, Massachusetts.
London. Don Mills, Ontario. Sydney

Science

RC
114.5
M4

ISBN 0-805-38340-9

ISBN 0-8053-8340-9
ABCDEFGHIJ-HA-7987654

TABLE OF CONTENTS

IV. VIRUSES IN CHRONIC CENTRAL NERVOUS SYSTEM DISEASE

V. WHERE IS THE VIRUS OF HUMAN HEPATITIS?

VI. MECHANISMS OF CELL TRANSFORMATION BY DNA TUMOR VIRUSES

VII. CELL TRANSFORMATION BY RNA TUMOR VIRUSES

VIII. CONTROL MECHANISMS FOR PHAGE

CONTENTS

IX. ONCOGENIC HERPES VIRUS

PREFACE

Mechanisms of Virus Disease was the final conference of the 1974 winter symposia on topics in molecular and cellular biology sponsored by ICN Pharmaceuticals, Inc. and organized through the Molecular Biology Institute of the University of California, Los Angeles. It is the first conference in this series which attempted to integrate research on biological problems at the basic and clinical levels.

The formal presentations in this conference focused on the basic biological and molecular processes that occur in virus infection and on their relation to the disease state. The factors that determine the course of virus infection in an intact host are complex and include multiple host-directed processes as well as the properties of the individual viruses. In an attempt to gain a more thorough understanding of the events following infection by disease-causing viruses, the program was constructed to include virologists working at the most fundamental level, those working with models of animal virus disease and those who encounter virus-mediated diseases at the clinical level. We hoped that in this way the conference might promote useful discussions and exchanges of ideas and stimulate research at all levels. We are indebted to the session chairpersons, Thomas Merigan, Frank Lilly, Alice Huang, Bernard Fields, Walter Eckhart, Hidesaburo Hanafusa, George Miller and Mark Ptashne, who designed and organized the individual sessions and are largely responsible for the success of the conference.

We are grateful to the Life Sciences Division of ICN Pharmaceuticals, Inc. for their continued support of this series, and to the National Cancer Institute for granting travel funds for speakers at this conference. We also express gratitude to Hans Neurath, editor of *Biochemistry* and to the editorial boards of the *Journal of Virology* and the *New England Journal of Medicine* for publishing announcements of this meeting in their respective journals. Finally, for extraordinary efforts in our behalf we thank Bettye Knutsen and George Sullivan of United Air Lines, Los Angeles for arranging travel; William Parson, Olive Nielson and the Olympic Village Hotel staff; Charlotte Miller and Fran Stusser of the ICN-UCLA conference staff; and Adrian Perenon of W.A. Benjamin, Inc.

William S. Robinson, Stanford University

C. Fred Fox, University of California, Los Angeles

I

IMMUNOLOGICAL INJURY IN VIRUS DISEASE

AUTOREACTIVITY AND LEUKEMOGENESIS

M. R. Proffitt,M. S. Hirsch, and P. H. Black

Department of Medicine,
Harvard Medical School;
Massachusetts General Hospital,
Boston, Massachusetts 02114.

ABSTRACT. In recent years there has been much circumstantial evidence for a close relationship among viruses,
autoimmune phenomena, and oncogenesis. A central defect
stemming from virus infection of host immunocytes might
alter the capacity of those immunocytes to distinguish
self from nonself antigens. In support of this, we review
evidence that during the couse of leukemogenesis induced
by Moloney murine leukemia virus (MuLV-M), thymus cells
from congenitally infected mice (carriers) exhibited a
vigorous cell-mediated reactivity against noninfected,
syngeneic target cells during both the preneoplastic and
neoplastic periods. Identically derived, but MuLV-M
infected, target cells were usually spared. Transplantable
thymic lymphoma cells retained this pattern of reactivity.
With spleen and lymph node lymphocytes from young carrier
mice, reactivity against MuLV-M infected target cells, but
not against noninfected target cells, was seen; like thymocytes, lymphocytes from older carrier mice were reactive
against noninfected target cells. The autoreactivity by
carrier thymocytes was apparently mediated by MuLV-M
infected, theta antigen positive, cortisone resistant cells.

INTRODUCTION

A number of mechanisms may account for the triggering
of autoimmune responsiveness in conjunction with virus
infections: First, virus infection of certain cells might
lead to the release of an antigen(s) with which host
immunocytes have never interacted because of "sequestering"
of the antigen(s) early in ontogeny. Second, a virus might

3

share antigenic determinants with normal host cell membrane constituents thereby causing an anti-viral response to be directed against normal host cells. This would be especially true for viruses which "bud" from cell membranes. Third, certain virus infections might lead to the expression on host cell membranes to antigens "masked" of "repressed" during ontogeny prior to the development of immunologic recognition of self. All of these mechanisms would reflect a pathological expression of normal immunocyte reactivity. A fourth mechanism by which a virus might initiate autoimmune responsiveness would constitute a central defect wherein virus-infected immunocytes no longer would be capable of functioning normally in distinguishing self from nonself antigens; that viruses can alter normal immunocyte functions is well established (1, 2,3). Both direct (4,5) and indirect (6) roles for virus in the induction of a central lymphocyte defect leading to autoimmunity and eventually malignant lymphoproliferation have been postulated. Despite their inherent attractiveness, the latter hypotheses have lacked necessary experimental support, although in recent years there has been much circumstantial evidence for a close relationship among viruses, autoimmune phenomena, immunodeficiency, and oncogenesis (5,7,8). Recently, we demonstrated that during the course of leukemogenesis induced by Moloney murine leukemia virus (MuLV-M), thymus cells from congenitally infected mice (carriers), exhibited a vigorous cell-mediated autoreactivity during both the preneoplastic and frankly neoplastic periods (9). We now review evidence that MuLV-M-infected, theta antigen bearing thymocytes are the mediators of this reactivity. Moreover, transplantable lymphoma cells established from a carrier mouse exhibit reactivity against uninfected syngeneic target cells, linking the malignancy to the proliferation of functionally aberrant lymphoid cells.

MATERIALS AND METHODS

For our studies we used male mice from a colony of C3H/HeJ mice carrying MuLV-M since birth (carriers). Normal C3H/HeJ mice served as controls. C3H/HeJ embryo cell lines of common origin infected with MuLV-M or not infected were used as target cells for thymocyte or lymphocyte microcytotoxicity assays. Whereas 90 to 100% of the infected target cells were producing infectious MuLV-M, uninfected target cells were negative for virus (10). Establishment of the carrier colony and the target cell lines, and the virus used have been described (10).

Thymocyte suspensions were prepared from the pooled thymuses of three to four carrier or normal mice. Both weanling (4 weeks old) and adult (12 weeks old) mice were used, depending on the experimental design. Lymphocyte suspensions were prepared from the spleen and lymph nodes of individual mice. Procedures for the preparation of thymocyte and lymphocyte suspensions have been described (9,10).

An in vitro microcytotoxicity assay (10) was used to determine the effect of MuLV-M induced lymphoma cells (9, 11) or of thymocytes or lymphocytes (effector cells) from normal or carrier mice at different ages when reacted against syngeneic target cells. Briefly, target cells were suspended in culture medium, then added to flat-bottom 96 well microtest plates. In early experiments approximately 100 target cells were added to each well; in later experiments, approximately 150 cells were added. Eighteen hours later, effector thymocytes, lymphocytes or lymphoma cells were added to each well. After incubation for 48 hours, the effector cells were removed and the target cells were fixed, stained and counted. Infected target cells usually plate less efficiently than non-infected target cells (9); this difference is reflected in Table 1. The reductions in number of target cells by carrier thymocytes should be compared with reduction of that same target cell by normal thymocytes (group comparison in Table 1 should be made horizontally).

RESULTS

Thymus cells from both weanling (3-4 weeks old) and adult (12-16 weeks old) carrier mice were vigorously reactive against normal, noninfected target cells (Table 1). The percent target cell reduction by adult carrier thymocytes (37-87%) usually was greater than that of weanling carriers. Thymus cells from normal mice, on the other hand, often had a stimulatory effect on the growth of noninfected target cells when compared to the same tar-

5

get cells cultured in medium alone. In most cases normal thymus cells were not stimulatory to infected target cells. In contrast to their reduction of noninfected target cells, carrier thymocytes usually had little, if any, effect on infected target cells.

Dose-response data (Table 2) showed that, relative to noninfected target cells grown in medium alone, carrier thymocytes caused a significant reduction (48-77%) of those target cells at thymocyte-to-target cell ratios of 1000:1 or greater; again, normal thymocytes significantly enhanced the growth of noninfected target cells. However, with respect to infected target cells grown in medium alone, carrier thymocytes caused a significant reduction of those cells only at a ratio of 5000:1. Even at that ratio, the reduction (38%) was less than the reduction of normal target cells (77%). As with normal target cells, normal thymocytes slightly enhanced the growth of infected target cells in this experiment.

Having previously observed that thymus cells from a carrier mouse with overt thymic lymphoma were reactive against syngeneic target cells in a pattern similar to that shown by thymocytes from preleukemic carriers (9), transplantable lymphoma cells derived from the thymus and lymph nodes of a lymphomatous carrier mouse (11) were tested for their ability to react against syngeneic target cells (Table 3). At ratios of 1000:1 or 100:1, the lymphoma cells caused a significant reduction of noninfected target cells when compared to the target cells grown in medium alone. Again, normal control thymus cells slightly stimulated the growth of noninfected target cells. Against infected target cells, however, the lymphoma cells were reactive only at a ratio of 1000:1; even at this ratio, the percent reduction was less than the percent reduction of normal target cells at a ratio of 100:1. Normal thymus cells were slightly stimulatory to the growth of infected target cells at ratios of 100:1 or less, whereas at 1000:1, there was a slight reduction of target cells. Whether this represents a low-level cell-mediated immunity against endogenous MuLV (crossreactive with MuLV-M) is not clear; however, the presence of humoral antibodies against endogenous MuLV in mice is well documented (12,13).

Recently, we showed that viable thymocytes are necessary to mediate carrier thymocyte reactivity against non-infected syngeneic target cells. Moreover, close thymocyte-target cell interaction rather than mediators apparently is responsible for the reaction (14). Further studies were done to characterize the thymocyte population(s) involved in these reactions (14). A summary of these studies is presented in Table 4. The reactive cells, present in a light buoyant density fraction of nonadherent cells when fractionated on Ficoll-Hypaque gradients (9), have a lymphoid morphology. Antisera directed against the H-2^K-histocompatability antigen of C3H mice and against the theta-C3H antigen, which serves as a marker for thymus-derived T cells (15), were effective in eliminating the reactive thymocyte population in the presence of rabbit complement. On the other hand, antiserum against mouse immunoglobulin determinants (IgG) present on bone marrow-derived lymphocytes (15) did not remove the reactive cells. In addition, antiserum with specificity against MuLV antigens was also effective in eliminating reactive carrier thymocytes, indicating that thymocytes infected with MuLV-M are directly involved in mediating reactivity against noninfected target cells. The reactive thymocyte population of carrier mice was not removed by treating the mice with hydrocortisone. In fact, the ratio of corticosteroid resistant to sensitive thymocytes was nearly five times greater in carrier than in normal mice (14).

Although most thymocytes in normal adult mice are immunologically immature, have a high representation of theta antigen, a low representation of H-2 histocompatibility antigens and are sensitive to corticosteroids, a small fraction of thymocytes ($<$ 5%) with a lighter buoyant density can respond immunologically. This small subpopulation of "mature" cells has a high representation of H-2 antigen, is corticosteroid resistant and mediates cellular immune responses (15,16,17,18,19,20). The thymocytes in the mature subpopulation can still be identified as thymus-derived T cells by the presence of surface theta antigen, although the antigen is present in much lower amounts than it is in the immature subpopulation (15,19,21). Our data indicate that the reactive carrier thymocytes probably belong to this normally small subpopulation of "mature" cells which has expanded during the course of infection by MuLV-M.

7

In view of these observations, we examined the effects of spleen and lymph node lymphocytes from early (8-12 weeks old) and late (16-17 weeks old) preleukemic carrier mice on infected and noninfected syngeneic target cells. As indicated in Table 5, lymphocytes from 7/10 preleukemic carriers (aged 8-12 weeks and showing no overt evidence of lymphoma) were reactive against infected target cells, while lymphocytes from only 1/10 of these mice reacted against noninfected target cells. In contrast, 3/3 older preleukemic carriers (aged 16-17 weeks; also not overtly lymphomatous, but having markedly involuted thymuses) reacted against noninfected target cells whereas lymphocytes from 0/3 of these mice were significantly reactive against infected target cells. The appearance in older preleukemic carriers of spleen and lymph node lymphocytes with reactivity against noninfected syngeneic target cells apparently reflects the spread of reactivity first evident in the thymus. This is coincident with the time at which lymphoma cells allegedly metastasize from the thymus (22, 23). Similarly, autoreactive lymphocytes appear in aging NZB mice (24), a strain noted for an increased incidence of autoimmune disease and lymphoma (reviewed in reference 25).

Since transplantable lymphoma cells from carrier mice were reactive against syngeneic target cells, we believe that the process of lymphomagenesis in carrier mice may represent a metastatic lymphoproliferation of autoreactive immunocytes. Figure 1 is a schematic representation of the events which may occur in the process of lymphomagenesis in carrier mice.

DISCUSSION

Our observations suggest that at least some lymphoproliferative disorders may result from expression of virus-induced clones of lymphocytes with autoreactivity; these disorders might or might not remain self-limited depending on the relationships between the autoreactive cells and host cells active in immune surveillance. We have shown that thymocytes of carrier mice from weanling age to adults react against noninfected, syngeneic target cells in vitro and that lymphoma cells derived from carrier mice also exhibit this pattern of reactivity. Furthermore, the

reactive thymocytes were sensitive to treatment with antisera against both MuLV and theta antigen, indicating that
they are virus-infected, thymus-derived cells. If autoreactive cells lead to the destruction of normal lymphocytes active in host defense, then unrestricted proliferation of the autoreactive clones might occur, culminating
in disseminated leukemia or lymphoma. In this context, we
have preliminary data which indicate that thymocytes from
leukemia virus carrier mice are cytotoxic when reacted
against normal syngeneic thymus cells (unpublished observations). If, on the other hand, immunologically compe-
tent host lymphocytes were not targets for destruction by
autoreactive cells, then they might themselves be able to
contain the spread of autoreactive clones. The results of
such an interaction might be a self-limited lymphoproliferative disorder.

All of this, of course, presupposes a selective, complex interaction among viruses and immunocytes. That such
complex interactions do occur is becoming increasingly
apparent (1,2,3,26,27). For example, it now appears that
a herpes virus, the Epstein-Barr (EB) virus, which is
closely associated with malignant Burkitt's lymphoma in
some populations and nasopharyngeal carcinoma in others,
also is present in the lymphocytes of patients with infectious mononucleosis (28). Antibodies against a variety of
autoantigens (29) including those common to thymocytes and
a subpopulation of lymphocytes occur in patients with
infectious mononucleosis (30). Moreover, their lymphocytes
are transiently hyporeactive to certain mitogens (29,31)
and antigens (29). Based on immunoglobulin producing capability of lymphoblastoid cell lines derived both from patients with infectious mononucleosis and from patients with
Burkitt's lymphoma, bone marrow-derived B lymphocytes
appear to be targets for EB virus infection (32). It is
unclear why infectious mononucleosis is self-limited whereas Burkitt's lymphoma is malignant (28). The course of EB
virus infection may be determined by a subtle interaction
between EB virus and the host's lymphoid cells. Environmental (33) and/or genetic (34,35) factors could be determinants in the type of disease that eventually occurs.

In addition to Burkitt's lymphoma and infectious mononucleosis, the evidence suggesting viral participation in
other human autoimmune and lymphoproliferative diseases is

9

increasing. Cytomegalovirus (CMV) can cause a mononucleosis syndrome very similar to EB virus-associated infectious
mononucleosis (36) with a variety of associated immuno-
pathologic disturbances (37). Although human patients
having systemic lupus erythematosis (SLE) display a pano-
rama of autoimmune disorders (38), it is unclear whether
they have an increased incidence of lymphoid neoplasia
(38,39,40). Virus-like structures appear in the lymphocytes of many SLE patients (41,42) and their offspring
(43). Other human autoimmune disorders such as Sjögrens
syndrome are associated with a higher than normal incidence
of lymphoma (44,45) and virus-like structures not unlike
those seen in the lymphocytes of SLE patients have been
observed in lymphocytes from these patients (42). A
variety of autoimmune disorders are commonly associated
with malignant lymphoproliferative diseases such as
Hodgkin's disease and chronic lymphocytic leukemia, in
which viral etiologies have been suggested (46,47). Thus,
it appears that similar sequences of events, i.e. virus
infections, autoreactivity and lymphoproliferative diseases
may be applicable for me as they appear to be for mice.

ACKNOWLEDGMENTS

We should like to thank Drs. B. Gheridian and I. F. C.
McKenzie for helpful advice and aid during the course of
these studies. We also thank Mr. D. A. Ellis and Ms. B.
Allitto for expert technical assistance and Ms. L. Parlee
for aid in preparation of the manuscript.

M. R. Proffitt is a Special Fellow of the Leukemia
Society of America. These studies were supported in part
by PHS grant CA 12464-03 and Contract NIH-NO1-CP-43222 of
the Virus Cancer Program of the National Cancer Institute.

REFERENCES

1. A.L. Notkins, S.E. Mergenhagen and R.J. Howard, Ann.
   Rev. Microbiol. 24, 525 (1970).
2. E.F. Wheelock and S.T. Toy. Adv. in Immunol. 16, 123
   (1973).
3. P. Häyry, D. Rago and V. Defendi, J. Nat. Cancer Inst.
   44, 1311 (1970).
4. N.F. Stanley and N.-I.M. Walters, Lancet 1966-I, 962
   (1966).

5. J.G. Sinkovics, et al, In: Genetic Concepts and Neo-plasia. Williams and Wilkins Co., Baltimore (1970), pp. 138-190.
6. P. Bretscher, Cellular Immunol. 6, 1 (1973).
7. F.M. Burnet,Cellular Immunology. Melbourne University Press,Melbourne (1969), pp. 255-285.
8. W. Dameshek, In: Carcinogenesis: A Broad Critique. Williams and Wilkins Co., Baltimore, (1967), pp. 141-155.
9. M.R. Proffitt, M.S. Hirsch, and P.H. Black, Science 182, 821 (1973).
10. M.R. Proffitt, M.S. Hirsch and P.H. Black, J. Immunol. 110, 1183 (1973).
11. M.R. Proffitt, M.S. Hirsch, B. Gheridian, I.F.C. McKenzie and P.H. Black, in preparation.
12. M.B.A. Oldstone, T. Aoki and F.J. Dixon, Proc. Nat. Acad. Sci. 69, 134 (1972).
13. M.G. Hanna, Jr., et al., Cancer Res. 32, 2226 (1972).
14. M.R. Proffitt,M.S. Hirsch, I.F.C. McKenzie, B. Gheri-dian and P.H. Black, in preparation.
15. M.C. Raff, Transplant. Rev. 6, 52 (1971).
16. H. Blomgren and B. Andersson, Exp. Cell Res. 57, 185, (1969).
17. M.A. Levine and H.N. Claman, Science 167, 1515 (1970).
18. M.C. Raff, Nat. New Biol. 229, 182 (1971).
19. D.E. Mosier and C.W. Pierce, J. Exp. Med. 136, 1484 (1972).
20. E. Leckband and E.A. Boyse, Science 172, 1258 (1971).
21. T. Aoki, et al., J. Exp. Med. 130, 979, (1969).
22. R. Siegler, Experimental Leukemia, M.A. Rich (Ed.) Appleton-Century-Crofts, New York, (1968), pp. 51-98.
23. D. Metcalf, The Thymus, Springer Verlag, New York, (1966), pp. 100-117.
24. C.R. Stiller, et al., Clin. exp. Immunol. 15, 445 (1973)
25. J. East, Progr. Exp. Tumor Res. 13, 84 (1970).
26. M.S. Hirsch, et al., Proc. Nat. Acad. Sci. 69, 1069, (1972).
27. S.B. Halstead, J.S. Chow and N.J. Marchette, Nature New Biol. 243, 24 (1973).
28. M.A. Epstein and B.G. Achong, Ann. Rev. Microbiol. 27, 413 (1973).
29. Editorial, Lancet 1973-II, 712 (1973).
30. D.B. Thomas, Lancet 1972-I, 399 (1972).
31. A.D. Rubin, Blood, 28, 602 (1966).

32. J.L. Fahey, et al., Science 152, 1259 (1966).
33. D. Burkitt, J. Nat. Cancer Inst. 42, 19 (1969).
34. A.O. Williams, J. Med. Genetics 3, 177 (1966).
35. R.S. Bar, et al., New Eng. J. Med. 290, 363 (1974).
36. T.H. Weller, New Eng. J. Med. 285, 203 (1971).
37. G.L. Kantor, et al., Ann. Internal Med. 73, 553 (1970).
38. H.R. Holman, In: Immunological Diseases M. Samter (Ed.), Little, Brown Co., Boston, 1971, pp. 995-1013.
39. G.J. Goldenberg, F. Paraskevas and L.G. Israels, Semin. Arthritis Rheum. 1, 174 (1971).
40. C.K. Smith, J.T. Cassidy and G.G. Bole, Amer. J. Med. 48, 113 (1970).
41. G.A. Andres, H. Spiele and R.T. McCluskey, Prog. Clin. Immunol. 1, 23 (1972).
42. P.M. Grimley, J.L. Decker, H.J. Michelitch and M.M. Frantz, Arthritis Rheum. 16, 313 (1973).
43. J.H. Klippel, P.M. Grimley and J.L. Decker, New Eng. J. Med. 290, 96 (1974).
44. K.J. Bloch and A.R. Myers, In: Immunological Diseases. M. Samter, (Ed.), Little, Brown and Co., Boston, 1971, pp. 1172-1177.
45. A.M.S. Mason, J.M. Gumpel and P.L. Golding, Semin. Arthritis Rheum. 2, 301 (1973).
46. R. Hehlmann, D. Kufe, and S.Spiegelman, Proc. Nat. Acad. Sci. 69, 435 (1972).
47. R. Hehlmann, D. Kufe, and S. Spiegelman, Proc. Nat. Acad. Sci. 69, 1727 (1972).

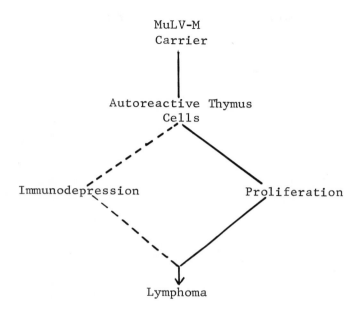

Fig. 1   Lymphoma in mice infected with MuLV-M as neonates may represent the culmination of a complex series of interactions between MuLV-M and the immune system. The virus may infect and nonspecifically activate a variety of cells in the thymus with potential reactivity against various antigens, including self. Moreover, noninfected immunocytes with reactivity against MuLV may specifically respond to virus antigens. A consequence would be "civil war" among virus-sensitized and self-sensitized, virus-infected immunocytes. Unrestrained proliferation of anti-self immunocytes might eventually be favored; this would be especially true if anti-self reactivity led to depression of normal immunocompetence or to a derangement of mechanisms controlling the immune response.

TABLE 1

Reactivity of thymocytes from MuLV-M Carrier and normal mice against MuLV-M infected and noninfected syngeneic target cells

		Mean no. of target cells remaining after reaction with the following thymocytes:[a]						
Experiment	Target cells	None	Adult normal	Adult carrier	% red.[b]	Weanling normal	Weanling carrier	% red.
A	Inf.	56	63	58	8	75	74	0
	Noninf.	84	108	26	76[c]	112	70	38[c]
B	Inf.	23[d]	18	21	0[c]	17	18	0[c]
	Noninf.	NT	38	8	79[c]	38	28	26[c]
C	Inf.	68	55	62	0[c]	NT	NT	
	Noninf.	NT	62	39	37[c]	NT	NT	
D	Inf.	37	45	40	11	NT	45	0[c]
	Noninf.	136	157	35	68[c]	NT	50	68[c]
E	Inf.	121	114	75	34[e]	NT	NT	
	Noninf.	143	164	22	87[c]	NT	NT	

a Each mean value was derived from at least 10 replicate observations. Thymocytes used in experiments A, B, C, and D were purified on Ficoll-Hypaque gradients; those used in experiment E were not purified. Effector cell to target cell ratio 5000:1.

b Percent reduction relative to the effect of normal thymocytes on infected or noninfected target cells.

c Significant reduction (p < 0.01 by paired t-tests) compared to the effect of normal thymocytes reacted against noninfected target cells.

d Not tested.

e Significant reduction (p < 0.05 by paired t-tests) compared to the effect of normal thymocytes reacted against infected target cells.

TABLE 2

Dose-response effect of thymocytes from MuLV-M carrier and normal C3H/HeJ mice against MuLV-M infected and noninfected syngeneic target cells

Mean no. of target cells remaining after reaction with the following thymocytes:[a]

Ratio[b]	Noninfected target cells					Infected target cells				
	None	Adult normal	% red.[c]	Adult carrier	% red.	None	Adult normal	% red.	Adult carrier	% red.
0	69(±3.2)					61(±4.3)				
10:1		62(±5.0)	11	76(±6.0)	<0		77(±6.0)	<0	78(±4.5)	<0
100:1		84(±7.1)	<0	56(±6.8)	19		79(±6.4)	<0	87(±4.0)	<0
1000:1		90(±9.1)	<0	36(±2.5)	48[d]		98(±4.7)	<0	71(±5.3)	<0
5000:1		102(±7.3)	<0	16(±1.2)	77[d]		88(±7.8)	<0	38(±3.9)	38[d]

a   Each mean value (± standard error) was derived from at least 10 replicate observations.

b   Ratio of thymocytes to target cells.

c   Percent reduction relative to target cells not reacted with thymocytes.

d   Significant reduction (p <0.01 by paired t-tests) compared to target cells grown in medium alone.

15

TABLE 3

Reactivity of transplantable lymphoma cells against MuLV-M infected and noninfected syngeneic target cells

Target cells	Ratio[b]	Mean no. of target cells remaining after reaction with the following effector cells:[a]				
		None	Normal thymus	% red.[c]	Lymphoma	% red.
Inf.	0	130($\pm$7.9)				
	10:1		145($\pm$14.5)	< 0	137($\pm$8.9)	< 0
	100:1		157($\pm$15.3)	< 0	140($\pm$11.3)	< 0[d]
	1000:1		101($\pm$17.5)	23	82($\pm$7.5)	37
Noninf.	0	144($\pm$6.3)				
	10:1		151($\pm$12.7)	< 0	158($\pm$7.0)	< 0[d]
	100:1		152($\pm$12.2)	< 0	69($\pm$4.2)	52[d]
	1000:1		168($\pm$8.5)	< 0	34($\pm$3.1)	77[d]

[a]   Each mean value ($\pm$ standard error) was derived from at least 10 replicate observations.

[b]   Ratio of effector cells to target cells.

[c]   Percent reduction relative to target cells not reacted with effector cells.

[d]   Significant reduction ($p < 0.01$ by paired t-tests).

TABLE 4

Characteristics of autoreactive
MuLV-M carrier thymocytes

Cell type		Sensitivity to various antisera	
Lymphoid morphology	yes	Anti-theta	yes
Nonadherent	yes	Anti-IgG	no
Corticosteroid resistant	yes	Anti-H-2^k	yes
MuLV-M infected	yes		

TABLE 5

Reactivity of lymphocytes from MuLV-M carrier mice of
different ages against MuLV-M infected and noninfected
syngeneic target cells

Target cells	No. of mice having demonstrable, significant reactivity[a]	
	Preleukemic carriers (8-12 weeks old)	Preleukemic carriers (16-17 weeks old)
Inf.	7/10	0/3
Noninf.	1/10	3/3

[a] Significant reactivity ($p < 0.05$) compared to the effect of lymphocytes from normal mice of the same age.

TISSUE INJURY AND DISEASES ASSOCIATED WITH CHRONIC VIRAL INFECTIONS: ROLE OF THE IMMUNE RESPONSE

Michael B.A. Oldstone

Department of Experimental Pathology
Scripps Clinic and Research Foundation
La Jolla, California 92037

The hypothesis that viruses may cause or be associated with chronic or degenerative diseases of man has been suggested by many investigators. Most exciting is the realization within the last few years that this hypothesis may, in fact, be true for certain diseases. With this realization, which is based mainly on experimental models in animals and partly on observations in humans (reviewed in 1,2), has come the understanding that viruses may infect tissues throughout the life of the host and usually not be cytopathic per se.

In virtually every such viral infection a significant and often disease producing immune response is elicited from the host. This immune response may cause disease by formation of antiviral antibodies and their subsequent interaction with virus or viral soluble antigens in the circulation forming immune complexes that deposit in various tissues and produce injury (1,3). Another mechanism of antiviral antibody caused injury is interaction of antibody with infected cells carrying virus induced antigens on their surfaces. For this reaction to result in injury, viral antigens must be accessible to bind with antibody and complement must be activated (reviewed in 4). Viruses may also stimulate aberrant immune responses, such as antibodies to nuclear antigens or DNA, which lead to autoimmune disorders (5). In contrast to enhancement of aberrant immune responses, viruses may also cause immunosuppressive effects (6, reviewed in 7,8).

Evidence for virus-antibody immune complex disease can be gathered by demonstrating virus-immunoglobulin (presumably antiviral antibody) complexes in the circulation and in showing localization of virus, antiviral antibody and complement at the site of tissue injury. That virus travels in the circulation complexed to immunoglobulin and complement can be demonstrated by several different techniques. The first demonstration of virus complexed to host immunoglobulin and complement occurred when immune specific removal of either immunoglobulin or complement from the serum of animals chronically infected with virus resulted in significant reduction of serum infectivity titers (reviewed in 2). In contrast, removal of albumin or fibrinogen did not lower the serum infectivity titer, which indicated that decreased serum infectivity was due to removal of an immunoglobulin-virus or complement-immunoglobulin-virus complex and not due to nonspecific coprecipitation and trapping. Precipitation of a virus-antibody complex with an antibody directed towards the antibody or complement bound with the virus has been used successfully to demonstrate circulating virus-antibody immune complexes in mice chronically infected with lactic dehydrogenase virus, lymphocytic choriomeningitis virus, Moloney leukemia and murine sarcoma viruses, mink infected with Aleutian disease virus, horses infected with equine infectious anemia virus, and man infected with Australian antigen (hepatitis B virus).

Other techniques employed to show circulating virus-antibody immune complexes are C1q agar precipitation, complement utilization, electron microscopy with direct visualization, analytical ultracentrifugation, monoclonal rheumatoid factor precipitation, platelet agglutination, and assays in which cultured cells having receptors for bound C3 are used (reviewed in 9). These findings imply that in chronic viral infection there is a deficiency in the humoral surveillance mechanism since virus can persist in the circulation in infectious form despite being bound to both antiviral antibody and complement.

Deposition of circulating virus-antibody complexes in tissues is best demonstrated by identifying virus or viral antigen products, immunoglobulin and complement in a granular pattern along the basement membranes of several tissues. Immunofluorescent and electron microscopic study of tissues containing immune complexes are characteristic (2,10). Studies of tissues from animals and man with immune complex disease indicate that the renal glomeruli, the choroid plexus in the brain and blood vessels throughout the body are the main sites of immune complex deposits. Other tissues in which immune complex deposits have been found include the joints, uvea, and heart valves. Of all these tissues the renal glomeruli are most frequently involved.

After demonstrating the presence of host immunoglobulin deposited in a tissue, it is necessary to immunochemically dissociate the antigen-antibody bonds, recover the immunoglobulin and determine its specificity. This is usually done by eluting the immunoglobulin from tissues in which immune complexes are deposited with 3 M potassium or sodium chloride buffers, 0.01 M citrate, or glycine hydrochloric buffers (pH 2.8 to 3.0). Although these studies have limitations, most notably loss of eluted antibody via recombination with antigens, incomplete elution and denaturation of antibody, they nevertheless provide the only direct identification and quantitation of antibodies present in injured tissues.

As immune complexes occur in most if not all viral infections in which there are both ongoing viral replication and continuous host immune response, tissues which trap and concentrate antigens and antibodies, e.g., renal glomeruli, may well be a fruitful source for markers identifying agents causing or associated with diseases presently of unknown etiology. For example, in the spontaneously occurring leukemia of AKR mice which is known to be caused by Gross leukemia virus, we have been able to demonstrate a high incidence of immune complex deposits in the renal glomeruli (11) and to elute, recover and identify several antibodies present in the deposits. These antibodies show specificity to Gross virus cell surface antigen and to Gross virus envelope antigen, as well as blocking activity for murine reverse transcriptase (12,13). Hence, there is much interest in reports of immune complex deposits being found in the kidneys of patients with cancer and leukemia (14) as well as in patients with chronic degenerative diseases of unknown

21

etiology, such as amyotrophic lateral sclerosis (15).

In addition to the combination of virions and soluble virus antigens with antibody in the circulation to form immune complexes, there is recent evidence from our laboratory that antibody can redistribute and concentrate viral antigens on the plasma membrane (capping) with the resultant extrusion of virus-antibody-plasma membrane complex in the fluid phase. This stripping of viral antigens from the plasma membrane of infected cells not only changes the distribution of virus antigens in and on the cell, but also affects the ability of antibody and complement to lyse such a cell and provides a ready source of fluid phase virus-antibody complexes. In this regard, the blocking factors found in many tumor systems usually are demonstrated to be antigen-antibody complexes (17,18). When these complexes become trapped in tissues, they provide the opportunity for detection and identification. The further elucidation of mechanisms of formation and deposition of immune complexes and their subsequent recovery and identification will not only define a number of diseases currently listed as being due to unknown mechanisms, but may also help to identify the etiologic agents of these disorders.

ACKNOWLEDGMENTS

This is publication number 829 from the Department of Experimental Pathology, Scripps Clinic and Research Foundation, La Jolla, California. This research was supported by USPHS grants AI-09484 and AI-07007, Contract No. NO1 CP 33204 within the Virus Cancer Program of the National Cancer Institute, and the Violet June Kertell Memorial Grant for research on Multiple Sclerosis from the National Multiple Sclerosis Society. The author is a recipient of Career Development Award AI-42580 AID from the USPHS.

REFERENCES

1. M.B.A. Oldstone and F.J. Dixon, Textbook of Immuno-pathology, P. Miescher and H. Müller-Eberhard (Eds.), Grune & Stratton, in press.
2. M.B.A. Oldstone, Progress in Medical Virology, J.L. Melnick (Ed.), S. Karger, in press.
3. M.B.A. Oldstone and F.J. Dixon, J. Exp. Med. 134, 32s (1971).
4. D. Porter, Ann. Rev. Microbiol. 25, 283 (1971).
5. G. Tonietti, M.B.A. Oldstone and F.J. Dixon, J. Exp. Med. 132, 89 (1970).
6. C. Von Pirquet, Dtsch. Med. Wochenschr. 34, 1297 (1908).
7. A.L. Notkins, S.E. Mergenhagen and R. Howard, Ann. Rev. Microbiol. 24, 525 (1970).
8. M.H. Salaman, Proc. Roy. Soc. Med. 63, 11 (1970).
9. J. Exp. Med. 134 (Supp.) (1971).
10. C.G. Cochrane and D. Koffler, Adv. Immunol. 16, 185 (1973).
11. M.B.A. Oldstone, A. Tishon, G. Tonietti and F.J. Dixon, Clin. Immunol. Immunopath. 1, 84 (1972).
12. M.B.A. Oldstone, T. Aoki and F.J. Dixon, Proc. Nat. Acad. Sci. 69, 134 (1972).
13. V.W. Hollis, T. Aoki, O. Barrera, M.B.A. Oldstone and F.J. Dixon, J. Virology 13, 448 (1974).
14. J.C. Sutherland and M. Martinez, J. Nat. Cancer Inst. 50, 633 (1973).
15. M.B.A. Oldstone, C.B. Wilson, D. Dalessio and F. Norris, Trans. Am. Neurol. Assoc. (1973).
16. B.S. Joseph, P.W. Lampert and M.B.A. Oldstone, J. Exp. Med., submitted.
17. B. Balwin, Adv. Biosciences, vol. 12, Vieweg, in press.
18. H. Sjögren, I. Hellström, S.C. Bansal and K.E. Hellström, Proc. Nat. Acad. Sci. 68, 1327 (1971).

An Approach to the Mechanism of Viral
Interaction with Lymphoid Cells

Barry R. Bloom, Maja Nowakowski and Shogo Kano

Department of Microbiology and
Immunology
Albert Einstein College of
Medicine
Bronx, New York 10461

25

In contrast to most of the laboratories represented
at this meeting, the basic interest of my own has been
rather far removed from virology, pathogenesis of disease
or molecular biology. Our interest is immunology, and
specifically the mechanism of cell-mediated immune responses. It has emerged over the past 10 years that there
are two principal arms of the immune response; one mediated
by circulating antibodies or immunoglobulins, and the other
by sensitized lymphocytes. Within lymphocyte populations,
there is a specialized dicotomy in that all antibody-
secreting cells arise from a bone marrow-derived or B-cell
population, while many of the cell-mediated immune reactions, such as rejection of grafts and tissues and resistance to intracellular parasites are mediated by thymus-
derived lymphocytes or T-cells.

Great progress in understanding the formation of antibodies has been made largely due to the Jerne plaque technique, a method which has permitted enumeration of individual antibody forming cells. Unfortunately, no such direct
technique has been available for enumeration of sensitized
T-cells, and it has been a major interest of my laboratory
to devise in vitro methods for doing so. In pursuit of
this goal, and, in point of fact, in sheer desperation when
other possibilities failed, we attempted to use viruses as
indicators of sensitized lymphocytes. From studies of
Wheelock (1) and Nahmias (2), to name but two, there was
abundant evidence indicating that resting lymphocytes were
rather poor producers of a variety of viruses, but upon
activation with mitogens such as PHA they rapidly acquired
the capacity to do so. The exquisite sensitivity of virological techniques was appealing, and we decided to try to
enumerate sensitized lymphocytes by an infectious centers
assay. The logic was simple: if resting lymphocytes are
non-permissive for viruses and become permissive upon
activation by specific antigens, following a period of
culture in the presence of antigen, activated lymphocytes,
following infection by an indicator virus, vesicular stomatitis virus, should be capable of producing infectious
centers. Because our interest was primarily in the cell-
mediated immune responses, we studied the activation of
lymphocytes from tuberculin sensitive guinea pigs and
humans over the course of 4 days in culture and found a
rise in infectious centers linearly with time reaching a

26

maximum in the case of guinea pig lymph node cells of 2/100 cells or in the case of highly sensitized human peripheral blood lymphocytes of approximately 5/1000 (3, 4). This was encouraging, and indicated that viruses might be useful tools for probing the activation and biology of lymphocytes.

There were two compelling questions to be considered. From the immunological point of view, it was necessary to ascertain which type of lymphocyte was being enumerated. From the point of view of the cell biology of the lymphocyte, it was of interest to understand the nature of the block in resting lymphocytes, which was overcome early upon antigen stimulation. The approach to delineating the lymphoid cell type producing virus was relatively straightforward. First, lymphoid cells were stimulated with antigens and mitogens, infected with vesicular stomatitis virus and infectious centers were compared with electron microscopical enumeration of cells associated with virus. The results indicated a reasonable degree of correlation, and the morphologic studies demonstrated that the virus producing cells were principally lymphocytes, and not other cell types (5). It has been established that selective activation of T-cells and B-cells in the mouse can be accomplished by judicious choice of mitogens, Con A stimulating essentially only T-cells, lipopolysaccharide (LPS) stimulating essentially only B-cells (6). Results of infectious center assays for cells activated by these two mitogens indicated that mouse spleens were activated only by T-cell mitogens to produce VSV infectious centers; activation of B-lymphocytes by LPS produced an almost negligible increase above background. To confirm this point, mouse spleens stimulated with Con A were treated both before and following stimulation with anti-thy.1 (anti-theta) serum, specific for a T-cell associated membrane antigen. Under these conditions, virtually all the T-cells were destroyed, and V-PFC cells were reduced by 97-99%. These studies indicate a restriction on replication of VSV by resting T- and B-leukocytes, which is removed upon antigen activation apparently only for T-lymphocytes, and that the "virus plque assay" may be a unique and useful method for enumerating activated T-cells.

The question of the nature of the restriction in non-

activated lymphocytes is a formidable one to approach.
One of the principal difficulties centers upon the fact
that even with highly sensitized cells and strong antigens
or mitogens, fewer than 10% of the lymphocytes can be activated. And it is extremely difficult to study molecular
changes in less than 10% of any cell population. Nevertheless, it has been possible to ask whether the failure of
resting lymphocytes to produce virus is caused by an inability of VSV to enter into the cell. An experimental
design similar to that employed by Wheelock and Edelman (7)
was used to provide indirect evidence on this point. In
contrast to the previous studies mentioned, in these
experiments lymphocytes were infected with VSV, washed
and cultured for 1-4 days in the absence of any mitogenic
or activating stimuli. At various periods of time,
aliquots of these virus treated cells were stimulated with
PHA, and infectious centers were counted. The results
(Fig. 2) show clearly that pretreatment with VSV initiates
a latent infection, which becomes manifest up to 4 days
later upon activation of the cells by mitogens. The results suggest that the restriction on VSV replication in
primary lymphocytes is not primarily at the level of adsorption or penetration.

In order to study more precisely the molecular basis
for this restriction, we chose to study viral replication
in cloned human lymphoblastoid cell lines as reasonable
models for primary lymphocytes to virus infection. We
have screened several lines for susceptibility to VSV,
polio and NDV, and have selected both a permissive line
(Wil-2) and a non-permissive (Raji) for these studies. In
terms of infectious centers, following infection for 24
hrs, the Wil-2 line produces 74% infectious centers while
the Raji line produces only 15%, and the restriction
applies to all 3 viruses so far tested.

The lines have an additional advantage in that they
can be synchronized, and the first question considered was
whether there was a restriction on virus replication by
the permissive cell during the cell cycle. As can be seen
from Fig. 3 infectibility was in fact a marked function of
cell cycle, maximal infectious centers being obtained when
infection was carried out during transition from G1 into
S phase of the cycle. Independent measurement of adsorp-

tion of labeled VSV to the cells showed that receptors were present throughout the cell cycle. It is interesting to note that in study of activation of latent Epstein-Barr virus in synchronized lymphoblastoid lines by Hampar et al (8), a peak of virus activation was similarly observed during G1-S transition.

VSV specific RNA synthesis in infected cells can be divided into two types: (i) primary transcription of multiple RNA species complementary to virion RNA resulting from the activity of virion associated RNA polymerase; and (ii) secondary transcription and replication of virion RNA which occurs by mechanisms not understood at present, but requiring virus specific protein synthesis (9). Therefore, uridine incorporation by VSV infected lymphoblastoid cells was examined in the presence of actinomycin D and cycloheximide as well as in the presence of actinomycin D alone (Fig. 4). In the producer line (Wil-2), incorporation of uridine was linear in the presence of actinomycin D alone for at least 10 hrs, similar to HeLa cells, while in the non-producer line, incorporation was markedly diminished. In the presence of actinomycin D and cycloheximide, the amounts of radioactivity incorporated by these two cell lines are approximately the same. Thus, inhibition of protein synthesis reduced the incorporation of ^3H uridine into VSV specific RNA by Wil-2 cells, presumably by preventing secondary transcription and replication, but had no effect on incorporation of radioactivity by VSV infected Raji cells suggesting that little secondary transcription occurred in these cells. The restriction to VSV replication in the Raji cell line was localized more precisely by means of velocity sedimentation on sucrose gradients. Figure 5 shows a sucrose gradient analysis of VSV specific RNA produced by 3 cell lines incubated with ^3H uridine between 2 and 7 hrs post-infection in the presence of actinomycin D. The 13S and 26S VSV RNAs are believed to have messenger RNA function, and the relative proportions are virtually identical in all 3 cell lines. In contrast, the relative amount of 42S virion RNA is different in each cell line, Raji being the poorest in virion RNA. Recent preliminary observations on the synthesis of the 4 major VSV proteins, as analyzed on SDS gradient acrylamide gel electrophoresis and autoradiography, indicate that the 4 major virus proteins are present even in the non-producer Raji line.

In sum, these results indicate that the restriction of RNA virus replication in these model lymphoblastoid lines occurs in late stages of infection, and is associated with secondary transcription and replication of virion RNA (14). We hope it will be possible to localize more precisely the molecular basis for the block in these cultured cells, specifically whether there is an enzymic defect or assembly block, and then to ascertain whether the same type of restriction occurs in primary lymphocytes as well.

It is interesting to speculate whether the behavior of lymphocytes towards infection by RNA viruses, which we are studying, could bear any relationship to the pathogenesis of disease. There are conceivably at least three levels at which this might occur. In the first, infection of resting lymphocytes, which themselves cannot replicate virus, might provide (i) a haven and focus for dissemination of virus, (ii) a medium for conferring latency on the virus and, (iii) upon activation with even irrelevant antigens, a source of infectious virus. The duration of latency of viruses in lymphocytes is not at all known, and is currently a subject of great interest in our laboratory. It is interesting to note, in this regard, the isolation of measles virus from tissues of patients with subacute sclerosing panencephalitis was accomplished years following measles by co-cultivation of lymph node lymphocytes (10).

The second level to which studies of virus lymphocyte interaction might have relevance concerns the immunosuppression, particularly of cell-mediated immunity, known to be associated with a variety of viral infections, the best examples being measles (11), influenza, varicella, etc. Very little is understood about the mechanisms involved; in some cases lymphocytes can be made unresponsive to antigens in vitro although they do not yield infectious virus. Nevertheless, since immunity is crucial to clearing viruses in vivo, more attention should be given to the basis for and consequences of this immunosuppression. Correlative is the question how once immunosuppression induced by viruses is manifest, it is possible for the immune system to overcome this and reassert itself.

Perhaps the most exciting possible relevance of this line of investigation pertains to the problem of viral carcinogenesis, and particularly leukemogenesis. In this regard, the demonstration of leukemia and lymphoma induction in mice undergoing graft versus host reactions or even allograft rejection by Black, Hirsch and Schwartz (13) lends credence to this possibility. It is tempting to argue that while infectious leukemia viruses may be necessary to leukemogenesis, they may not be sufficient causes; the state of permissiveness or activation of the lymphocyte target cell may be an equally crucial feature.

References

1. R. Edelman and E.F. Wheelock. Science 154:1053(1966).

2. A.J. Nahmias, S.Kibrick, R.C. Rosan. J. Immunol. 93: 69(1964).

3. Bloom, B.R., L. Jimenez, P.I. Marcus. JEM 132:16 (1970).

4. L.Jimenez, B.R. Bloom, M.R. Blume, H.F. Oettgen. JEM 133:740(1971)

5. M. Nowakowski, J. Feldman, S.Kano, and B.R. Bloom. JEM 137:1042(1973).

6. S. Kano, B.R. Bloom, M.L. Howe. PNAS 70: 2299(1973).

7. E.F. Wheelock and R. Edelman. J. Immunol. 103:429 (1969).

8. Hampar, B., Derge, J.G., Martos, L.M., Tagomets, M.A., Chang, S.Y. and Chakrabarty, M. Nature NB 244:214 (1973).

9. A.S. Huang and E.K. Manders. J. Virol. 9:909(1972).

10. Horta-Barbosa, L., Hamilton, R., Wittig, B., Fuccilo, D.A., Sever, J.L. Science 173:840(1971).

11. Von Pirquet, C.E. Arch. Int. Med. 7:259(1911).

12. A.L. Notkins, S.E. Mergenhagen, and R.J. Howard. Ann. Rev. of Microbiol. 24:525(1970).

13. M.S. Hirsch, S.M. Phillips, C. Solnik, P.H. Black, R.S. Schwartz, and C.B. Carpenter. PNAS 69:1069(1972).

14. Nowakowski, M., Bloom, B.R., Ehrenfeld, E. and Summers, D.F. J. Virol. 12:1272(1973).

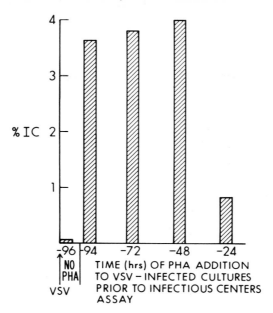

Fig. 1. Virus plaque forming cells in mitogen-stimulated
mouse spleens.

    Normal C57 B1/10 spleen cells, at 15×10^6 viable
cells/ml were stimulated by Concanavalin A (Con A) (2.5 µg/
ml), pokeweed mitogen (PWM) (1:10) or E. coli lipopolysaccharide (LPS) (100 µg/ml) for 2 days in medium RPMI 1640
supplemented with 5% heat-inactivated fetal calf serum,
2 mM L-glutamine, penicillin (100 U/ml) and streptomycin
(100 µg/ml). Con A-stimulated cells recovered from cultures were treated twice with 0.1M ⋏-methyl-D-mannoside at
37° for 10 min to remove Con A. Stimulated and control
cells were infected with vesicular stomatitis virus (VSV)
at a multiplicity of infection (moi) of 100 PFU/cell for
2 h at 37°. After adsorption cells were washed once and
treated with 0.02 ml of guinea pig anti-VSV serum for 1 h
at 4° to neutralize free virus. After three washings,
duplicate aliquots of virus-infected cells were plated in
a thin layer of agar monolayers of indicator L-cells in
60 mm plastic culture dishes; three log dilutions of each
sample were plated. The plates were incubated for 2 days
at 37° in 5% CO_2 in air, and the virus plaques were counted
after staining with neutral red. (from Ref. 6)

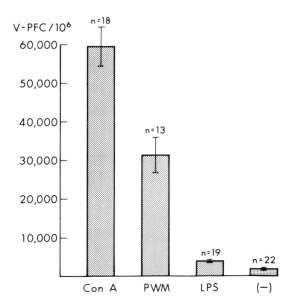

Fig. 2. PHA stimulation of virus-producing cells in pre-infected cultures.

Human peripheral blood lymphocytes were isolated by ficoll-hypaque density centrifugation. A set of cultures (1-2x10^6 cells) was prepared and all were infected with VSV at a multiplicity of infection (moi) of 10PFU/cell. One was left untreated, and to the remaining cultures PHA was added on consecutive days to a final concentration of 50 μg/ml, so that the mitogen was present for the last 24 h, 48 h, 72 h or 94 h after addition of virus. All cultures were harvested at 96 h postinfection, washed, treated with guina pig anti-VSV serum to remove free virus, and the proportion of productively infected cells was determined by the infectious centers assay.

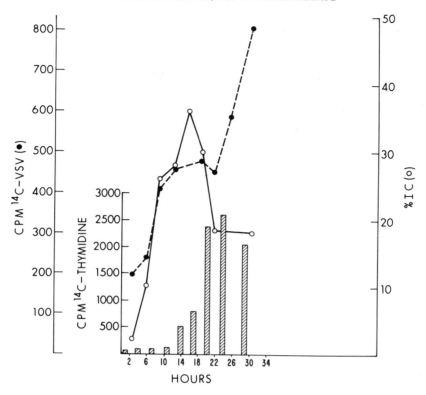

Fig. 3. Effect of cell cycle on VSV replication in Wil-2 cells.

Wil-2 cells were synchronized by medium depletion (R.A. Lerner and L.D. Hodge, J. Cell. Physiol. 77:265, 1971). At indicated times after resuspension in fresh medium, synchronized cells (2 x 10⁶) were examined for susceptibility to VSV infection in the infectious centers assay (o——o).In parallel, samples were tested for attachment of radiolabeled VSV. 3 x 10⁶ cells were incubated at 37° for 2 h with 3 x 10⁷ PFU of VSV (which had been radiolabeled with ¹⁴C-amino acids) washed, and cell-associated acid precipitable radioactivity was determined (●---●). DNA synthesis was monitored by incubating aliquots of 1 x 10⁶ cells in 1 ml of medium with 0.5 μCi of ¹⁴C-thymidine for 1 h at 37° at indicated times after refeeding, and determining the amount of radioactivity incorporated into acid-insoluble material (bars).

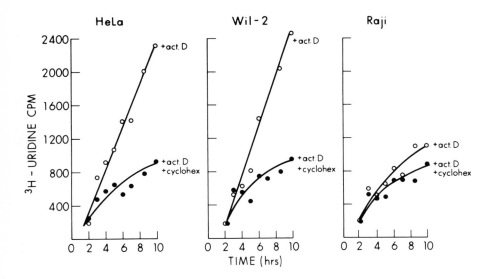

Fig. 4. Incorporation of ^{3}H-uridine by VSV-infected cells.

HeLa, Wil-2 or Raji cells (3 x 10^6 ml) were infected with VSV at an moi of 10 PFU/cell. One hour after addition of virus, actinomycin D was added to 4 µg/ml, and in duplicate samples cycloheximide was also included at a final concentration of 100 µg/ml. Incubation at 37° was continued for another hour, and ^{3}H-uridine (28 Ci/m mol) was added to a final concentration of 10 µCi/ml. At indicated times duplicate 0.1 ml samples of infected cells were transferred into 2 ml of cold Earle's salt solution, collected by centrifugation, and resuspended in 1 ml of distilled water, and 1 ml of 10% trichloroacetic acid was added. The precipitate was collected on Whatman GF/A glass fiber filters, and acid-insoluble radioactivity was determined in a Beckman L5200 scintillation counter using toluene-based scintillation fluid. (from Ref. 14)

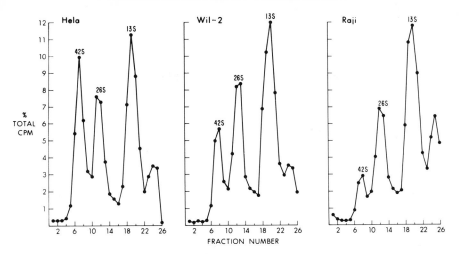

Fig. 5. Sucrose gradient analysis of VSV-specific RNA produced in HeLa, Wil-2 and Raji cells.

3×10^7 cells of each cell line (5 x 10^6 cells/ml) were infected and radiolabeled with ^{3}H-uridine as described in legend to Fig. 4. At 7 h postinfection cells were washed in cold Earle's salt solution, collected by centrifugation, and resuspended in 1.5 ml of RSB (0.01 M Tris [pH 7.2], 0.01 M NaCl, 0.0015 M Mg Cl$_2$). The cells were allowed to swell for 15 min at 4°C and were disrupted in a stainless steel Dounce homogenizer; cell disruption was monitored by phase microscopy. Nuclei were removed by centrifugation, and the supernatant cytoplasmic extracts were collected. Sodium dodecyl sulfate (SDS) was added to 0.5%, and cytoplasmic extracts were layered on 37 ml 15 to 30% linear sucrose gradients prepared in NETS buffer (0.1 M NaCl, 0.001 M EDTA, 0.01 M Tris [pH 7.0], 0.1% SDS). The gradients were centrifuged at 20°C for 17 h at 22,000 rpm in a Spinco SW27 rotor. Fractions were collected through a Guilford recording spectrophotometer to monitor optical density (OD), with cellular ribosomal RNA (28S and 18S) serving as internal OD markers in each gradient. Acid-precipitable radioactivity in each fraction was determined by scintillation counting, and plotted as % of total radioactivity. Total radioactivity per gradient was: 47,368 CPM (HeLa), 40,754 CPM (Wil-2), and 27,052 CPM (Raji). (from Ref. 14)

37

II

INFLUENCE OF HOST GENETIC FACTORS
ON VIRUS DISEASE

MURINE LEUKEMIA VIRUS

AND SPONTANEOUS LEUKEMIA IN AKR MICE

Frank Lilly, Maria L. Duran-Reynals and Wallace P. Rowe

Departments of Genetics and Pathology
Albert Einstein College of Medicine, Bronx, N.Y. 10461
Laboratory of Viral Diseases
National Institute of Allergy and Infectious Diseases
Bethesda, Maryland 20014

ABSTRACT. Tissue extracts from six-week old mice of the high leukemic AKR strain contain a high level of infectious murine leukemia virus. In F_1 mice of the cross, BALB/c × AKR ($H-2^k/H-2^d$), both the virus and the spontaneous leukemia are suppressed, due largely to the presence of the $Fv-1^b$ allele inherited from the BALB/c parent. Mice of the F_1 × AKR backcross generation were observed for possible correlations between virus expression, $H-2$ type and leukemia incidence. Only a slight correlation between virus expression and $H-2$ type was seen, but there was a very strong correlation between virus expression and leukemia and a strong correlation between $H-2$ type and leukemia.

Mice of the inbred AKR strain, which show a near 100% incidence of spontaneous leukemia occurring mostly at 8-11 months of age, also show high levels of infectious, N-tropic murine leukemia virus (MuLV) in extracts of their tissues from soon after birth *(1)*.

The transmission of each of these characteristics of AKR mice (spontaneous leukemia and presence of MuLV) has been shown in crosses of AKR with various low-leukemia, low-MuLV strains of mice to be subject to complex host genetic control. The expression of infectious MuLV is governed by at least two sorts of genes: (a) a pair of dominant genes, *Akv-1* and *Akv-2*, sometimes referred to as the "inducibility" genes, the presence of either one of which renders mice capable of expressing infectious virus *(2)*; and (b) a regulatory gene, *Fv-1 (3)*, which, depending on its type,

TABLE 1

Characteristics of parental and F_1 hybrid mice of the cross, BALB/c × AKR

Trait	AKR	(BALB/c × AKR) F_1	BALB/c
H-2 type	H-$2^k/H$-2^k	H-$2^k/H$-2^d	H-$2^d/H$-2^d
Fv-1 type	Fv-$1^n/Fv$-1^n	Fv-$1^n/Fv$-1^b	Fv-$1^b/Fv$-1^b
Akv-1 and Akv-2	Akv-$1/Akv$-1	Akv-$1/$-	-/-
	Akv-$2/Akv$-2	Akv-$2/$-	-/-
Leukemia incidence	90% (8-11 mo.)	4% (>1 yr.)	low (>1 yr.)
MuLV expression	100% (10^{3-4}) (4)	83% ($10^{1.7}$) (4)	20-60% (low titer late in life)

permits or suppresses the spread of MuLV, and hence its expression, in *Akv-1*- and/or *Akv-2*-positive mice *(4)*. The occurrence of spontaneous leukemia is also influenced by at least two sorts of genes: (a) *Rgv-1*, a gene located within the complex *H-2* region of linkage group IX, the effects of which may be mediated by immunologic mechanisms *(5)*; and (b) a pair of dominant genes, presumably identical with *Akv-1* and *Akv-2*, which govern the expression of MuLV group-specific antigen in outcrosses of AKR mice *(6)*.

THE EXPERIMENT

The present study was undertaken in order to examine the relationship between MuLV expression, *H-2* type and the occurrence of leukemia in mice of the cross, BALB/c × AKR, which has not previously been studied in these respects. Mice of the BALB/c strain ($H-2^d/H-2^d$, $Fv-1^b/Fv-1^b$) show only a low incidence of N-tropic MuLV in their tissues, invariably expressed at low titers late in life *(7)*. F_1 hybrids of the cross BALB/c × AKR ($H-2^k/H-2^d$, $Fv-1^n/Fv-1^b$) show a markedly reduced titer of the virus by comparison with parental strain AKR mice ($H-2^k/H-2^k$, $Fv-1^n/Fv-1^n$) *(4)*. Both BALB/c and (BALB/c × AKR) F_1 mice show only a very low incidence of spontaneous leukemia, occurring much later in life than that in AKR mice *(7,8)*. These characteristics of mice of this cross are summarized in Table 1.

Backcross mice from the mating (BALB/c × AKR) $F_1♀$ × AKR♂ were raised in our own colonies. At six weeks of age, a 1 cm. segment of the tail was clipped from each mouse and stored at -70°; after prolonged storage, individual tail samples were extracted in cold saline, and the extracts were assayed for MuLV activity by the XC cell method *(9)*, using NIH Swiss mouse embryo cells as targets. (Due to the prolonged storage of the tail segments before the virus assays were performed, the titers of MuLV were lower than those expected from fresh preparations.) At 2-3 months of age the animals were tested individually for *H-2* type by the hemagglutination method *(10)*, using erythrocytes obtained by eye-bleeding and a hemagglutinating alloantiserum [(C57BL/6 × AKR) F_1 anti-BALB/c normal tissues] specific for antigens governed by the $H-2^d$ haplotype of the BALB/c grandparent. Thereafter the backcross animals were observed for the development of leukemia, as scored by the detection of markedly enlarged lymphoid organs (thymus,

TABLE 2

Leukemia incidence among mice of the (BALB/c × AKR) × AKR backcross generation, according to MuLV expression (presence or absence at six weeks of age) and *H-2* type

MuLV	*H-2* type	N	Leukemic	Number of mice dead: Nonleukemia	Not autopsied	Alive
+	*kk*	94	61 (65%)	3	5	25
	kd	79	35 (44%)	7	6	31
	subtotal	173	96 (56%)	10	11	56
–	*kk*	72	10 (13%)	15	2	45
	kd	90	5 (6%)	6	3	76
	subtotal	162	15 (9%)	21	5	121
Total		335	111 (33%)	31	16	177

spleen and/or lymph nodes) prior to death and at autopsy.
The experiment was terminated and the remaining mice
(52.8%) were sacrificed when the youngest reached the age
of 19 months, at which time deaths from leukemia had become
extremely rare.

Of the 335 mice for which complete $H-2$ and MuLV typing
data were obtained, 166 (49.6%) were homozygous $H-2^k/H-2^k$
and the rest were heterozygous $H-2^k/H-2^d$. 173 mice (51.6%)
showed detectable infectious MuLV in their tail extracts.
A small but only marginally significant association was
apparent between $H-2$ type and the presence of MuLV: 94/166
(56.6%) of $H-2^k/H-2^k$ homozygotes showed virus, whereas 79/
169 (46.7%) of $H-2^k/H-2^d$ heterozygotes did so (P≈0.08).
Thus $H-2$ type can be only a minimally important factor in
the control of virus expression in these mice.

The occurrence of leukemia among these backcross mice
is summarized in Table 2. 111 clearly leukemic deaths occurred, for an overall leukemia incidence of 33.1%. 47
mice (14.0%) died before the completion of the experiment
either from nonleukemic causes (31, 9.3%; most of these
were males severely damaged by fighting) or from unknown
causes (16, 4.8%) because no autopsy was performed.

The disease was very closely correlated with the presence of MuLV among these mice: 96/173 (55.5%) MuLV-posi-
tive mice developed leukemia, whereas only 15/162 (9.3%)
MuLV-negative mice did so (P<<0.001). Table 3 indicates

TABLE 3

Relation between MuLV titer at 6 weeks of age
and leukemic incidence in mice of the
(BALB/c × AKR) × AKR backcross generation

Virus Titer ($\log_{10}$)	Leukemia Incidence	
3.9 - 3.0	22/25	(88.0%)
2.9 - 2.0	47/80	(58.8%)
1.9 - 1.0	16/38	(42.1%)
0.9 - 0.3	11/30	(36.7%)
total positive	96/173	(55.5%)
negative	15/162	(9.3%)
Total	111/335	(33.1%)

that there was also a clear correlation between virus titer and death from leukemia: the higher the level of virus detected at 6 weeks of age, the higher the incidence of leukemia later in life.

The disease was also markedly influenced by the $H-2$ type of the mice, although this correlation was less pronounced than that with MuLV. 71/166 (42.8%) $H-2^k/H-2^k$ mice developed the disease, whereas 40/169 (23.7%) $H-2^k/H-2^d$ mice did so (P<0.001).

Another factor examined for a possible correlation with leukemia incidence was sex, but in this case the small difference observed (34.8% of females and 29.3% of males developed the disease) was not statistically significant.

DISCUSSION

In the backcross population, (BALB/c × AKR) × AKR, the amount of MuLV detectable in tail extracts of six-week old mice is very strongly indicative of the animals' risk of developing leukemia much later in life. These data provide strong genetic evidence that MuLV is associated with the disease syndrome: either the virus is the etiologic agent that gives rise to the disease or the virus is induced in these animals by the same factor(s) that give rise to the disease.

The details for the genetic basis for this close association between leukemia incidence and MuLV titer remain to be elucidated. Presumably the $Akv-1$ and $Akv-2$ genes are not involved in this particular case, since all members of the backcross under consideration carry at least one dominant allele for the virus at each of these loci. Based upon the previous findings of Rowe and Hartley (4), it seems likely that the $Fv-1$ gene is the major determinant of the titer of MuLV and therefore also of the leukemia incidence, although direct proof of this is still lacking.

Since $H-2$ type showed a marked correlation with leukemia but only a slight correlation with MuLV, it is reasonable to conclude that the $H-2$-linked effect on leukemogenesis is exerted at a relatively late stage in the disease syndrome. This conclusion is compatible with the hypothesis (11) that the fundamental mechanism of this $H-2$-linked gene is that of an immune response gene, i.e., it may govern the capacity of the animal to reject leukemic or potentially leukemic cells by immunologic means.

These findings lead us to the following hypothetical scheme for leukemogenesis in AKR mice. Because they carry the *Akv-1* and *Akv-2* genes, these mice have access to the information needed for the production of infectious MuLV. Because they lack $Fv-1^b$ (or any other known gene capable of suppressing the expression of the viral information), the production of infectious virus takes place, and the virus is expressed at a high titer. By an unknown mechanism, the virus favors the neoplastic transformation of lymphoid cells into leukemia cells. Because the mice lack $H-2^d$, the transformed cells have a high probability of growing progressively to the death of the host. (BALB/c × AKR) F_1 mice also possess the complete viral information, as conferred by the *Akv-1* and *Akv-2* genes, but here the $Fv-1^b$ allele exerts a strong suppressive effect on the production of infectious virus by interfering with its spread. In addition, the $H-2^d$ allele provides a barrier to the progressive growth of those leukemia cells which might occur at this low level of virus, and the consequence is that these F_1 mice show a very low incidence of leukemia.

REFERENCES

1. Rowe, W.P., and Pincus, T., *J. Exp. Med. 135:* 429 (1972)
2. Rowe, W.P., *J. Exp. Med. 136:* 1272 (1972)
3. Lilly, F., *J. Nat. Cancer Inst. 45:* 163 (1970)
4. Rowe, W.P., and Hartley, J.W., *J. Exp. Med. 136:* 1286 (1972)
5. Lilly, F., *Bibl. haemat. 36:* 213 (1970)
6. Meier, H., Taylor, B.A., Cherry, M., and Huebner, R.J., *Proc. Nat. Acad. Sci. U.S. 70:* 1450 (1973)
7. Peters, R.L., Hartley, J.W., Spahn, G.J., Rabstein, L.S., Whitmire, C.E., Turner, H.C., and Huebner, R.J., *Int. J. Cancer 10:* 283 (1972)
8. Lilly, F., and Duran-Reynals, M.L., *J. Nat. Cancer Inst. 48:* 105 (1972)
9. Rowe, W.P., Pugh, W.E., and Hartley, J.W., *Virology 42:* 1136 (1970)
10. Gorer, P.A., and Mikulska, Z.B., *Cancer Res. 14:* 651 (1954)
11. Lilly, F., *Cellular Interactions in the Immune Response*, G. Cudkowicz *et al.* (Eds.), Karger, Basel, 1971, p. 103

CELLULAR REGULATION OF BIOLOGICALLY DISTINGUISHABLE ENDOGENOUS MOUSE TYPE C RNA VIRUSES

Stuart A. Aaronson and John R. Stephenson

Viral Carcinogenesis Branch
National Cancer Institute
Bethesda, Maryland 20014

SUMMARY. Mouse cells contain the inherited genetic information for multiple type C RNA viruses. In the inbred BALB/c strain, loci for two biologically distinguishable viruses have been demonstrated. These viruses are shown to be subject to different restrictions by the host cell at levels affecting their activation and persistence. Two classes of chemicals, halogenated pyrimidines and inhibitors of protein synthesis, are highly efficient inducers of one BALB/c endogenous virus (BALB:virus-2). However, the kinetics of virus activation in response to these drugs differs markedly. The other virus, BALB:virus-1, is induced only by halogenated pyrimidines. These results indicate that the cellular control of induction of these viruses must differ as must the mechanisms of action of the chemical inducers. A genetic locus, Fv-1, is shown to play an important role in the cellular restriction to persistence of BALB:virus-1. In contrast, Fv-1 has no effect on BALB:virus-2, which is unable to persist in cells with any of the known alleles at Fv-1. The presence of this latter virus in Fv-1 nonpermissive cells, however, helps BALB:virus-1 to overcome the cellular restriction at Fv-1. Further study of genetic controls over endogenous type C virus expression and the molecular processes involved should lead to understanding of factors that influence the malignant potential of these viruses in vivo.

The inherited basis for factors involved in leukemogenesis in mice was established many years ago with the development by MacDowell (1) and Furth (2) of inbred strains having extremely high susceptibility to the

49

natural occurrence of leukemia. The first evidence that viruses were etiologically involved in this disease was provided by Gross (3), who demonstrated transmission of leukemia to mice by filtrates from tumors of high leukemia incidence strains. Subsequent studies in vivo have confirmed and extended these observations, documenting the intimate association of type C RNA virus with the mouse and the etiologic role of the virus in leukemia.

The question as to whether these viruses were horizontally transmitted or vertically, through infection within the reproductive tract, or whether the viruses were naturally-transmitted within the gamettes, themselves, has been extensively investigated in recent years. Early immunologic studies demonstrated subviral expression in mouse strains which did not yield infectious virus (4). In tissue culture, the first suggestive evidence for genetic transmission of the virus was provided by the discovery that mouse cells could be spontaneously induced to produce type C virus after growth for many generations in the absence of detectable virus production (5). The subsequent discoveries of highly efficient chemical virus activators (6,7,8) led to the demonstration that endogenous type C viruses could be induced from their unexpressed state from every cell of many strains of mice.

Accumulating genetic and biochemical evidence strongly argues that endogenous viruses naturally reside within the DNA of the host cell. Several laboratories have demonstrated the segregation of loci for virus induction in inbred mouse strains (9-12). Further, one virus inducibility locus has genetically been mapped (13). Evidence that inducibility loci represent virus structural genes rather than regulatory genes affecting virus expression comes from studies showing the mendelian segregation of biologically distinguishable viruses of one parental strain in backcrosses with a noninducible strain (14). Hybridization of type C viral DNA probes to normal mouse cell DNA has revealed the presence of multiple copies of viral-specific information within the high molecular weight DNA of the cells (15). These findings have been confirmed by several laboratories (16,17). The above studies provide overwhelming evidence in favor of the concept that type C viruses are genetically transmitted within the mouse cell

DNA.

The present review summarizes our current knowledge concerning the regulation of different endogenous viruses. Particular emphasis is placed on the experimental model provided by the inbred BALB/c mouse strain, a strain characterized by a low incidence of naturally-occurring leukemia. Factors influencing the induction and persistence of biologically distinguishable viruses of BALB/c mouse cells have been analyzed by a biologic assay utilizing cells nonproductively transformed by murine sarcoma virus (MSV) (18). Spontaneous or chemical activation of these cells results in rescue of the sarcoma virus genome in the envelope of the cell's endogenous helper viruses (19,20). While assays for helper leukemia viruses invariably require multiple cycles of replication, transformation by MSV requires only a single cycle of infection. Thus, this technique provides one of the most sensitive and quantitative biologic techniques available for studying endogenous viruses (8,35).

Biologic Properties of BALB/c Endogenous Viruses. Some of the biologic properties of two inducible viruses of BALB/c cells are summarized in Table 1. BALB:virus-1 is preferentially infectious for NIH Swiss mouse cells but does grow, although less efficiently, in both BALB/c mouse and normal rat kidney (NRK) cultures. A second endogenous BALB/c virus, designated BALB:virus-2, that has previously been shown to segregate independently from BALB:virus-1 in appropriate genetic crosses (14), transmits to NRK cells in the absence of detectable infectivity for cells of either mouse strain. Serologically, the two viruses can also be distinguished by the fact that BALB:virus-2, but not BALB:virus-1, is neutralized by sera obtained from normal BALB/c mice (Table 1). The very low leukemia incidence NIH Swiss strain has also been used in some of the genetic studies described here. Embryo cells of this strain are not virus inducible in tissue culture (22), but recent evidence indicates that this strain does contain a virus resembling BALB:virus-2 in some of its characteristics. However, these two viruses can be distinguished by some differences in host range and on the basis of the immunologic characteristics of at least one of their viral structural polypeptides (23,24) (Table 1).

Spontaneous Activation of BALB/c Endogenous Viruses in vitro. When exponential phase cultures of different MSV nonproducer clones and subclones were assayed for virus activation in the absence of chemical activation, the frequency of spontaneously virus-induced cells ranged from 1.1×10^{-6} to 4.5×10^{-6} among different clones (Table 2). Since the frequency of virus activation in subclones tested many generations later was very similar, these findings support the conclusion that BALB/c cells undergo a constant but very low frequency activation of a virus that is incapable of spread to other cells. This conclusion has been substantiated by the demonstration that the host range of the spontaneously released virus is identical to that of BALB:virus-2 (35).

Activation of BALB/c Endogenous Viruses by Chemical Inducers. Two classes of chemicals, halogenated pyrimidines and inhibitors of protein synthesis, have been shown to be highly efficient inducers of type C virus from BALB/c cells (7,8). Evidence that their mechanisms of action differ comes both from knowledge of their dissimilar biochemical effects on cells and from observed differences in the virus induction response to these agents. The kinetics of virus release following exposure of a clone of KiMSV-transformed BALB/c nonproducer cells (K-BALB) to representatives of each class, iododeoxyuridine (IdU) and cycloheximide, are shown in Figs. 1 and 2. In these experiments, virus activation was measured both by the release of virus into tissue culture fluids, and by the ability of activated cells to register as infectious centers on a monolayer of susceptible assay cells. Following exposure to IdU, virus release reached a peak at around 3-4 days and persisted at this level for several days (Fig. 1). The kinetics of virus induction following exposure to cycloheximide were strikingly different (Fig. 2). Virus release was maximal within the first 12 hours following drug treatment and declined rapidly thereafter. By 72 hours, virus-positive cells were no longer detectable. These results indicate that the induction response to cycloheximide was much more labile than that observed with IdU (8,35).

In the above studies, NRK cells were utilized for virus assays in order to allow detection of either or both

BALB/c endogenous viruses (Table 1). Further evidence of dissimilarities in the effects of the two inducers was obtained by comparison of their abilities to induce the two BALB/c viruses As shown in Table 3, IdU and bromo-deoxyuridine each caused cells to register as virus-positive both on NRK and NIH/3T3 cells, indicating that BALB:virus-1 and probably BALB:virus-2 were activated from a similar high fraction of cells. Since BALB:virus-1 also transmits at low efficiency to NRK cells (Table 1), additional evidence, obtained from induction of cells containing only BALB:virus-2, has confirmed that IdU does, in fact, activate this virus at high frequency (21). Two inhibitors of protein synthesis, cycloheximide and puromycin, each induced cells to register as virus-positive when plated to NRK assay cells at a frequency higher than that observed with the halogenated pyrimidines (8). However, activation of NIH Swiss-tropic virus (BALB:virus-1) was not detectable with either of these chemicals (Table 3). The above studies, thus, demonstrate that two classes of chemical inducers of type C virus have very dissimilar effects on different endogenous viruses. These drugs should be useful in defining the mechanisms by which the cell regulates the expression of its naturally-integrated viruses.

Genetic Factors Influencing Expression of BALB/c Endogenous Viruses. In studies of cellular regulation of mouse type C viruses, tissue culture lines with genetically defined properties have been established (10,12). Continuous lines from backcross embryos involving BALB/c and NIH Swiss strains [NIH Swiss x (NIH Swiss x BALB/c)F_1] contain different numbers of activatable viruses. These cell lines have also been characterized with respect to their genotypes at a regulatory locus, Fv-1 (10). This latter gene is known to affect cell susceptibility to exogenous infection by many strains of MuLV (25-27) and appears to act at a step in virus replication beyond adsorption or penetration (28-30). The effect of Fv-1 on activation and persistence of two BALB/c endogenous viruses following exposure to IdU has been determined by study of representative clonal MSV-transformed nonproducer lines having the appropriate virus and regulatory gene properties (21). As shown in Fig. 3a, IdU induction of an Fv-1 permissive clone, containing both BALB:virus-1 and 2, resulted in early release of virus infectious for NRK cells; peak virus production was observed at four days with a decline to a level below detection by the 8th day. In contrast, when the same tissue culture fluids were assayed on NIH/3T3, infectious virus was first detected at 4-6 days and subsequently increased in titer to around 10^4 focus-forming units/ml by day 16. These results indicate that the early peak of focus-forming activity was due to BALB:virus-2, while the later activity was that of BALB:virus-1. The virus that transmitted to rat cells at day 16 was found to be BALB:virus-1 by the fact that it was preferentially infectious for NIH/3T3 cells (21).

When an Fv-1 nonpermissive clone containing both viruses was chemically induced, the kinetics and magnitude of early virus release were very similar to that observed with the permissive clone (Fig. 3b). However, the titer of virus infectious for NIH/3T3 cells was, at each time point tested, around 100-fold lower than that observed with the Fv-1 permissive clone. Thus, while the Fv-1 genotype markedly influenced activation and persistence of BALB:virus-1, it had no apparent affect on BALB:virus-2. These conclusions with regard to BALB:virus-2 were corroborated by examination of the influence of Fv-1 on the induction of BALB:virus-2 from clonal lines containing this virus in the absence of BALB:virus-1 (Figs. 4a and b). IdU treatment of both Fv-1 permissive and nonpermissive clones resulted in very similar kinetics of BALB:virus-2 activation. In each case, peak virus production occurred at around 4 days, and by 8-10 days, virus was no longer detectable.

The effects of Fv-1 genotype on the kinetics of virus activation from clonal lines containing BALB:virus-1 in the absence of BALB:virus-2 are shown in Fig. 5. Cells permissive at Fv-1 first released detectable virus infectious for NIH/3T3 cells at around 4-5 days following exposure to IdU; subsequently, the virus titer gradually increased and reached a level of around 10^4 focus-forming units/ml by 16 days (Fig. 5a). Virus infectious for NRK cells showed a very similar pattern of appearance but at a 50-100-fold lower magnitude. This virus was demonstrated by subsequent passage to NIH/3T3 and NRK cells, to be BALB:virus-1. The results of chemical induction of an MSV-transformed nonproducer line containing BALB:virus-1 but nonpermissive at Fv-1 were strikingly different. This line yielded no more than an occasional infectious virus transmissible to NIH/3T3 at any time following exposure to IdU (Fig. 5b). These results provide further evidence of the influence that Fv-1 exerts on persistence of induced BALB:virus-1. In addition, the block to expression of BALB:virus-1 in Fv-1 nonpermissive cells was found to be much more pronounced in cells lacking BALB:virus-2. It should be noted that the results in Figs. 3-5 have been confirmed by tests of several independent clonal lines from different embryo cultures of each genotype (21).

The above findings demonstrate the differential effect of one regulatory gene, Fv-1, on two BALB/c endogenous viruses. While Fv-1 has little or no effect on the activation or persistence of BALB:virus-2, it markedly influences BALB:virus-1. These studies also show that the nonpermissiveness at Fv-1 can be partially overcome by the interaction of BALB:virus-1 with a second endogenous virus. The mechanism by which the presence of BALB:virus-2 in Fv-1 nonpermissive cells favors the establishment of BALB:virus-1 is not yet known. However, the fact that the titers of BALB:virus-1 at early time points were low but similar in clones with each genotype supports the possibility that the interaction occurs at a late rather than a very early step in BALB:virus-1 activation.

In Vivo Expression of Endogenous Viruses. The above studies indicate that the BALB/c mouse cell exerts different controls over the spontaneous expression of its two endogenous viruses at levels affecting both virus activation and persistence. At the level of activation, BALB:virus-1 is more tightly restricted than BALB:virus-2. In contrast, cellular restriction to the persistence of BALB:virus-2 is absolute, while it is only relative for BALB:virus-1. The restriction to BALB:virus-1 persistence appears to be primarily due to the Fv-1 gene. The nature of the cellular block to persistence of BALB:virus-2 is not yet known.

The findings from in vitro investigations can be correlated with information available concerning the in vivo expression of the two viruses. Evidence has recently become available that BALB:virus-2 is spontaneously activated in vivo as well as in vitro. As shown in Table 4,

sera obtained from normal BALB/c mice of different ages
contain antibodies that specifically neutralize this virus.
The antibody titers against BALB:virus-2 are very high,
ranging from 1:500 to 1:2500; the same sera have no
detectable neutralizing activity against either BALB:virus-
1 or other representative mouse leukemia virus strains.
Sera from NIH Swiss mice, whose embryo cells are noninducible in culture, have been found to lack detectable antibodies to viruses serologically related to BALB:virus-2
(31). There is evidence that BALB:virus-1 is also activated in vivo. An increasing fraction of mice become virus-
positive with age, and the virus isolated from these
animals has been shown to have biologic properties indistinguishable from those of BALB:virus-1 (32,33). Even
though its frequency of spontaneous activation is much
lower than that of BALB:virus-2, the relative rather than
absolute restriction to its persistence at the Fv-1 locus
apparently is insufficient to prevent BALB:virus-1, once
activated, from persisting and growing to high titer in an
increasing proportion of animals.

Recently, an endogenous type C virus, chemically
activatable from virus-negative mouse cells in culture, has
been demonstrated to be leukemogenic when inoculated into
newborn animals of a low leukemic incidence strain (34).
Since this virus is activated from cells containing the
genetic information of the C58 strain, a strain characterized by a very high incidence of leukemia, it seems
apparent that inability of C58 cells to control the
expression of this naturally-integrated virus must be a
primary factor in the development of leukemia in the C58
strain. While the in vivo biologic activities of the
BALB/c endogenous viruses described in these studies are
not as yet known, further investigation of cellular
controls over their expression may help in understanding
their roles in naturally-occurring disease. Such studies
may also provide insight into the molecular processes involved in gene regulation in eukaryotic cells.

ACKNOWLEDGEMENT

These studies were supported by Contract no. NCI-73-
3212 of the Special Virus Cancer Program of the National
Cancer Institute.

REFERENCES

1. MacDowell, E.C. and Richter, M.N. Arch. Path. 20, 709 (1935).
2. Furth, J., Seibold, H.R. and Rathbone, R.R. Am. J. Cancer 19, 521 (1933).
3. Gross, L. Proc. Soc. Exp. Biol. Med. 78, 342 (1951).
4. Huebner, R.J., Kelloff, G.J., Sarma, P.S., Lane, W.T. and Turner, H.C. Proc. Nat. Acad. Sci. U.S.A. 67, 366 (1970).
5. Aaronson, S.A., Hartley, J.W. and Todaro, G.J. Proc. Nat. Acad. Sci. U.S.A. 64, 87 (1969).
6. Lowy, D.R., Rowe, W.P., Teich, N. and Hartley, J.W. Science 174, 155 (1971).
7. Aaronson, S.A., Todaro, G.J. and Scolnick, E.M. Science 174, 157 (1971).
8. Aaronson, S.A. and Dunn, C.Y. Science 183, 422 (1974).
9. Taylor, B.A., Meier, H. and Myers, D.D. Proc. Nat. Acad. Sci. U.S.A. 68, 3190 (1971).
10. Stephenson, J.R. and Aaronson, S.A. Proc. Nat. Acad. Sci. U.S.A. 69, 2798 (1972).
11. Rowe, W.P. J. Exptl. Med. 136, 1272 (1972).
12. Stephenson, J.R. and Aaronson, S.A. Science 180, 865 (1973).
13. Rowe, W.P., Hartley, J.W. and Bremner, T. Science 178, 860 (1972).
14. Aaronson, S.A. and Stephenson, J.R. Proc. Nat. Acad. Sci. U.S.A. 70, 2055 (1973).
15. Gelb, L.D., Milstien, J.B., Martin, M.A. and Aaronson, S.A. Nature New Biol. 244, 76 (1973).
16. Scolnick, E.M., Parks, W., Kawakami, T., Kohne, D., Okabe, H., Gilden, R. and Hatanaka, M. J. Virol. 13, 363 (1974).
17. Chattopadhyay, S.K., Lowy, D.R., Teich, N.M., Levine, A.S. and Rowe, W.P. Proc. Nat. Acad. Sci. U.S.A. 71, 167 (1974).
18. Aaronson, S.A. and Rowe, W.P. Virology 42, 9 (1970).
19. Aaronson, S.A. Proc. Nat. Acad. Sci. U.S.A. 68, 3069 (1971).
20. Klement, V., Nicolson, M.O. and Huebner, R.J. Nature New Biol. 234, 12 (1971).
21. Stephenson, J.R., Crow, J.D. and Aaronson, S.A., Virology, in press.
22. Stephenson, J.R. and Aaronson, S.A. J. Exptl. Med.

136, 175 (1972).
23. Stephenson, J.R., Tronick, S.R., Reynolds, R.K. and Aaronson, S.A. J. Exptl. Med. 139, 427 (1974).
24. Stephenson, J.R., Aaronson, S.A., Arnstein, P., Heubner, R.J. and Tronick, S.R., submitted for publication.
25. Axelrad, A. Nat. Cancer Inst. Monogr. 22, 619 (1966).
26. Lilly, F. Science 155, 461 (1967).
27. Pincus, T., Rowe, W.P. and Lilly, F. J. Exptl. Med. 133, 1234 (1971).
28. Eckner, R.J. J. Virol. 12, 523 (1973).
29. Huang, A.S., Bermer, P., Chu, L. and Baltimore, D. J. Virol. 12, 659 (1973).
30. Krontiris, T., Soeiro, R. and Fields, B.N. Proc. Nat. Acad. Sci. U.S.A. 70, 2549 (1973).
31. Aaronson, S.A. and Stephenson, J.R. Proc. Nat. Acad. Sci. U.S.A., in press.
32. Hartley, J.W., Rowe, W.P., Capps, W.I. and Huebner, R.J. J. Virol. 3, 126 (1969).
33. Peters, R.L., Hartley, J.W., Spahn, G.J., Rabstein, L.S., Whitmire, C.E., Turner, H.C. and Huebner, R.J. Int. J. Cancer 10, 283 (1972).
34. Stephenson, J.R., Greenberger, J.S., Aaronson, S.A. J. Virol. 13, 237 (1974).
35. Aaronson, S.A. and Dunn, C.Y. J. Virol. 13, 181 (1974).

TABLE 1

Properties of Endogenous Type C RNA Viruses of
BALB/c and NIH Swiss Mouse Cells

Properties	BALB:virus-1	BALB:virus-2	NIH virus
replication on:			
NIH mouse	++	-	-
BALB/c mouse	+	-	-
rat	+	++	+
human	-	+	++
neutralized by:			
anti-R-MuLV	-	-	-
anti-AKR-MuLV	++	++	++
natural BALB/c sera	-	++	++
p12 antigenic determinants:			
MuLV group specific	++	++	++
AKR-MuLV type-specific	++	-	-
R-MuLV type-specific	-	-	+

TABLE 2

Spontaneous Virus Activation from BALB/c-derived
MSV-transformed nonproducer clones

Cell line	MSV-infectious centers/total cells[1]
K-BALB	
Clone 1	4.5×10^{-6}
Subclone 1	2.8×10^{-6}
Subclone 2	5.1×10^{-6}
K-BALB	
Clone 2	3.2×10^{-6}
Subclone 1	7.3×10^{-6}

[1]Growing cultures of each cell line were exposed to
mitomycin C (25 µg/ml x 1 h) and then transferred at
10-fold cell dilutions in duplicate to petri dishes containing 10^5 NRK cells for infectious center assay.
K-BALB/Cl 1 and Cl 2 are clonal nonproducer lines derived
from different foci of Ki-MSV-transformed BALB/3T3 cells
(35). The results are the average of two experiments with
each line.

TABLE 3

Comparison of Induction of Two BALB/c
Endogenous Viruses by Inhibitors of
Protein Synthesis and Halogenated Pyrimidines

Inducer	Amount (μg/ml)	Induction frequency (% virus-activated cells)[1]	
		NRK	NIH/3T3
Cycloheximide	10	8.3	<0.001
Puromycin	10	12	<0.001
IdU	30	3.8	2.4
BrdU	30	1.6	0.8

[1]Growing cultures (5×10^5 K-BALB cells) were exposed to the appropriate inducer for 18 hours at 37°C. The cells were then treated with mitomycin C (25 μg/ml) for 1 hour and transferred for infectious center assay on either NRK or NIH/3T3 cells as described in the legend to Table 1. The results are the average of two experiments with each inducer (8).

TABLE 4

High Titered Neutralizing Activity Against BALB:virus-2 in Sera of Normal BALB/c Mice

Source	Dilution	MuLV pseudotype of Ki-MSV:[1] (% reduction of focus formation)			
		R-MuLV	Ki-MuLV	BALB:virus-1	BALB:viru
Rat					
anti-Rauscher	1:100	95	<10	<10	<10
anti-AKR	1:100	<10	95	95	95
BALB/c					
2 months	1:20	<10	<10	<10	97
	1:20	-	-	-	90
6 months	1:20	<10	<10	<10	98
	1:200	-	-	-	92
24 months	1:20	<10	<10	<10	100
	1:200	-	-	-	92

[1]Neutralization tests were performed by the focus-reduction method. Arc 100 focus-forming units (FFU) of each MuLV pseudotype of KiMSV were incubated with the appropriate dilution of neutralizing antisera for 30 min at 37°. BALB:virus-2 pseudotypes were assayed on polybrene (2 µg/ml)-treated NRK cells whereas each of the other pseudotypes were assayed on polybrene-treated NIH/3T3 cells. The number of MSV foci was scored at 7 days. Results are expressed as mean values of 3 separate experiments (31).

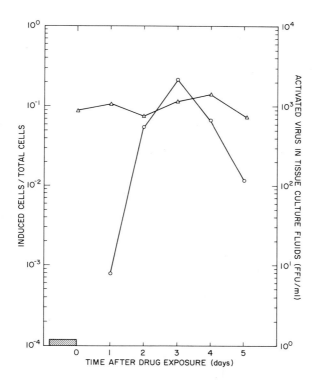

Fig. 1.   Kinetics of IdU induction of K-BALB.
Cultures containing 5 x 10⁵ cells were exposed to 30 μg/ml
IdU for 20 hr at 37°C and then washed twice. At subsequent 24 hr intervals, the cells were transferred for
infectious center assay on NRK cells (35).   In addition,
tissue culture fluids were assayed for focus-forming virus
on NRK cells. △ , induced cells/total cells; ○ , activated
virus fluids 10⁶ cells.

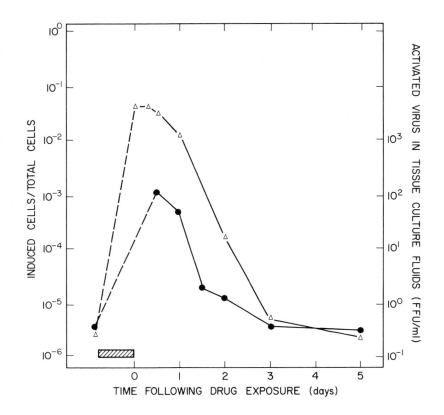

Fig. 2. Kinetics of cycloheximide induction of
K-BALB. Cultures containing 5 x 10^5 cells were exposed to
10 µg/ml cycloheximide for 20 hours at 37°C, and then
washed twice. At subsequent times, the cells were transferred for infectious center assays on NRK cells (8). At
12 hour intervals for the first 48 hours, and at 24 hour
intervals thereafter, tissue culture fluids were assayed
for focus-forming virus on NRK cells. △ , induced cells/
total cells; ● , activated virus/ml/10^6 cells.

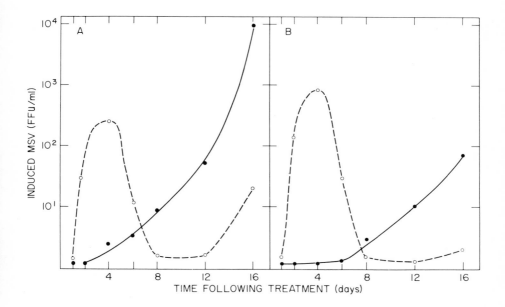

Fig. 3. Kinetics of KiMSV activation from Nx(NxB)F₁ nonproducer clonal lines containing BALB:virus-1 and 2 (21). Cells in exponential growth phase were treated with IdU (30 μg/ml) for 24 hrs. Culture fluids were collected at the indicated times, filtered, and assayed for trans-mission of focus-forming virus to ●, NIH/3T3 and ○, NRK cells. The genotype at Fv-1 was A) nn; B) nb.

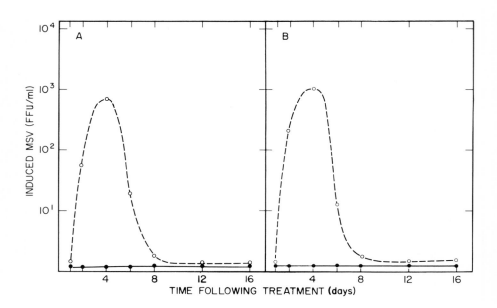

Fig. 4. Activation of KiMSV from Nx(NxB)F₁ nonproducer clonal lines containing BALB:virus-2 alone (21).
Cells were treated with IdU, and assayed for focus formation on ●, NIH/3T3 and ○, NRK as described in the
legend to Fig. 3. The genotype at Fv-1 was A) nn; B) nb.

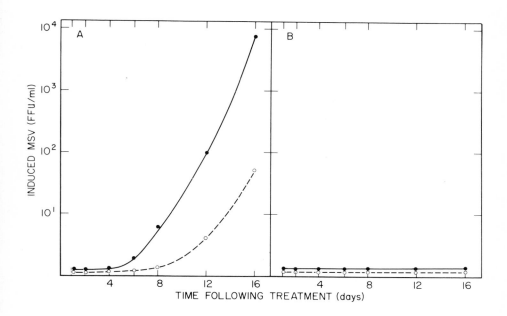

Fig. 5.   Activation of KiMSV from Nx(NxB)F$_1$ nonproducer clonal lines containing BALB:virus-1 alone (21).
Cells were treated with IdU and culture fluids and assayed
for focus formation on ●, NIH/3T3 and ○, NRK as in
Fig. 1.   The genotype at Fv-1 was A) nn; B) nb.

HOST RESTRICTION OF FRIEND LEUKEMIA VIRUS

Ruy Soeiro, Michael M. Sveda,
Theodore G. Krontiris and Bernard N. Fields

Departments of Medicine, Cell Biology
and Microbiology
Albert Einstein College of Medicine
Bronx, New York   10461

ABSTRACT. Host restriction of oncogenesis by RNA tumor viruses may be studied in vitro by measuring the replication of the lymphatic leukemia component of the Friend Virus Complex (LLV-F) in either NIH-Swiss or Balb-C mouse' embryo cells. These cells derive from mice which differ at the Fv-1 locus which controls the replication of all murine RNA leukemia viruses. Studies of early events in the replication of LLV-F were carried out by following the infection of permissive and restrictive mouse embryo cells by ^{32}P labelled LLV-F. The results demonstrate that ^{32}P labelled viral genome RNA rapidly becomes associated with cell nuclei, and may be found integrated to the same extent with high molecular weight host DNA of either permissive or restrictive cells. The results suggest that Fv-1 mediated host restriction of LLV-F occurs at a step following integration of viral genome RNA into host DNA.

INTRODUCTION

The factors that govern the ultimate result of the interaction of RNA tumor viruses with their host are complex and poorly understood. In the case of murine oncornaviruses, the host response to infection is mediated by at least five host genes (1,2). One mouse gene in particular, the Fv-1 locus, plays a major role since it controls susceptibility to most natural strains of murine leukemia virus. This gene governs the host range of the lymphatic leukemia virus of the Friend virus

complex (LLV-F). The original LLV-F is an N-tropic virus,
that is, it replicates 100-1000 fold better in NIH Swiss
(N-type; $Fv-1^N/Fv-1^N$) than in Balb-C mice. The expression
of the Fv-1 locus is retained by cultured mouse embryo
cells, that is, the degree of replication of LLV-F in
vitro depends upon whether the source of cells is from a
permissive or a restrictive host (3). Lilly and Steeves
(1973) have produced a B-tropic LLV-F, a strain of Friend
LLV which replicates better in Balb-C cells which are
normally restrictive for N-tropic LLV-F. The reciprocal
inability of N-tropic strain (N-LLV-F) to grow in Balb-C
cells (B-type or $Fv-1^B/Fv-1^B$) or of the B-tropic strain
(B-LLV-F) to grow in NIH cells has been demonstrated and
forms the basis of a system in which host restriction may
be studied in vitro.

Our earlier studies (4) followed the fate of
infectious input virus particles and demonstrated that
host restriction of LLV-F was not associated with virus
coat properties, and appeared to occur after uncoating of
the virion took place. In those studies it was shown
that N-tropic LLV adsorbed to the same extent, and with
the same kinetics to mouse embryo monolayers of either
permissive (NIH-Swiss) or restrictive (Balb-C) cells.
The reciprocal experiment with B-tropic LLV confirmed
these results. Furthermore, by superinfection of mouse
embryo monolayers which were producing either N-tropic
or B-tropic LLV with Vesicular Stomatitis Virus (VSV), it
was possible to produce phenotypically mixed virions
which contained a core of VSV genetic information within
a coat containing LLV-F neutralizing antigen(s). It was
shown that VSV enclosed by either N-tropic or B-tropic
LLV coat protein(s) adsorbed, penetrated and replicated
equally well on N-type or B-type mouse embryo cells. It
was found therefore that LLV-F coat protein(s) containing
neutralizing antigen did not effect the uncoating process
of phenotypically mixed VSV virions. A tentative conclusion therefore was made, consistant with the apparent
absence of antigenic differences between the two strains
(5) that LLV-F coat protein(s) played no role in host
restriction of the replication LLV-F.

In the experiments to be presented, we have now
investigated early events in virus replication by
following the fate of labelled input virions in permissive

and restrictive mouse embryo cells. Analysis of labelled input viral RNA associated with the cell nucleus reveals that N and B tropic LLV-F genome RNA becomes integrated with host DNA to the same extent in both permissive and restrictive cells. These results confirm earlier studies which suggested that restriction was an intracellulr event (6) and suggest that Fv-1 host restriction is determined at a step in viral replication following integration.

RESULTS

1. ADSORPTION AND INTRACELLULAR DISTRIBUTION OF RADIO-LABELLED VIRIONS. The initial experiments were designed to measure the kinetics of adsorption to and penetration of mouse embryo cells by ^{32}P labelled LLV-F which had been purified by isopycnic banding in a sucrose density gradient (7). In each case, a comparison was made between the adsorption of N or B tropic virus to both permissive and restrictive sub-confluent mouse embryo cell monolayers. Adsorption of labelled virions was allowed to take place for 30-45 min, following which the medium containing unadsorbed virions was removed, the cell monolayer was washed, fresh medium was added, and the infected cells were incubated for varying periods of time. At harvest, the cell monolayer was mechanically suspended in Earles buffer, washed by centrifugation, and nuclear and cytoplasmic fractions were prepared. The results in Table 1 indicate that equal numbers of labelled virions adsorbed to each cell type. At all periods of incubation studied, the majority of cell associated ^{32}P labelled virus material remained in the cytoplasm, but both the absolute amount of nuclear associated radioactivity and the relative proportion of radioactivity associated with the nuclei of each cell type was the same. These results confirm and extend our earlier studies which demonstrated that infectious N and B tropic virions adsorbed equally to permissive and restrictive cells.

It is important to point out that in earlier studies only the adsorption of infectious plaque forming units was measured. In those studies, approximately 80% of infectious virions adsorbed to the cell monolayer (4).

71

In the present analysis of the adsorption of radioactively labelled virions, only 20-30% of the labelled
particles were adsorbed over the same time period. The
apparent discrepancy in the percentage adsorption of
infectious units versus radioactively labelled virions is
most likely attributable to the fact that not all virus
particles are infectious. The ratio of particles to
plaque forming units for FLV has not been determined. In
studies of this type, the possibility that the fate of
labelled but non-viable particles within the cell will
obscure the true biological pathway of infectious virions
must always be considered. The validity of this approach
has been demonstrated in another animal virus system (8)
and will be commented upon below.

2. DENSITY ANALYSIS OF NUCLEAR ASSOCIATED VIRION NUCLEIC
ACID. At the end of each incubation period, infected
cell nuclei were purified and nucleic acids were
extracted by phenol-chloroform-isoamyl alcohol. The
extracted nucleic acids were denatured according to the
method of Boedtker (1968) (9) in 3% formaldehyde, and
analyzed by equilibrium density centrifugation in Cs_2SO_4
density gradients. Labelled RNA from purified virions
extracted and treated in this manner banded isopycnically
exclusively at the density characteristic of purified RNA
in Cs_2SO_4 (ρ 1.67 gm/cc). Fig. 1a shows that after 60
min. of incubation following the period of adsorption,
nuclear associated N type virus nucleic acid in both N
or B type mouse embryo cells demonstrated a second peak
of radioactivity at a density of 1.55 gm/cc. Since this
nucleic acid was denatured, this banding density suggested a molecule composed of both DNA and RNA which was
covalently linked. Furthermore, when material isolated
from the Cs_2SO_4 density gradient at ρ 1.55 gm/cc was
pooled, treated with DNAse, and rebanded on Cs_2SO_4, a
quantitative shift of ^{32}P labelled nucleic acid to the
density of RNA (1.67 gm/cc) occurred (not shown). At
3.5 hrs. post adsorption (Fig. 1b), ^{32}P labelled nucleic
acid appeared also at a density of 1.44 gm/cc, characteristic of DNA. After 7.5 hrs, ^{32}P material at ρ 1.44
gm/cc represented the predominant nuclear species. At
all times, ^{32}P labelled nucleic acid isolated from the
cytoplasm banded solely at ρ 1.67 gm/cc. In the case of
either N or B tropic virus at each time point tested, the

distribution in either the permissive or the restrictive cell type was the same. Since no DNA associated ^{32}P was found in the cytoplasmic fraction, this data further suggests that the activation and viral DNA synthesis is predominantly a nuclear event.

3. ANALYSIS OF NUCLEAR ASSOCIATED VIRAL RNA BY VELOCITY SEDIMENTATION. The sedimentation coefficient of the RNA subunit of the denatured murine oncornavirus genome is approximately 32s-35s when analyzed by velocity sedimentation through sucrose density gradients (10). Polyacrylamide gel analysis in buffered formaldehyde reveals this 32s species to be 2.3×10^6 daltons (11). In order to analyze the molecular weight of the ^{32}P labelled nucleic acid, a sample of the denatured nuclear associated ^{32}P labelled material pooled from each density peak shown in Fig. 1 was analyzed by velocity sedimentation in sucrose density gradients. Fig. 2(a) shows that ^{32}P labelled nucleic acid banding at ρ 1.67 gm/cc after 3.5 hrs of incubation contains some species which sediment as high as 32s, but the majority of nucleic acid species have lower S values. Similarly, material banding at ρ 1.55 gm/cc (Fig. 2b) sediments heterogeneously with sedimentation values ranging from 4s to 32s. However, after 7.5 hrs of incubation, material banding at ρ 1.44 gm/cc sediments with a range of values up to 100s (Fig. 2c). No such high molecular weight species were ever observed when cytoplasmic fractions were similarly analyzed. The distribution at 3.5 hrs of incubation of material banding at ρ 1.44 was essentially the same as at 7.5 hrs. When a sample of each fraction was hydrolyzed in alkali, all of the ^{32}P labelled nucleic acid banding at ρ 1.67 (not shown) and at ρ 1.55 was rendered acid soluble, suggesting that all the ^{32}P nucleic acid was RNA (Fig. 2b). However, while 80% of the ^{32}P nucleic acid from the ρ 1.44 region was similarly solubilized by alkali, 20% remained acid precipitable (Fig. 2c). This result suggested that a transfer of some ^{32}P radioactively into material other than RNA had occurred.

4. ANALYSIS BY CHEMICAL AND ENZYMATIC DEGRADATION. Table 2 summarizes the results of analysis of ^{32}P labelled nucleic acids pooled from the putative DNA-RNA hybrid

73

regions. Radiolabelled material banding at ρ 1.55 was rendered completely soluble by nuclease S$_1$ (indicating a completely single stranded structure), pancreatic RNAse, or KOH, and was completely resistant to DNAse. These findings confirm the results of simple alkali treatment of material banding at ρ 1.55 shown in Fig. 2b. Although physically linked to DNA (see results of DNAse treatment noted above) all the ^{32}P radioactivity of the ρ 1.55 material appears to be in RNA. However, material banding at ρ 1.44, while completely solubilized by nuclease S$_1$, is only 80% sensitive to RNAse or KOH, and reciprocally 20% sensitive to DNAse. Single strand ^{32}P labelled RNA at ρ 1.44 is therefore linked to high molecular weight DNA (see Fig. 2c) but in this case, some radioactivity appears to be in DNA.

The possibility that degradation of ^{32}P labelled viral RNA with reutilization for the synthesis of new DNA or RNA was considered. Although the infection with labelled virions was carried out in the presence of un-labelled purine and pyrimidine nucleosides to prevent potential reutilization for nucleic acid synthesis of any ^{32}P labelled viral material, this possibility cannot be eliminated. However, both host RNA and DNA species should derive from such a pathway, and no clear host RNA (ribosomal or heterogeneous nuclear RNA) species were produced (Fig. 2 a,b,c). Furthermore, no acid soluble ^{32}P was found in either the nuclear or cytoplasmic cellular fractions of cells infected with labelled virus, again suggesting an absence of recycled nucleotides.

5. ANALYSIS OF NUCLEAR ASSOCIATED INPUT DNA-RNA MOLECULAR HYBRIDIZATION. The product of the endogenous RNA directed DNA synthesis reaction of oncornavirions synthesized in the presence of Actinomycin D represents 80-90% of the sequences of the viral genome (12). As such, it forms an excellent molecular probe for the detection of genomic RNA. The data in Table 3 demon-strates that after hybridization of ^{32}P labelled viral genome RNA with single-stranded reverse transcriptase product (FLVssDNA), 80% of viral genome was protected from digestion by nuclease S$_1$. Self annealing of virus genome RNA, FLVssDNA or RNA isolated from a Cs$_2$SO$_4$ gradient at ρ 1.44 gm/cc resulted in little to no

protection from digestion by this single strand-specific nuclease. In confirmation of its assumed source as ^{32}P labelled input viral RNA, ^{32}P labelled nucleic acid, pooled from material banding in Cs_2SO_4 density gradients at ρ 1.44 and ρ 1.55 after 7.5 hrs. of incubation, was between 56-60% protected from nuclease S_1 digestion after hybridization to FLVssDNA. These results indicated that ^{32}P labelled input virion nucleic acid, isolated from infected cell nuclei, bands at densities in Cs_2SO_4 which indicate covalent linkage with DNA. The complete sensitivity to digestion by the single strand specific nuclease; the shift in isopycnic banding density after treatment with DNAse; plus the distribution of sedimentation values of the RNA banding at ρ 1.44, allow this conclusion.

DISCUSSION

Earlier studies by Hartley et al (1970) (6) on the mechanism of the Fv-1 gene host restriction phenomenon suggested that restriction of viral replication in the non-permissive cell occurred at a step subsequent to penetration and uncoating. Our studies (4) confirmed and extended these results, and demonstrated clearly that the virus coat proteins are not involved in host restriction. These same results were obtained by Huang et al (1973) (13) and by Yoshikura (1973) (14) using similar methods.

The data reported here again demonstrate that there is no difference in binding, penetration or nuclear appearance of input viral RNA in permissive or restrictive cells. Our data further indicate that within 60 min. after adsorption, viral specific RNA initially becomes covalently associated with low molecular weight DNA (Fig. 2b), (nucleic acid banding isopycnically at ρ 1.55 gm/cc in Cs_2SO_4 - suggests molecules whose average composition is approximately 50% RNA and 50% DNA), and only later is covalently linked (Fig. 1b,c and 2c) to high molecular weight DNA (ρ 1.44 gm/cc in Cs_2SO_4). This latter form suggests strongly the integration of input virion RNA into the host cell DNA as a presumed "provirus" structure. The annealing of this RNA to FLVssDNA defines it as virus specific.

75

Bolognesi and Graf (1970) (15) demonstrated by the use of ^{32}P labelled avian myeloblastosis virus that viral RNA became cell associated and was distributed mainly in the cytoplasm. Dales and Hanafusa (1972) (16) found that radioactively labelled Rous Sarcoma Virions 60s RNA became associated with the cell nucleus within one hour after infection. Our results showing the integration of labelled input RNA into host cell DNA are an extension of these studies and are directly comparable to the results of Leis et al (1974) (17) using ^{3}H uridine labelled Rous sarcoma virus infection of chick embryo fibroblasts.

A direct comparison of both N tropic and B-tropic LLV-F infection of permissive and restrictive cells shows that no difference in the rate or degree of integration of input LLV-F genome RNA into permissive or restrictive cell DNA can be observed. Of importance here is the fact that the multiplicity of infection of input virions was monitored and maintained at approximately 0.2 pfu/cell since at high multiplicities of infection the Fv-1 restriction effect is overcome (Rowe, pers com.). These results suggest that the mechanism of Fv-1 host restriction is at the level of transcription, translation, or assembly, steps in virus replication subsequent to integration of the provirus. Since, in the non-permissive host, complete infectious virions are produced but at a reduced level, it is less likely that integration of an incomplete pro-virus has occurred. However, what has not been excluded by these studies, is the possibility that unstable integration occurs in the non-permissive host. All of these possibilities are open to experimental verification.

The initial RNA-DNA covalent hybrid molecules (ρ 1.55 gm/cc in Cs_2SO_4) are predominantly low molecular weight species (Fig. 2b). Since on alkaline hydrolysis, no transfer of label to acid precipitable DNA is found (Table 2), the DNA moiety must be at the 3' end. Once input viral RNA becomes covalently integrated into high molecular weight DNA (Fig. 1c, 2c), then, when digested with alkali, approximately 20% of the ^{32}P label is transferred to DNA, suggesting that linkage at the 5' end has now occurred. Analysis of this ^{32}P labelled DNA is currently underway. These facts are consistant with the model postulated by Leis et al (1974) (17) that the provirus is formed through the combined action of the two virus associated enzymes, reverse transcriptase and RNAse H. Furthermore, the data presented here showing the covalent linkage of input RNA with DNA are consistant with data obtained in vitro with the reverse transcriptase reaction (12). 1) The direction of DNA synthesis is from 5'——> 3'; 2) the initial DNA made is a low molecular weight species covalently linked to the 3' end of primer RNA; 3) only low molecular weight DNA species are synthesized in vitro. All these features of the in vitro DNA product are similar to those of the 32_p material banding at ρ 1.55 gm/cc. However, some ρ 1.55 gm/cc labeled material may derive from RNAse H hydrolysis of genome RNA coupled with its ligation to newly synthesized DNA.

Two possibilities have been proposed for the fate of the DNA-RNA hybrid molecule produced by these enzyme activities. The first is that the hybrid might be integrated with host DNA directly, and the second that only subsequent to complete elimination of the RNA moiety and the production of a DNA-DNA hybrid might integration occur. Our results suggest that a DNA-RNA hybrid is integrated directly into host cell DNA, and that the provirus is, at least transiently, a DNA-RNA hybrid.

The use of labelled input virus has proven very useful in following early events in the replication cycle of reovirus (8). In vitro studies have supported the biological validity of this approach (18). In the data reported here, our constant concern was that the true biological pathway of input virion was being followed. To this effect. we have obtained data to be presented elsewhere, which demonstrated that by drug induced inhibition of DNA synthesis or by modification of cell growth conditions known to inhibit virus replication (19, 20) the production of DNA-RNA hybrid molecules, and the integration of viral RNA with host DNA did not occur. Furthermore, these events described here occurred only in infected cell nuclei and not in the cytoplasm. This data suggests strongly that the localization of the activation step for oncornavirions reverse transcription is in the nucleus. The exclusive location of DNA-RNA hybrids found here suggests but do not prove the validity of this conclusion and this approach.

ACKNOWLEDGEMENTS

This work was supported in part by grants, NIH R01 AI-10326 and NIH R01 CA010993. We were also supported as follows: Ruy Soeiro, NIH Career Development Award, 1-K04 CA-70850; Bernard N. Fields, American Cancer Soceity Faculty Research Award, PRA 63 and Irma T. Hirschl Scholar Award; Michael M. Sveda, NIH GM 2209, and Theodore G. Krontiris, 5T5 GM-167409.

REFERENCES

1. Lilly, F., J. Natl. Cancer Inst. 45, 163 (1970).
2. Lilly, F. and Steeves, R., Virology 55, 363 (1973).
3. Pincus, T., Hartley, J.W. and Rowe, W., J. Exp. Med. 133, 1219 (1971).
4. Krontiris, T., Soeiro, R. and Fields, B.N., Proc. Natl. Acad. Sci. USA 70, 2549 (1973).
5. Steeves, R.A. and Eckner, R.J., J. Natl. Cancer Inst. 44, 587 (1970).
6. Hartley, J.W., Rose, W. and Huebner, R.J., J. Virol. 5, 221 (1970).
7. Stewart, M., Summers, D.F., Soeiro, R., Fields, B.N. and Maizel, J.V., Proc. Natl. Acad. Sci. USA 70, 1308 (1973).
8. Astell, S.C., Silverstein, D.H., Levin, H. and Acs, G., Virology 48, 648 (1972).
9. Boedtker, H., J. Mol. Biol. 35, 61 (1968).
10. Duesberg, P.H., Proc. Natl. Acad. Sci. USA 60, 1511 (1968).
11. Sveda, M., Maizel, J.V. and Soeiro, R. (in prep.).
12. Temin, H. and Baltimore, D., Adv. in Virus Res. 17, 129 (1972).
13. Huang, A., Besmer, P., Chu, L. and Baltimore, D., J. Virol. 12, 659 (1973).
14. Yoshikura, H. J. Gen. Virol. 19, 321 (1973).
15. Bolognesi, D. and Graf, T. In The Biology of Large RNA Viruses, Eds. Barry, R.D. and Mahy, B.W.J., p. 221, Academic Press (1970).
16. Dales, S. and Hanafusa, H., Virology 50, 448 (1972).

17. Leis, J., Hurwitz, J., Shincariol, T. and Joklik, W., Symposium on Biology of Tumor Viruses, 34th Annual Biology Colloquium, Oregon State Univ., Ed. George Beandreau (in press) (1974).
18. Shatkin, A.J. and La Fiandra, A.J., J. Virol. 10, 698 (1972).
19. Temin, H.M., In The Biology of Large RNA Viruses, Eds. Barry, R.D. and Mahy, B.W.J., p. 233, Academic Press (1970).
20. Bader, J., Virology, 48, 485 (1972).
21. Borun, T.W., Scharff, M.D. and Robbins, E., Biochim. Biophys. Acta 149, 302 (1967).
22. Soeiro, R., Birnboim, H.C. and Darnell, J.E., J. Mol. Biol. 19, 362 (1966).
23. Leis, J. and Hurwitz, G., Proc. Natl. Acad. Sci. USA 69, 2331 (1972).
24. Penman, S., J. Mol. Biol. 17, 117 (1966).

TABLE 1

Kinetic Analysis of Adsorption and Sub-Cellular Distribution of $32P$ Labelled Friend Leukemia Virus.

Virus	Cells	TIME (Hrs Post Adsorp)	NUCLEI CPM	NUCLEI %	CYTOPLASM CPM	CYTOPLASM %	C/N	% ADSORBED Acid Precipitable Radioactivity
Exp I								
N → N		1.0	79,520	(8%)	846,000	(92%)	11/1	32%
N → B		1.0	77,940	(8.5%)	842,000	(91.5%)	10/1	32.4%
Exp. II								
B → B		3.5	52,590	(14%)	317,700	(86%)	6/1	25%
B → N		3.5	50,050	(16.5%)	250,250	(83.5%)	5/1	22%
B → B		7.5	58,200	(25%)	232,800	(75%)	4/1	22%
B → N		7.5	50,500	(19.5%)	211,100	(80.5%)	4/1	25%

$32P$ labelled LLV-F was adsorbed to monolayers of permissive or non-permissive secondary mouse embryo (ME) cells in the presence of DEAE (25 µg/ml) according to Hartley et al (1970) (6) for 30-45' at 37°C. At the end of the adsorption period, the adsorption medium containing unattached virus was removed and the cell monolayer rinsed twice with buffer. The radioactivity present in the medium removed at the end of adsorption plus the virus in the two rinses together represented unadsorbed radioactive virus particles. The cytoplasmic fraction was obtained by NP40 treatment of the cells (21). Nuclei were obtained by previously described methods (22).

TABLE 2

ANALYSIS OF DNA-RNA HYBRID REGIONS

	Control	+KOH	+DNAse	+RNAse	+S_1 Nuclease
ρ 1.44	692	135	542	114	43
ρ 1.55	618	29	604	36	18

A sample of material pooled from the Cs_2SO_4 density gradients shown in Fig. 1c at ρ 1.55 (fractions 9-13) and ρ 1.44 gm/cc (fractions 17-20) was dialyzed to eliminate Cs_2SO_4. The dialyzate was then digested chemically with alkali or enzymatically with the enzymes noted, and the remaining material acid precipitated and assayed for radioactivity. In each case shown, the numbers represent acid precipitable radioactivity in counts per minute after the treatment indicated.

TABLE 3

HYBRIDIZATION OF NUCLEAR INPUT RNA

	INPUT CPM	NUCLEASE S_1 RESISTANT HYBRID
FLVssDNA	600 (H^3)	50 (H^3)
ρ 1.44 input	4,150 (P^{32})	215 (P^{32})
FLVssDNA + Balb-C DNA (uninfected)	620 (H^3)	45 (H^3)
ρ 1.44 P^{32} + FLVssDNA	3,660 (P^{32})	2,190 (60%)
ρ 1.55 P^{32} + FLVssDNA	3,740	2,085 (56%)
60-70s P^{32} RNA	3,185	135
60-70s P^{32}RNA + FLVssDNA	3,375	2,675 (80%)

Single stranded FLV specific DNA (FLVssDNA) was
synthesized in vitro by the endogenous reverse transcriptase reaction in the presence of Actinomycin D
(according to the method of Leis and Hurwitz (1972)
(23). The single stranded nature of this product, and
its specificity for viral genome RNA are demonstrated
by self annealing, or annealing with ^{32}P labelled viral
genome. At the end of the annealing reaction, the incubation mixture was diluted, digested enzymatically
with Nuclease S_1 (single strand-specific) and the acid
precipitable radioactivity remaining was assayed by
liquid scintillation counting.

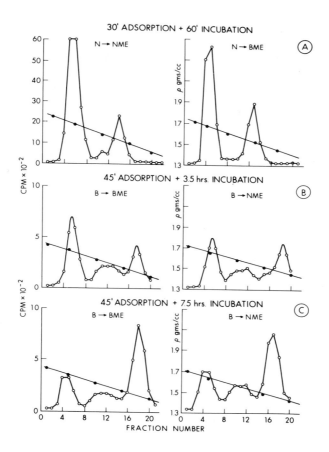

Fig. 1. Analysis of Nuclear Associated Radioactive Input Material by Cs_2SO_4 Isopycnic Density Gradients. Material isolated from detergent washed nuclei from each incubation period shown in Table 1 was deproteinized according to the method of Penman (1966) (24). The extracted nucleic acids were denatured by exposure to 3% formaldehyde at 65°C for 15 minutes. Following this treatment, the material was analyzed for its distribution in Cs_2SO_4 density gradients as described by Leis and Hurwitz (1972) (23). A sample of each fraction was assayed for acid precipitable radioactivity. ^{32}P counts per min o——o
Density, gm/cc ●——●

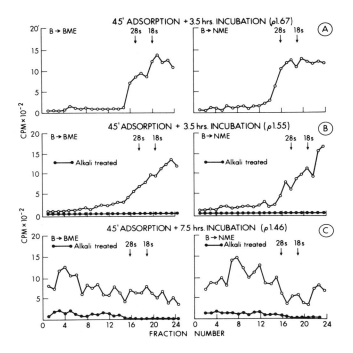

<u>Fig. 2</u>. Analysis of Nuclear Associated Radioactive
Nucleic Acid by Scurose Gradient Velocity Sedimentation.
A sample of material pooled from each peak of radioactivity in Fig. 1 was dialyzed to eliminate Cs_2SO_4.
The dialysate was re-treated with HCHO (3%) for 15 min
at 65°C to ensure its single stranded form, and layered
over 15-30% sucrose density gradients (22). Sedimentation was carried out at 14,000 RPM for 24 hrs at 22°C
in a SW27 rotor. Hela cell ribosomal 28 + 18s RNA
species were cosedimented and served as an optical
density marker for molecular weight. A sample of each
fraction was assayed for acid precipitable radioactivity before and after treatment with 0.3N KOH for
16 hrs. at 37°C.

III

DEFECTIVE VIRUSES: THEIR FORMATION AND INFLUENCE ON THE COURSE OF INFECTION

VESICULAR STOMATITIS VIRUS: DEFECTIVENESS AND DISEASE

Alice S. Huang and Eduardo L. Palma*

Department of Microbiology and Molecular Genetics
Harvard Medical School
Boston, Massachusetts 02115

ABSTRACT. Vesicular stomatitis virus and its defective interfering T particle have been used in reconstruction experiments with Chinese hamster ovary cells. The results indicate that genome RNA replication, and not transcription, is the direct site of interference by defective interfering particles. When cells are producing a maximum amount of defective interfering particles nucleo-capsids, or inclusion bodies, build-up intracellularly. These nucleocapsids contain RNA of the size found in defective particles, but the RNA is both virion-like and complementary. The production of intracellular nucleo-capsids is highly pH-dependent. At more acid pH values, overall nucleocapsid synthesis is inhibited, but nucleo-capsids the size of T particle nucleocapsids are preferentially synthesized over those the size of B particle nucleo-capsids.

INTRODUCTION

Defective interfering (DI) viruses are a special class of deletion mutants which are capable of inter-

---

*Present address: Centro de Investigaciones Microbiologicas, Universidad de Buenos Aires, Facultad de Ciencias Exactas y Naturales, Buenos Aires, Argentina.

fering with the growth of their helper standard virus
(see 1). The initial detection of such deletion mutants
in virus preparations was made with influenza virus
in the 1950's and the interference called the von Magnus
phenomenon (2). Gradually, over the years, each group
of animal virus was found to generate their own DI particles (see 1). The latest addition to the catalogue of
viruses found to make their own DI particles are herpesvirus (3) and coronavirus (Bradburne, personal communication). We have postulated that the generation of
DI particles provides a natural control of the viral population explosion and that exploitation of DI particles may
permit us to alter the course of viral infections (4).

The properties of DI particles and their molecular
biology was recently reviewed (1). Once DI particles
have been identified in a virus system, there are the
following important questions concerning them. First,
we would like to know about their genesis - that is, the
mechanism of formation of the initial DI particle in a
cloned virus population. Little is known about the genesis except that different groups of viruses and different
strains within the same group have different frequencies
for the generation of their DI particles (see 1). Also,
virus strains appear to generate specific and different
DI particles (5, 6, 7).

The second question concerns the growth and amplification of DI particles. In order for us to detect
them, they must grow to a relatively large number in
cells co-infected with helper virus and, generally, in
competition with their helper standard virus. How this
amplification or enrichment occurs may be different for
different viruses. For instance, tandem duplications of
the region of the SV40 genome containing the initiation
site for DNA synthesis may indeed give such a defective
molecule a competitive advantage during DNA synthesis
(8, 9, 10). Enrichment necessarily involves interference
and the mechanism of how DI particles interfere with the
growth of their helper virus is another important ques-

tion. Because the strategy of viral multiplication differs for virus groups, the mechanism of interference may be different, but they all appear to involve nucleic acid synthesis in one way or another.

Concerning enrichment and interference is the question of how other parameters affect the degree of enrichment or interference. It has been known for some time that cells from different species or from different tissues within a species will cause differing degrees of interference when infected with the same preparation of standard and DI particles (11, 12, 4). More recently, congenic strains of mice have been shown to have a dominant gene resistant to West Nile virus. The gene appears to affect the degree of interference caused by DI particles (13). Such host effects must necessarily act intracellularly. Possible effects on interference by other parameters should be sought for.

Finally, we would like to find out if DI particles play any role in vivo -- either in ameliorating virus disease or in the biology of chronic and latent virus infections. Such possibilities have been suggested (4) and supporting evidence was recently published by Holland and his colleagues (14, 15).

THE VESICULAR STOMATITIS (VSV) SYSTEM

Our studies on DI particles utilizes the VSV system ever since it was found that its DI particles are readily separated from standard bullet-shaped (B) virions and purified by rate zonal centrifugation (16). Although VSV can generate several DI particles of different sizes, a DI particle, one-third the length of B virions are used throughout these studies. This DI particle is called the T particle or DI-T particle.

Advantages in using the VSV system lie in the absence of interferon induction (17, 18) and intrinsic interference (Marcus, unpublished observations) by the DI-T particles. Also, DI-T particles are incapable of synthesizing any functional messenger RNA or any viral proteins (19). Thus, interference caused by DI-T particles is easily studied in the absence of any other interference phenomena and in the absence of any gene products of DI-T particles.

THE MOLECULAR MECHANISM OF INTERFERENCE BY DI-T PARTICLES

Ever since DI-T particles were first separated from the standard B particles of VSV (16) there has been the question of how these particles interfered with or inhibited the growth of B particles. Initial studies showed that the interference, 1) occurs intracellularly, 2) is not mediated by interferon, 3) is prevented by prior ultra-violet irradiation of the DI-T particles, and 4) is quite specific for the serotype from which DI-T particles are derived (18). These criteria for interference by DI-T particles have held true for subsequent studies on other virus systems.

Examination of intracellular VSV-specific macromolecular synthesis showed that interference occurs during RNA synthesis (20). To define the exact step it was first necessary to study RNA synthesis by purified B particles alone. Figure 1 summarizes currently available knowledge regarding VSV RNA synthesis. The genome RNA sediments at 40S and is negative-stranded (21, 22). It functions not as naked RNA but in a helical nucleocapsid structure sedimenting at 120S (23). The virion associated transcriptase transcribes the genome RNA into complementary smaller pieces of RNA sedimenting at 28S and 13-15S (24, 19). The smaller RNA's function as messenger RNA and contain poly(A) apparently at their 3' ends (25, 26). Transcription off of the incoming genomes is called primary transcription and is the only VSV-specific RNA synthesis detected in infected cells when cycloheximide is added at the beginning of infection (19, 27).

The genome is also copied into a complete strand of complementary 40S RNA which contains poly(A) and is also found in helical nucleocapsids (28, 23). This complementary RNA, in turn, acts as template for the replication of minus-stranded 40S RNA. Intracellularly, the ratio of plus-stranded 40S RNA to minus-stranded 40S RNA is 20-30% to 70-80%. Newly synthesized minus-stranded 40S RNA has several functions: it can participate in additional rounds of replication; it can become template for secondary transcription, and it can mature into extracellular progeny virions.

There are, apparently, two separate pathways for VSV RNA synthesis: one, the transcriptive pathway and the other, the replicative pathway. They are thought to be separate because inhibition of one pathway appears not to affect the products of the other pathway in any way. This type of dissociation of one pathway from the other is accomplished by the use of temperature-sensitive mutants (29) and by the use of cycloheximide added after the initiation of infection (30). Despite the separation of these two synthetic pathways, they both appear to utilize a common core enzyme, which has been postulated to be the virion-associated transcriptase or L protein (30, 31, 32).

When cells are co-infected with temperature-sensitive B particles and DI-T particles it was found that the RNA species synthesized from DI-T RNA are synthesized via the replicative pathway (33). Previously, it was found that the presence of interfering amounts of DI-T particles has no effect on primary transcription by standard B virions (19, 27). Therefore, it can be concluded that interference by DI-T particles occurs during replication and not transcription. How DI-T RNA competes advantageously against B RNA for replicative enzymes is not known.

BUILD-UP OF NUCLEOCAPSIDS IN CELLS PRODUCING DI-T PARTICLES

Because inclusion bodies are major diagnostic aids in viral infection and because inclusion bodies are often made-up of masses of nucleocapsids, we tested for the effects of DI-T particles on the production and retention of nucleocapsids by infected cells. The detection of any intracellular build-up of VSV antigens or nucleocapsids occurs only when infected cells are producing large amounts of DI-T particles extracellularly (34). These nucleocapsids contain both plus and minus single-stranded 19S RNA (Table 1). DI-T particles, in contrast, contain only minus-stranded 19S RNA. How this selection is made during the maturation of DI-T particles is not known.

POSSIBLE EFFECTS OF pH ON INTERFERENCE CAUSED BY DI-T PARTICLES

Recently, Fiszman et al (35) pointed out the strong dependence on alkaline pH for the production of infectious VSV. Using the organic buffers suggested by Eagle (36) media was made up at different pH values; the molar content of organic buffers was kept constant among the different batches of media. Figure 2a shows that production of intracellular 120S B nucleocapsids (BNC) was very much dependent on pH with an optimum for production at pH 7.4. Higher pH values than the ones shown in Figure 2 have been tested. There was a direct correlation between the amounts of intracellular BNC and infectious extracellular B particles. When cells were co-infected with B and DI-T particles, the profile of pH dependence for the production of intracellular BNC and 70S DI-T nucleocapsids (TNC) was altered. The optimum pH became pH 7.0 (Fig. 2a). When the ratio of intracellular TNC to BNC is plotted versus pH, it is apparent that the synthesis of TNC was favored at the lower pH values even though overall nucleocapsid synthesis was inhibited. How pH affects extracellular production of B and DI-T particles by co-infected cells remains to be determined.

DISCUSSION

The study of VSV DI-T particles has shown that in vitro reconstruction experiments can provide insights into the virus-host interaction. We conclude that, 1) a variety of host responses on the cellular level exists, dependent on the relative concentrations of standard and DI particles in a virus preparation; 2) that inclusion bodies may be diagnostic of the presence of DI particles and finally, 3) that the molecular basis of interference, quite specifically, involves genome replication although other steps during viral maturation may be involved, also.

ACKNOWLEDGMENTS

This work was supported by research grants from the American Cancer Society VC-63Z, from the U.S. Public Health Service AI-10100 and from the National Science Foundation GB 34266. A. S. H. is a Research Career Development Awardee of the U.S. Public Health Service, National Institute of Allergy and Infectious Disease. E. L. P. is a World Health Organization-Pan American Health Organization Fellow on leave from the University of Buenos Aires, Argentina.
We thank Norma Hewlett for excellent technical support.

REFERENCES

1. A. S. Huang, Ann. Rev. Microbiol. 27, 101-117 (1973).
2. P. von Magnus, Acta Pathol. Microbiol. Scand. 28, 278-293 (1951).
3. D. L. Bronson, G. R. Dreesman, N. Biswal and M. Benyesh-Melnick, Intervirol. 1, 141-153 (1973).
4. A. S. Huang and D. Baltimore, Nature 226, 325-327 (1970).

93

5. M. E. Reichmann, C. R. Pringle and E. A. C. Follett, J. Virol. 8, 154-160 (1971).
6. K. Yoshiike, Virology 34, 391-401 (1968).
7. K. Yoshiike, Virology 34, 402-409 (1968).
8. W. W. Brockman, T. N. H. Lee and D. Nathans, Virology 54, 384-397 (1973).
9. M. A. Martin, L. D. Gelt, G. C. Fareed and J. B. Milstein, J. Virol. 12, 748-757 (1973).
10. G. Khoury, G. C. Fareed, K. Berry, M. A. Martin, T. N. H. Lee and D. Nathans, J. Mol. Biol. in press (1974).
11. P. W. Choppin, Virology 39, 130-134 (1969).
12. D. W. Kingsbury and A. Portner, Virology 42, 872-879 (1970).
13. M. B. Darnell and H. Koprowski, J. Infect. Dis. in press (1974).
14. J. J. Holland and M. Doyle, Infect. & Immunity 7, 526-531 (1973).
15. M. Doyle and J. J. Holland, Proc. Nat. Acad. Sci. U.S. 70, 2105-2108 (1973).
16. A. S. Huang, J. W. Greenawalt and R. R. Wagner, Virology 30, 161-172 (1966).
17. R. R. Wagner, A. H. Levy, R. M. Snyder, G. A. Ratcliff and D. F. Hyatt, J. Immunol. 91, 112-122 (1963).
18. A. S. Huang and R. R. Wagner, Virology 30, 173-181 (1966).
19. A. S. Huang and E. K. Manders, J. Virol. 9, 909-916 (1972).
20. M. Stampfer, D. Baltimore and A. S. Huang, J. Virol. 4, 154-161 (1969).
21. F. L. Schaffer, A. J. Hackett and M. E. Soergel, Biochem. Biophys. Res. Commun. 31, 685-692 (1968).
22. A. S. Huang, D. Baltimore and M. Stampfer, Virology 42, 946-957 (1970).
23. M. Soria, S. P. Little and A. S. Huang, submitted for publication (1974).

24. D. Baltimore, A. S. Huang and M. Stampfer, Proc. Nat. Acad. Sci. U.S.A. 66, 572-576 (1970).
25. E. Ehrenfeld and D. F. Summers, J. Virol. 10, 683-688 (1972).
26. M. Soria and A. S. Huang, J. Mol. Biol. 77, 449-455 (1973).
27. J. Perrault and J. J. Holland, Virology 50, 159-170 (1972).
28. T. G. Morrison, M. Stampfer, H. F. Lodish and D. Baltimore, Proceedings Negative Strand Virus Mtg., Cambridge, England, in press (1973).
29. S. M. Perlman and A. S. Huang, Intervirology, in press (1974).
30. S. M. Perlman and A. S. Huang, J. Virol. 12, 1395-1400 (1973).
31. S. M. Perlman and A. S. Huang, in Virus Research (Second ICN-UCLA Symp. on Mol. Biol.) ed. C. F. Fox and W. S. Robinson, Academic Press, N.Y., 97-104 (1973).
32. S. U. Emerson and R. R. Wagner, J. Virol. 12, 1325-1335 (1973).
33. E. L. Palma, S. M. Perlman and A. S. Huang, J. Mol. Biol. 84, in press (1974).
34. E. L. Palma and A. S. Huang, J. Infect. Dis., in press (April) (1974).
35. M. Fiszman, J. B. Leaute, C. Chany and M. Girard, J. Virol. 13, 801-808 (1974).
36. H. Eagle, Science 174, 500-503 (1971).
37. A. S. Huang and D. Baltimore, J. Mol. Biol. 47, 275-291 (1970).

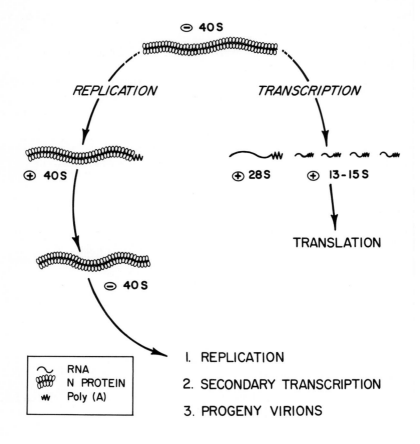

Figure 1. Graphic summary of VSV RNA synthesis.

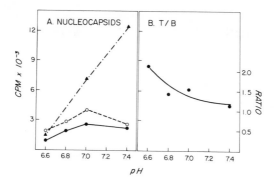

Figure 2. The effect of pH on the intracellular synthesis of nucleocapsids in Chinese hamster ovary cells infected with B particles alone or co-infected with B and
DI-T particles. Two samples of 2.4×10^7 CHO cells in
6 ml of medium were either infected with B particles at
an input multiplicity of 50 PFU/ml or co-infected with B
particles at the same multiplicity plus T particles at an
estimated multiplicity of 3. After attachment at 4°C for
40 min each sample was divided into 4 aliquots containing
6×10^6 infected cells. The aliquots were centrifuged at
400 x g for 3 min and the pellets resuspended in 3 ml of
the medium which was organically buffered at the desired
pH and containing 15 µg of Actinomycin D. After 30 min
of incubation at 35°C 15 µCi of H^3-uridine was added and
the infected cells further incubated for 4.5 hours. At the
end of the incubation cytoplasmic extracts were made
with 1% Nonidet P-40 and then treated with 1% sodium de-
oxycholate. Each sample was layered on a 15-30% su-
crose-NEB gradient and centrifuged at 45,000 x g for 15
hours at 4°C in the Beckman SW27 rotor. Sucrose gradient fractions were collected and acid-precipitated. Details of procedures and materials are published elsewhere
(19, 20, 37). The results were plotted and the areas under peaks at 120S (BNC) and 70S (TNC) were added up to
yield the data shown here. (▲·-·-▲) BNC made in cells
infected with B particles alone; (o---o) TNC made in
cells co-infected with B and DI-T particles; (●—●) BNC
made in cells co-infected with B and DI-T particles.

Table 1

Annealing of 19S RNA from T particles and from intracellular nucleocapsids to virion RNA or to messenger RNA.*

SOURCE OF LABELED RNA	PER CENT RIBONUCLEASE RESISTANCE
19S RNA from intracellular nucleocapsids**	
annealed to virion RNA	41.9
annealed to 13-28S mRNA	67.0
not annealed	5.7
19S RNA from a cytoplasmic extract**	
annealed to virion RNA	40.8
annealed to 13-28S mRNA	71.9
not annealed	3.2
19S RNA from T particles***	
annealed to virion RNA	8.5
annealed to 13-28S mRNA	106.7
not annealed	5.4
40S RNA from B virions***	
annealed to virion RNA	6.4
not annealed	2.8
13-15S mRNA from a cytoplasmic extract***	
annealed to virion RNA	101.0
annealed to 13-28S mRNA	3.1
not annealed	2.4

*Different samples of ^{3}H-labeled RNA, containing 3,000 cpm or greater, were resuspended in 0.3 ml of 2 x SSC containing 20% sucrose and 0.1% sodium dodecyl sulfate

(SDS). The samples were annealed either with 8 µg/ml of nonradioactive 40S virion RNA or with 300 µg/ml of unlabeled 13-28S intracellular RNA or not annealed. The annealing was performed by incubation at 70°C for 3.5 hr. Then, all the samples were diluted with 2 x SSC to 2 ml and divided into two aliquots one of which was treated with ribonuclease as previously described (19).

**Intracellular 19S RNA was prepared either from 70S nucleocapsid material which was labeled and isolated as shown for Figure 4a or from whole cytoplasmic extracts as shown for Figure 2 . The RNA was extracted by treatment with 1% SDS and centrifuged in a 15-30% sucrose gradient in SDS buffer containing 0.1% SDS (20). Analysis of the 70S nucleocapsid in parallel experiments showed that all of the RNA was ribonuclease-resistant prior to SDS treatment. After deproteinization all of the RNA migrated as a single 19S species on polyacrylamide gels and was completely sensitive to ribonuclease.

***Preparation of 19S RNA from T particles, 40S RNA from B particles and messenger RNA species were done as described (19).

TEMPERATURE SENSITIVE MUTANTS OF VESICULAR STOMATITIS VIRUS AND INTERFERENCE

M. E. Reichmann, R. N. Leamnson

Department of Microbiology
University of Illinois
Urbana, Illinois 61801

ABSTRACT. RNA species of different sizes were isolated from defective interfering (DI) particles generated in infections with vesicular stomatitis virus (VSV) (Indiana) wild types of different origin, temperature sensitive (ts) mutants and a heat resistant (HR) mutant. The relationship of some of these RNA to various viral cistrons was investigated by means of annealing experiments. Advantage was taken of the fact that VSV mRNA contain nucleotide sequences complementary to the viral RNA and to DI particle RNA. Two tentative maps of the DI particle RNAs relative to the cistronic regions are suggested. In either map difficulties are encountered if an attempt is made to explain the specificity of interference on the basis of nucleotide sequences common to all DI particles.

The annealing data have also shown that none of the short DI particle RNAs carry information for a complete viral cistron while the HR DI particle RNA contains information for all the cistrons except one (30S).

INTRODUCTION

Defective interfering (DI) virus particles are generated during repeated high multiplicity passages of nearly all the major groups of animal viruses (1, 2). DI particles have been compared to deletion mutants because they lack part of the viral genome and as a result of this deficiency are incapable of autonomous replication in the absence of their homologous nondefective virion. Their ability to interfere with infection is presumably linked in some way to a requirement for a viral function which they inherently lack and for which they are successfully competing with the complete virion. Neither the mechanism of interference nor the events leading to the generation of these particles are well understood.

101

The DI particles of polyhedral viruses differ from their virion by a small deletion in the genome which in most cases results in only a minor change in physical properties. For this reason separation of the DI particles is difficult and incomplete. (However, polio virus is an exception because its DI particle exhibits an unusually low density, which cannot be fully accounted for by the deletion.) In bullet shaped viruses like vesicular stomatitis virus (VSV) the deletion in the RNA is accompanied by a shortening of the entire particle (3) (see also Fig. 1), resulting in significantly different sedimentation properties. Isolation of these particles by zonal centrifugation was therefore feasible and the physical and biological properties were studied on purified preparations (4). It was found that wild type VSV (Indiana) generated only one type of DI particle which corresponded to approximately 1/3 the size of the virion. Later Prevec and Kang showed that a heat resistant mutant (HR) of VSV (Indiana) generated a longer DI particle which corresponded to 1/2 the size of the virion (5). The relative sizes of the particle RNA also follow the same size relationship (6).

Temperature sensitive (ts) mutants of VSV (Indiana) which were obtained after application of chemical mutagens (7) were shown to generate other size groups of DI particles, some of which are shown in Fig. 1 (8). No correlation was found between complementation group and the size of DI particle generated; furthermore, all attempts to use the genetic information stored in DI particles for complementation purposes have so far failed (8). These results pose questions about the nature of the genetic information stored in the DI particles and about the ability of the system to express this information. Since it is the RNA of the DI particles of VSV which is responsible for the phenomenon of interference (9, 10), an answer to these questions may also be basic to the understanding of the mechanism of interference (14).

The following features of the VSV system provide a convenient means for the correlation of DI particle RNA to various viral cistrons. The single stranded nonfragmented viral RNA is transcribed in vivo into a defined population of complementary messenger RNA (mRNA) molecules (11, 12). The complementarity of these mRNA molecules to the DI particle RNA (13) suggested to us that annealing experiments could establish the nature of the information stored in DI particle RNA relative to viral cistrons. From the relative sizes of these mRNA molecules their relationship to the individual viral proteins can be deduced (12). The work described below deals with these problems.

MATERIALS AND METHODS

The detailed experimental procedures dealing with cell growth, virus infection, isolation and purification of virion and DI particles, preparation of particle RNA and virus induced intracellular RNA, polyacrylamide gel electrophoresis and analysis of the gels have been described (8, 15). Annealing was carried out as described by Huang, Baltimore and Stampfer (16).

The three wild types MS, HU and HOW originated in Drs. Summers' (11), Huang's (16) and Howatson's (22) laboratories and were obtained from Dr. Holland. In addition to these, we used our own wild type which originated in Dr. Pringle's laboratory (8) and from which all the Indiana ts mutants were originally derived (7). The HR mutant was a gift from Dr. Prevec (5).

RESULTS

The RNA species obtained from purified DI particles generated by different mutants and by wild type VSV were analyzed by polyacrylamide gel electrophoresis. The composite profile shown in Fig. 2a demonstrates the wide range of sizes and lack of any apparent pattern in the size groups of the DI particle RNA. These sizes range from approximately 10% (DI ts 31) to 70% (DI ts 11) of the viral genome. The results of the analysis of DI particle RNA generated by wild type VSV (Indiana) obtained from various laboratories suggested that a selection of a special DI particle may have taken place in each laboratory. This is demonstrated in Fig. 2b which represents a composite profile of three wild type DI particle RNAs obtained from inocula which originated in three different laboratories.

We have shown previously that the various ts mutant virions generated reproducibly their characteristic DI particles after repeated clonal isolations (8). Similar experiments with clonally purified wild types have shown

the same reproducible generation of DI particles whose RNA
species exhibited the typical polyacrylamide profiles
shown in Fig. 2b.

In order to investigate the relationship between the
various DI particle RNA species and the viral cistrons,
annealing experiments were carried out with viral mRNA
species which are complementary in their nucleotide sequences to VSV and DI particle RNAs. The various size
groups of VSV mRNA exhibit a characteristic profile following sucrose gradient centrifugation or polyacrylamide gel
electrophoresis (Fig. 3a and b respectively). The 30S RNA
component is probably the mRNA which is translated into the
L protein (190,000 daltons) (17) while the 18-13S components carry information for the other VSV encoded proteins
(G, N, NS and M) (18). The 30S mRNA was isolated by repeated sucrose gradient centrifugation followed by collection of peak fractions of this component. The 18 and 13S
fractions were also isolated from sucrose gradients and
were further separated into an 18S fraction and 13S fraction by means of preparative polyacrylamide gel electrophoresis (19).

Using the separated RNA size fractions, annealing
experiments were performed with the long HR, short ts 31
and three wild type DI particles RNAs. In one set of experiments a constant amount of ^{3}H labelled particle RNA
was annealed to increasing amounts of ^{14}C weakly labelled
mRNA. Following ribonuclease digestion, the percentage
complementarity of nucleotide sequences was determined
from the undigested ^{3}H label (corrected for the small [14]C
spillover). In the reverse experiments a constant amount
of ^{3}H labelled mRNA was annealed with increasing amounts
of unlabelled particle RNA and the ribonuclease resistant
mRNA label was monitored. Characteristic results of experiments of the first type are shown in Fig. 4. These
data also demonstrate the difference between the RNAs of
the HR (4a) and wild type (4b) DI particles. While annealing with increasing amounts of the 18S-13S mRNA
species rendered close to 90% of the HR DI particle RNA
ribonuclease resistant (solid circles in Fig. 4a), very
little annealing seemed to have taken place with a comparable concentration of the wild type HU DI particle RNA
(Fig. 4b, open circles). On the other hand, the latter
RNA annealed almost 100% to the 30S mRNA (Fig. 4b solid
circles) while very little of the HR RNA annealed to this

message (Fig. 4a open circles). The dotted lines in Fig. 4 are based on annealing with unlabelled BHK cellular RNA.

Analogous data obtained with other DI particle RNA in combination with the various mRNA size fractions are summarized in table 1. The percent ribonuclease resistance obtained when increasing amounts of various mRNA were annealed with the labelled MS DI particle RNA showed that the latter behaved very much like the HU DI particle RNA (Fig. 4b) in that 100% annealing took place with excess 30S mRNA while virtually no annealing was observed with the 18 + 13S mRNA species. On the other hand, the HOW DI particle RNA seems to have complementary sequence to the 30S as well as the 18 + 13S mRNA size groups (last column table 1). Unfortunately, the relative distribution of the nucleotide sequences of this particle RNA among the two mRNA fractions cannot be derived from the data, because the saturating annealing values add up to more than 100%. This is probably due to some cross contamination of the mRNA preparations.

Annealing data obtained from the reverse experiments are also consistent with the above conclusions. With increasing concentrations of HR DI particle RNA in the annealing mixture virtually all the 18S and 13S mRNA nucleotide sequences were made ribonuclease resistant whereas most of the 30S mRNA sequences remained ribonuclease sensitive. On the other hand, 29.7, 35.4 and 13.6 percent of the nucleotide sequences of the 30S mRNA were made ribonuclease resistant following annealing with MS, HU and ts 31 DI particle RNAs respectively (table 2). These percentages also correspond very closely to the respective sizes of the particle RNA species relative to the 30S mRNA (Fig. 2). The experiments at the bottom part of table 2 again indicate qualitatively that the HOW DI particle RNA has sequences complementary to all the mRNA size groups.

In order to examine whether the nucleotide sequences of DI particle RNA complement the same or different regions of the 30S mRNA, annealing experiments with mixtures of HU + MS and HOW + MS were performed (20). Had the DI particle RNAs corresponded to different regions, the plateau values of the mixtures would exceed the values obtained with the longest particle RNA in the mixture (table 2). This was not the case and the annealing data at any RNA concentration of the mixture were indistinguishable from the corresponding data obtained with the longest particle in the mixture. It must therefore be concluded that the

longer of these DI particle RNA's contain all the nucleotide sequences of the shorter ones.

DISCUSSION

The specificity of interference by DI particles of
VSV would suggest that the particle RNA contain a specific
interference site which could be related to a specific
nucleotide sequence. This sequence should be conserved in
all VSV DI particles regardless of the size of its RNA.
Based on this assumption, however, the interpretation of
the annealing data becomes difficult. Fig. 5a shows a
hypothetical map of the DI particle RNA which is consistant
with the annealing data. In this drawing the HR DI particle RNA corresponds primarily to the 18S and 13S mRNA
region on the virion, and it is also assumed that it contains a short sequence inside the 30S mRNA domain which is
too short to be detectable with any degree of confidence
by annealing experiments. The other DI particle RNAs, also
share this nucleotide sequence and except for HOW are fully
contained in the 30S domain as dictated by the annealing
data. However, a complication arises because the common
nucleotide sequence would be at the opposite ends of the
DI particles. Thus, if the site is assumed to involve the
3' end of the HR particle it can be seen from Fig. 5a that
the overlap would correspond to the 5' of the other DI particle RNA and vice versa. Moreover, in the case of HOW the
sequence would not coincide with either end. It may be
difficult to explain interference in terms of increased
affinities for RNA replicating enzymes (2) acting on two
nonequivalent ends of an RNA template.

Fig. 5b shows an alternate assignment of the DI particle RNA on the viral genome. In this assignment the
short DI particle RNAs initiate at a fixed point in the
30S mRNA domain with the shorter molecules being fully
contained inside the longer molecules. Since the HU RNA
is fully located in the 30S mRNA region, the initiation
point must be removed from the intercistronic border by at
least a nucleotide sequence corresponding in length to
this DI particle RNA. This hypothetical map suggested a
possible mechanism of the generation of various DI particle RNA. It could be assumed that the DI RNA species
are replicated from a fixed point on the viral genome but
the termination is variable either due to direct mutation

106

in the termination signal or due to a change in the secondary structure brought about by the mutation. In the case of the HR mutant it would have to be postulated that the initiation site itself was affected. The two maps suggested in Fig. 5 are not the only possible assignments consistent with the annealing data and other intermediate locations of the DI particles are also feasible. A more detailed investigation of nucleotide sequences would be required to narrow down the possibilities.

The unique capacity of the HR DI particle RNA to interfere heterotypically with the New Jersey serotype of VSV may be related either to its different origin on the viral genome or to the fact that it contains complete viral cistrons. Further work is in progress in order to correlate the ability for heterotypic interference with either DI particle size or the type of information contained in its RNA.

ACKNOWLEDGEMENTS

This work was supported by grants USNSF GB 34171 from the National Science Foundation and by the Jessie Guth Memorial Grant VC 92 of the American Cancer Society. We thank Drs. Huang, Holland, Howatson, Prevec and Pringle for the HU, MS, HOW, HR, and ts 31 virus incula respectively.

REFERENCES

1. Huang, A. S., and Baltimore, D., Nature 226, 325 (1970).
2. Huang, A. S., Ann. Rev. Microbiol. 27, 101 (1973).
3. Hackett, A. J., Virology 24, 51 (1964).
4. Huang, A. S., Greenawalt, J., and Wagner, R. R., Virology 30, 161 (1966).
5. Prevec, L., and Kang, C. Y., Nature 228, 25 (1970).
6. Huang, A. S., and Wagner, R. R., J. Mol. Biol. 22, 381 (1966).
7. Pringle, C. R., J. Virol. 5, 559 (1970).
8. Reichmann, M. E., Pringle, C. R., and Follett, E. A. C., J. Virol. 8, 154 (1971).
9. Huang, A. S., and Wagner, R. R., Virology 30, 173 (1966).
10. Sreevalsan, T., Science 169, 991 (1970).

11. Mudd, J. A., and Summers, D. F., Virology 42, 958 (1970).
12. Kang, C. Y., and Prevec, L., Virology 46, 678 (1971).
13. Schaffer, F. L., Hackett, A. J., and Soergel, M. E., Biochem. Biophys. Res. Comm. 31, 685 (1968).
14. Palma, E. L., Perlman, S. M., and Huang, A. S., J. Mol. Biol. In press, 1974.
15. Unger, J. T. and Reichmann, M. E., J. Virol. 12, 570 (1973).
16. Huang, A. S., Baltimore, D., and Stampfer, M., Virology 42, 946 (1970).
17. Stampfer, M., and Baltimore, D., J. Virol. 11, 520 (1973).
18. Wagner, R. R., Prevec, L., Brown, F., Summers, D. F., Sokol, F., and MacLeod, R., J. Virol. 10, 1228 (1972).
19. Uzunov, P., and Weiss, B., Biochem. Biophys. Acta 284, 220 (1972).
20. Leamnson, R. N., and Reichmann, M. E., J. Mol. Biol., In press, 1974.
21. Huang, A. S., and Manders, E. K., J. Virol. 9, 909 (1972).
22. Schincariol, A. L., and Howatson, A. F., Virology 49, 766 (1972).

TABLE 1

Annealing of VSV mRNA to labelled DI particle RNA.

Unlabelled[1] DI RNA		Percent ribonuclease resistance after annealing with labelled[3] RNA	
type	amount[2]	MS	HOW
30S	0	7.8	8.5
	10 μl	32.9	59.2
	20 μl	61.8	78.4
	50 μl	102.0	86.2
	100 μl	100.0	99.2
18S + 13S	0	7.8	8.5
	10 μl	8.0	18.5
	20 μl	8.0	28.5
	50 μl	8.0	44.6
	100 μl	8.3	75.4

[1] The mRNA was actually weakly labelled with ^{14}C for purposes of identification in the purification process. The ^{3}H counts in columns 3 and 4 were corrected for the ^{14}C spillover from the mRNA.

[2] The presence of large amounts of cellular RNA in the preparation made it impossible to determine absolute concentrations of mRNA. The relative concentration range given here in μl was selected in such a way that annealing with virion RNA of a concentration comparable to MS and HOW RNA showed the mRNA to be in excess at the 100 μl level.

[3] The ^{3}H label was in the range of 1,000-2,000 cpm.

TABLE 2

Annealing of DI particle RNA with labelled VSV mRNA.

Unlabelled DI RNA		Percent ribonuclease resistance after annealing with labelled[1] mRNA		
type	amount	13S	18S	30S
HR	0	4.8	7.4	5.0
	0.1 µg	74.7	59.2	6.7
	0.2 µg	83.8	81.5	9.0
	0.5 µg	87.3	84.3	11.2
	1.0 µg	90.0	86.0	17.9
MS	0	10.7	8.9	12.6
	0.1 µg	10.7	--	22.9
	0.2 µg	9.7	14.4	24.0
	0.5 µg	14.0	14.0	28.6
	1.0 µg	15.0	13.0	29.7
HU	0	6.7	7.0	12.6
	0.1 µg	6.7	7.0	35.4
	0.2 µg	8.0	7.0	--
	0.5 µg	13.4	8.0	32.0
	1.0 µg	10.7	8.0	35.4
ts 31	0	4.7	6.9	3.3
	0.1 µg	4.7	7.0	6.5
	0.2 µg	5.0	7.0	8.7
	0.4 µg	6.5	8.3	9.8
	0.9 µg	6.5	8.5	11.0
	1.8 µg	--	--	13.6
HOW	0	7.0	7.0	12.6
	0.1 µg	14.9	13.4	42.3
	0.2 µg	19.1	20.8	45.7
	0.5 µg	28.1	30.9	50.9
	1.0 µg	49.1	41.6	51.4

[1] 1,000-2,000 cpm H labelled mRNAs were used.

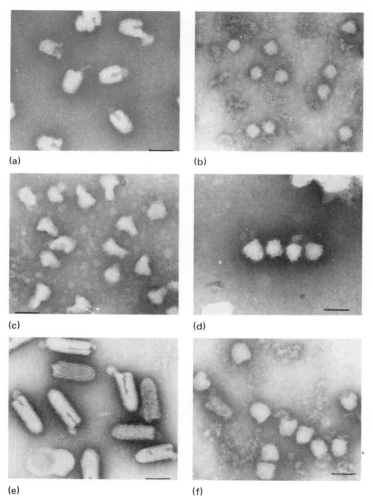

Fig. 1.   Electron micrographs of negatively stained purified preparations of VSV virion and DI particles. Ammonium molybolate (2%) was used as the negative stain and the photographs were taken with a Siemens Elmiskop IA at x 40,000 magnification; (a) ts 11 DI particle; (b) ts 31 DI particle; (c) ts 12 DI particle; (d) same as (c) but pretreated with 2% glutaraldehyde in 0.2 M tris buffer pH 7.4; (e) VSV wild type virion; (f) wild type DI particle bar = 100 nm [from Reichmann, et al., J. Virol. 8, 154 (1972)].

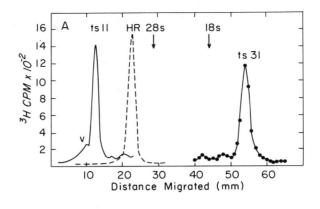

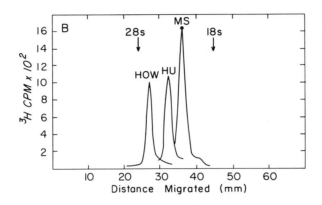

Fig. 2. Polyacrylamide gel electrophoresis of DI particle RNA species. The drawings are composites of superimposed gel profiles obtained with RNA preparations from purified DI particles. The purification procedures were described previously (8). The 28S and 18S markers were prepared from ^{14}C labelled uninfected BHK cells (15). Electrophoresis in 3E buffer (8), was from left to right at 10 mA per gel for 3 hrs. (A) The RNA species were isolated from DI particles generated by mutant VSV virions. ts 11, ts 31 were temperature sensitive mutants (7) and HR was a heat resistant mutant (5). (B) The RNA species were isolated from DI particles generated by wild type VSV obtained from three different laboratories (see Materials and Methods).

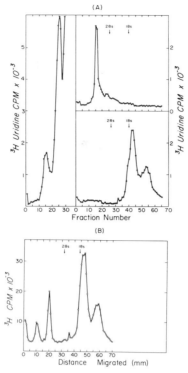

Fig. 3. Separation of VSV-induced cytoplasmic RNA species. RNA was extracted from infected cells as described previously (15). Ultracentrifugation was at 200,000 x g for 5 hr at 4° C using a 5-20% sucrose gradient in 3E (8) buffer. Polyacrylamide gel electrophoresis was performed as described in Fig. 2. Centrifugation is from right to left and electrophoresis is from left to right. (a) The left hand drawing presents a characteristic sucrose profile of the VSV induced cytoplasmic RNA in the presence of cycloheximide. Repeated purifications of the 10-20 and 25-30 fractions by sucrose gradient centrifugation resulted in a separation of the 30S and 18-13S size classes. A polyacrylamide gel profile of these species is shown in the right hand drawing, top and bottom respectively. (b) Polyacrylamide gel electrophoresis of VSV-induced cytoplasmic RNA. These RNA species were obtained from VSV-infected cells in the absence of cycloheximide. Therefore, in addition to the mRNA size classes shown in Fig. 3A, this preparation also contained the virion RNA (42s).

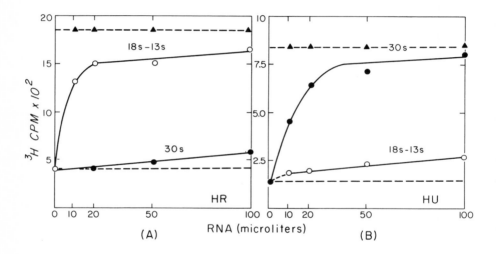

Fig. 4. Annealing of DI particle RNAs to variable amounts of purified viral mRNA. Annealing was carried out in 2.5 x SSC buffer (16) at 75° C for two hours. After dilution to 1 x SSC the RNA was digested with 10 μg/ml ribonuclease A and 2 units/ml of ribonuclease T₁ for 45 min at 37° C. Undigested RNA was precipitated with 10% cold TCA in the presence of 2 μg of carrier RNA per sample, filtered and counted in a liquid scintillation counter. The lines with solid triangles indicate the particle RNA counts added to each tube. The dotted lines indicate results obtained after annealing of the labelled particle RNA with non-labelled cellular RNA. (a) HR DI particle RNA. (b) HU DI particle RNA.

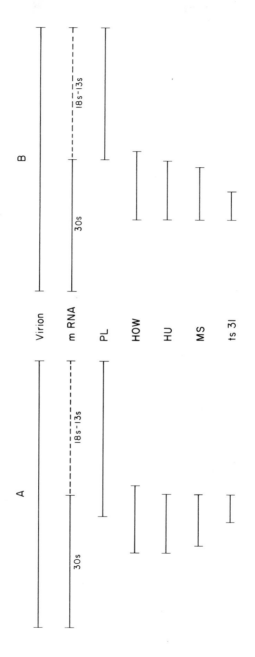

Fig. 5. Two tentative maps of DI particle RNA species on the viral genome. Both locations are consistent with the annealing data (for details see Discussion).

115

POLIOVIRUS DEFECTIVE
INTERFERING PARTICLES

David Baltimore, Charles N. Cole[*],
Lydia Villa-Komaroff and Deborah Spector

Department of Biology
Massachusetts Institute of Technology
Cambridge, Massachusetts 02139

Poliovirus, like many other animal viruses, spawns
defective interfering (DI) particles during multiple
cycles of growth at high multiplicities of infection (1).
Such particles have been characterized physically (1), the
nature of their defect has been elucidated (2), the
mechanism by which they interfere with the growth of standard virus has been investigated (3) and their ability to
be enriched at the expense of standard virus has been
studied (3, 4).

In the present paper the known properties of poliovirus DI particles will be briefly reviewed followed by
discussions of the mechanisms of interference and enrichment. Most of the experimental data on poliovirus DI
particles has been published in four papers from this
laboratory (1-4).

What is the defect in poliovirus DI particles?

Poliovirus DI particles contain about 15% less RNA
than standard poliovirus particles but a normal amount of
polyadenylic acid (1; Spector, unpublished results).
Because of this deficit in RNA, the particles can be purified to homogeneity using cesium chloride density gradi-

[*]Present address: Department of Biochemistry,
Stanford University School of Medicine, Palo Alto,
California 94305.

ents. When a purified preparation of DI particles infects
HeLa cells, there is a normal amount of virus-specific RNA
synthesis and virus-specific protein synthesis. However,
no new virions are formed by the infected cells. Only
when cells are co-infected by standard virus and DI particles are new DI particles produced.

The reason for the lack of virion production when
cells are infected only by DI particles has been traced to
the inability of DI RNA to code for the synthesis of the
protein which is the precursor to all of the capsid proteins in the virion (2). This protein, called NCVP 1, is
totally absent in polyacrylamide gel electropherograms of
the induced viral protein. It is replaced by a partially
deleted protein which is unstable in the infected cell
and rapidly degrades after its synthesis. There is no detectable synthesis of any of the four viral capsid proteins
in cells infected only by DI particles. It appears that
part of the information for NCVP 1 synthesis is deleted in
DI RNA and that this deletion corresponds to 15% of the
viral RNA. Use of poliovirus standard and DI RNA in mammalian cell-free protein-synthesizing systems has indicated that the same initiation is present on both RNA's,
so the deletion would appear to be internal (Villa-
Komaroff, unpublished results).

Mechanism of interference

An analysis of the yields of particles from cells co-
infected by standard and DI particles has led to the conclusion that the defect in capsid protein synthesis is
sufficient to explain the ability of DI to interfere with
the growth of standard virus. The yield of standard and
DI particles is determined by analyzing progeny particles
from infected cells labeled with radioactive uridine by
centrifugation of the particles to equilibrium in gradients of CsCl. Figure 1 shows the types of patterns observed. Cells infected by standard poliovirus yield a
single large peak of virions, cells infected by DI particles (examples of two DI particle populations are shown
in Fig. 1) give rise to little or no progeny; cells infected by a mixture of DI plus standard virions yield two
peaks, one of standard progeny and one of less dense DI
particles. The sum of the radioactivity in the two types
of particles in the co-infected cells is less than the

amount produced by the standard virus alone.

Cells infected by DI particles, standard virus or any mixture of the two all synthesize the same amount of virus-specific RNA (2). This amount of RNA must therefore be apportioned between standard RNA and DI RNA. While direct measurement of the ratio of intracellular standard RNA to DI RNA has not yet been experimentally feasible, we can assume that the two RNA's are found in approximately the same ratio as they occur in the inoculum which initiated the infection.

The fact that only a limited amount of RNA is made by infected cells has two consequences:

(a) There will be two kinds of polyribosomes in cells co-infected by standard virus and DI particles. One type of polyribosomes will contain standard viral messenger RNA and these polyribosomes will synthesize their normal complement of capsid proteins. The second kind of polyribosomes will have DI messenger RNA and this messenger RNA, while producing a normal amount of the non-virion proteins, will produce no capsid proteins. The consequence of having these two types of polyribosomes in co-infected cells is that the percentage of the normal amount of capsid protein made in co-infected cells will be determined by the relative percentages of standard RNA and DI RNA in the cell. The ratios of these two RNA's, we have assumed above, is determined by the percentage of standard virus in the inoculating mixture. This analysis predicts that there will be a linear relationship between the total amount of virus particle formation (which will be limited by the amount of capsid protein) and the percentage of standard virus in the inoculum. Such a linear relationship is evident in the data of Figure 2 (open circles) where the total yield of standard plus DI virions from co-infected cells are plotted versus the percentages of standard virions in the inoculum. This linear relationship validates the assumption made about the relative ratios of the two RNA's in the intracellular RNA pool.

(b) When the capsid protein which is made in co-infected cells starts to encapsidate viral RNA, it will have two types of molecules to choose from. Assuming that the capsid protein cannot tell the difference between standard RNA and DI RNA, the percentage of the total virus particle yield which is standard virus will again be determined by the percentage of standard virus in the inoculum since it is that percentage which determines the relative ratios of the two kinds of RNA in the pool. The analysis predicts a linear relationship between the percentage of standard virus in the inoculum and the percentage of standard virus in the yield. Such a relationship is evident in Figure 2 (crosses), again validating the assumptions used to predict it.

The above analyses indicate that there are two points of interference between standard virus and DI particles: one point at protein synthesis and the other point at encapsidation. If we focus on the yield of infectious particles from co-infected cells, then the percentage of the normal amount of infectious particles formed should be determined by multiplying the percentage of total virus formed by the percentage of that virus which is standard virus. Both of these factors are linear functions of the percentage of standard virus in the inoculum and therefore we can predict that the percentage of infectious virus formed should be related directly to the square of the percentage of standard virus in the inoculum. Again, experimental determination of the percentage of infectious virus formed (Fig. 3, triangles) has confirmed the square relationship.

It would thus appear that the mere existence of particles which are defective in capsid protein formation but carry out all other aspects of virus-specific function are sufficient to explain the ability of these particles to interfere with standard virus production. Because this interference is a function of the square of the proportion of standard virus in the inoculum, interference becomes a very potent check on virus production as the percentage of defective particles in the population increases.

Mechanism of enrichment

The process of interference is the way that defective particles limit the amount of virus produced. But the ability of defective particles to become a large percentage of the total virus population requires that defective particles replicate more efficiently than standard virus particles. This process we call enrichment and it is probably the most characteristic property of a DI particle.

If a DI particle arose which was unable to enrich itself at the expense of standard virus then, although it might slightly cut down the yield of virus in co-infected cells, it could never become a dominant factor in the population of virus particles and probably its existence would not be detected.

We have thus far been unable to completely elucidate the mechanism of enrichment but we have been able to perturb the levels of enrichment in a number of different ways which have suggested models by which enrichment can occur. The level of normally occuring enrichment is small, having been variously estimated at 5-8% (1, 3). This is evident from Figure 3 which compares the virions in a ^{14}C-uridine-labeled inoculum with the ^{3}H-uridine-labeled progeny by CsCl centrifugation. When the heights of the peaks of standard virus in the input and output are normalized, an excess of about 5% in the DI peak of the progeny virus is observed.

Two potential levels of enrichment have been un-covered:

(a) Enrichment by preferential encapsidation: As indicated above, when capsid proteins encapsidate stan-dard and DI RNA it would appear that they cannot select one or the other RNA. Analysis of the total yield of virus supports such a conclusion (Fig. 2). If cells are labeled with uridine for a very short period of time, how-ever, and therefore only the most recently made virus particles are labeled, in co-infected cells there is a hyperenrichment of DI particles among these recently-labeled progeny. Figure 4 shows an analysis of progeny after various times of labeling. It is evident that the hyperenrichment rapidly decays to an equilibrium value. Such behavior is consistent with the ability of DI to be more rapidly encapsidated than standard virus. Whether this more rapid encapsidation could lead to an enrichment or not would depend on the detailed kinetics of the pro-duction of virus particles. It has thus far been im-possible to prove whether or not this mechanism plays any important role in the ordinary level of enrichment but it is doubtful that it does play a major role.

(b) Enrichment by preferential replication does not occur: It seems plausible that enrichment might be a natural consequence of the fact that DI RNA is shorter than standard RNA because then DI RNA should replicate

121

more rapidly than standard RNA. A short RNA, however, will not necessarily replicate more rapidly than a long RNA--the rate of RNA synthesis will be determined by the rate of <u>initiation</u> of progeny RNA strands and this rate should be independent of the length of an RNA molecule.

For DI RNA to replicate more rapidly than standard RNA, DI RNA would have to have a more efficient binding site for the RNA replicase than does standard RNA. If that were true, then during a one step growth cycle, DI RNA should <u>continually</u> increase relative to standard RNA. Such a continual enrichment has been sought and was not found (3). The amount of enrichment was found to be independent of the time after infection--early progeny are as enriched in DI particles as are the last progeny made during a single cycle of infection. Therefore, DI RNA does not appear to have a selective advantage for the binding of replicase.

(c) <u>Enrichment as an early event</u>: If enrichment is complete before the first progeny are formed then either it is a process which occurs throughout infection at a constant rate or else it occurs very early in the growth cycle. The possibility of enrichment by preferential encapsidation could be a process occuring throughout infection but, as mentioned above, it is only evident in pulse-labeled progeny and probably plays at most a minor role in enrichment.

There is no obvious continuing process other than encapsidation which could produce an enrichment, so we sought evidence for an early event as the cause. Working on the hypothesis that if enrichment occurs early, extension of the early part of the growth cycle might produce a hyperenrichment, we attempted to extend the early phase by treating cells with cycloheximide (4). Cells were pulsed for 60 minutes with this inhibitor of protein synthesis at various times after infection, and then the total yield of particles formed throughout the ensuing infection cycle was analyzed for its content of standard and DI particles. Figure 5 shows that pulsing with cycloheximide from 13 to 73 minutes post-infection caused the most marked hyperenrichment. Treatment for other 60 minute periods also caused a hyperenrichment but the system was most affected by treatments during the early times.

This result suggests that events occuring early are

most responsible for enrichment. Exactly how cycloheximide is able to cause hyperenrichment is not known but it may be that by limiting the amount of replicase, enrichment can be achieved (4). More likely, however, enrichment may occur during the first cycles of RNA synthesis because DI RNA progeny will appear before standard progeny if both begin replication synchronously. Such an advantage would rapidly be lost as a steady-state condition was established. Cycloheximide might then effectively reset the infection clock so the earliest stage of infection is repeated.

Enrichment and interference

It would seem that enrichment should be evident in the data of Figure 2 where the relationship of input and progeny virus was studied. Although it was not indicated previously (see section on Interference), enrichment is evident in that data because, on the average, the points for total particle production fall a bit above the 45°-slope line and the points for percentage of the yield as standard virus fall a bit below the 45°-slope line. These small deviations measure the amount of enrichment which, as noted previously, is only 5–8% in one infection cycle.

Conclusion

It was argued previously that DI particle formation is a natural, evolutionarily programed aspect of the life cycle of most, if not all, animal viruses (5). In the case of poliovirus, the mode of DI formation appears to be internal deletion of part of the information for synthesis of the capsid. By leaving the other genes of the virus intact, the deletion provides a DI particle able to replicate normally. The DI particle thus interferes with the amount of standard RNA produced causing less virions to be made and causing many of those made to be new DI particles. The DI also is able to enrich itself at each cycle of virus growth so that it ultimately dominates the population of virions (1). The major cause of the enrichment appears to be an early event during the infection cycle and probably involves a transient, more rapid, synthesis of DI RNA than of standard RNA. If, in fact, DI particle generation is "purposefully" programed into viral structure, poliovirus appears to have found an elegantly simple solution to the formation of particles which are defective, interfering and able to enrich themselves.

Acknowledgements

This work was supported by grant AI-08388 from the National Institutes of Health. D. B. is an American Cancer Society Research professor. D. S. is a pre-doctoral fellow of the National Science Foundation.

References

1. Cole, C.N., Smoler, D., Wimmer, E. and Baltimore, D., J. of Virol. 7, 478 (1971).
2. Cole, C.N. and Baltimore, D., J. Mol. Biol. 76, 325 (1973).
3. Cole, C.N. and Baltimore, D., J. Mol. Biol. 76, 345 (1973).
4. Cole, C.N. and Baltimore, D., J. of Virol. 12, 1414 (1973).
5. Huang, A.S. and Baltimore, D., Nature 226, 325 (1970).

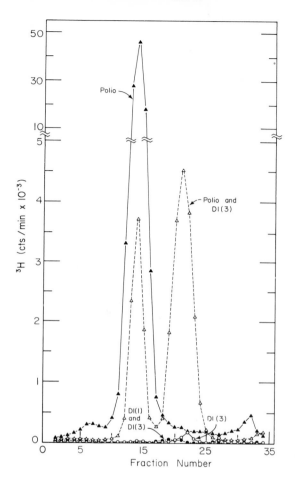

Fig. 1.   Demonstration and quantitation of interference.
HeLa cells were infected with multiplicities of 10 plaque-
forming particles per cell of either standard poliovirus,
DI particles or a mixture of the two (the definition of
plaque-forming unit equivalents for DI particles is
given in ref. 2).   The infected cells were labeled from
1.5–7 hours post-infection with ^{14}C–uridine, the labeled
virions were harvested and the virions were centrifuged
to equilibrium in gradients of CsCl.   The peak at fraction
14 is standard virus (ρ = 1.34gm/cc); the peak at fraction
22 is DI particles (ρ = 1.325 gm/cc).   Reprinted from ref.
2 with permission.

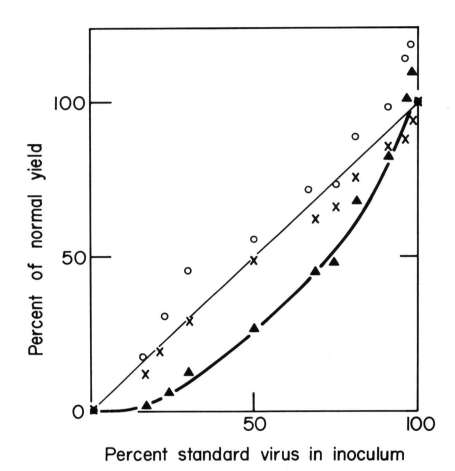

Fig. 2. Interference with standard virus growth by DI particles as a function of their relative input multiplicities. (0) Total yield of particles from cells infected by different relative multiplicities of standard and DI particles; (X) percentage of standard virions among the progeny; (▲) yield of plaque-forming virus (percentage of control). Reprinted from ref. 3 with permission.

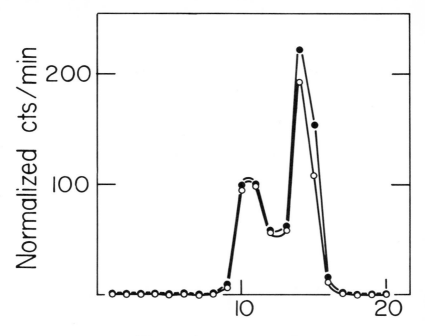

Fig. 3. Enrichment of DI particles during one growth
cycle. A culture of 4 x 10⁷ cells in 10 ml was infected
by a mixed stock of standard and defective particles. One-
quarter of the culture was exposed to [¹⁴C]uridine (2.5
µCi) beginning 60 minutes after infection. Infection was
halted in both labeled and unlabeled cultures 7 hours
after infection by 3 cycles of freezing and thawing. A
portion of the unlabeled culture was used to infect a culture of 4 x 10⁷ cells in 10 ml, and this was labeled with
[³H]uridine (10 µCi) beginning 60 minutes after infection.
Infection was halted after 7 hours by 3 cycles of freezing
and thawing. A portion of the [¹⁴C]uridine-labeled culture was added and the progeny virus examined by centrifugation in CsCl as described in Cole et al. (1). Radioactivity in all samples was normalized by setting one
point in the peak of standard virus equal to 100 for both
[¹⁴C]- and [³H]uridine-labeled virus. -O-O-, [¹⁴C]uridine-
labeled parental virus; -●-●-, [³H]uridine-labeled progeny
virus. Reprinted from ref. 3 with permission.

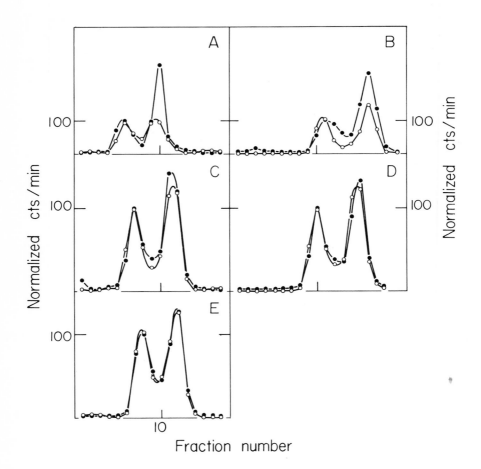

Fig. 4. CsCl density gradients of the progeny of standard
and DI particle co-infected cells labeled for various times
with ³H-uridine. (O) Progeny labeled with ¹⁴C-uridine
throughout one cycle of co-infection by standard and DI
particles. (●) Progeny pulse-labeled with ³H-uridine
starting at 2.75 hours after infection and continuing for
(A) 7 minutes, (B) 16 minutes, (C) 24 minutes, (D) 36
minutes and (E) 145 minutes. Reprinted from ref. 4 with
permission.

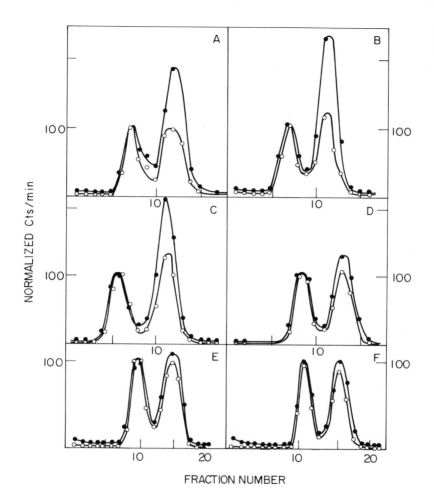

Fig. 5. CsCl density gradients of the progeny of standard
and DI(1) particle co-infected cells transiently treated
with cycloheximide. (O) Progeny of an unperturbed co-
infected culture labeled with ^{14}C-uridine. (●) Progeny
of cultures treated for 60 minute periods with cycloheximide (100 µg/ml) then labeled with ^{3}H-uridine and harvested at 7 hours after infection. The time of addition
of cycloheximide was : (A) 0; (B) 13 minutes; (C) 30
minutes; (D) 45 minutes; (E) 120 minutes and (F) 180
minutes. Reprinted from ref. 4 with permission.

129

DEFECTIVE INTERFERING PARTICLES AS MEDIATORS OF SLOWER, AND PERSISTENT NONCYTOCIDAL VSV INFECTIONS *IN VIVO* AND *IN VITRO*.

John J. Holland, Louis Perez Villarreal and
James R. Etchison

Department of Biology
University of California, San Diego
La Jolla, Ca. 92037

ABSTRACT. Vesicular stomatitis virus has been employed as a model system for normally virulent enveloped RNA viruses which can cause, under certain conditions, persistent non-cytocidal (carrier) infection of cells *in vitro*, and slowly progressive or persistent disease *in vivo*. We present evidence that defective interfering particles (T particles) are necessary for the establishment and maintenance of persistent noncytocidal infection of BHK_{21} cells in culture. In the absence of T particles, B virions (infectious full-size virions) of VSV are completely virulent and cause 100% death of BHK_{21} cells. A temperature-sensitive B virion strain was required along with homologous short T particles to initiate persistent noncytocidal infection, but as the carrier culture became established a new long T particle arose to displace the short T particle. These long T particles, when purified are capable of establishing persistent noncytocidal carrier infection even in combination with virulent (non-temperature-sensitive) wild type VSV. These long T particles have the unique ability to depress B virion transcriptase activity, and this regulatory effect on viral transcription could be largely responsible for the establishment and maintenance of persistent noncytocidal infection.

Defective interfering T particles can protect mice against otherwise fatal challenge by low doses of VSV B virions, but against high challenge doses they mediate slowly progressive viral disease which usually terminates fatally. The implications of these findings for persistent, slowly progressive, and noncytocidal infections caused by other enveloped RNA viruses are discussed.

INTRODUCTION

In 1970 Huang and Baltimore (1) speculated that defective interfering virus particles might play an important part in slow virus diseases *in vivo*. In this review we outline our continuing investigation of this possibility. We have employed VSV as a model system because it is presently the best understood of the enveloped RNA viruses from the standpoint of its biochemistry, genetics and cell biology (1,2,3) and because its T particles are readily purified on sucrose gradients (4). VSV is not yet known to be responsible for slow, persistent virus disease in man or animals although it causes persistent noncytocidal infection of insects and their cells in culture (5,6). However the closely related rabies virus and other Rhabdoviruses regularly cause slowly-progressing and latent infections of man and animals (7,8) and persistent noncytocidal infection of cells in culture (9). In 1963 Wagner *et al.* (10) showed that a small plaque mutant of VSV could establish persistent slowly-cytopathic carrier infection of L cells in culture. These carrier cells exhibited frequently-recurring crises of severe cytopathology with alternating periods of recovery. The molecular mechanisms of persistence could not be explored extensively at that time, but a possible role for interferon was suggested. Mudd *et al.* (6) recently showed that VSV Indiana routinely causes persistent noncytopathic infection of Drosophila cells in culture but the mechanism has not yet been examined.

Measles virus is an enveloped RNA virus which may be a latent agent of slow neurologic diseases such as subacute sclerosing panencephalitis (11,12) and multiple sclerosis (13). Also it readily establishes persistent noncytocidal carrier infections of cells in culture, and the presence of antibody facilitates the conversion of carrier cultures to latently infected (non-virus-yielding) cells (14,15). These latently infected cells in culture can be made to yield infectious virus after cocultivation with susceptible cells (16). This is the same process by which latent virus can be activated from brain cells of victims of subacute sclerosing panencephalitis (11), but little is known of the mechanism of establishment of persistent, noncytocidal and latent infection by measles or any other normally virulent RNA virus. Temperature sensitivity of the persistent virion appears to be a factor in both NDV and measles persistent infection (17,16). Our observations suggest that defective interfering particles may be a prerequisite for persistent noncytocidal infection *in vitro* or *in vivo*. *In vivo*, of course, the immune response of the host is crucial in determining the nature of the noncytocidal virus disease process. This review will present a narrative account of our recent studies, the detailed data are presented elsewhere (18-23).

METHODS

Materials and methods are described in detail elsewhere (18-23). Unless it is stated otherwise, VSV refers to the virulent wild type Indiana serotype of vesicular stomatitis virus. Homologous defective T particles of all VSV strains were produced by repeated high multiplicity passage of cloned B virions on BHK_{21} cells (except for the carrier long T particle whose origin is described below). All B virion preparations were cloned several times on BHK_{21} cells to free them of T particles, and all virus preparations and virus assays were carried out with BHK_{21} cells. Purified T particles completely freed of infectious virus were prepared by repeated sucrose gradient separation as described elsewhere (19).

RESULTS

1. *Highly purified T particles completely freed of infectious B virions are noncytotoxic, non-lethal and immunizing.* In his earliest studies of defective interfering particles of influenza virus, von Magnus showed a slight and variable *in vivo* prophylactic effect of these particles against simultaneously inoculated standard virus (24). Our first attempts,with M. V. Doyle, to confirm and extend these findings showed very little protective effect (18) due to infectious virus contaminating T particles. Therefore we devised a technique for preparing T particle preparations in milligram quantities completely free of infectious virus (19). These highly purified T particles showed the following characteristics (19): They do not kill most cells in culture at a multiplicity of 10^5 particles per cell

although most of the cells are killed at an overwhelming multiplicity of 10^6 particles per cell. They are not lethal or visibly toxic to mice when inoculated intracerebrally, but because they carry all virion proteins they act as good immunizing components and provide immunity to later challenge to homologous virus but not to heterologous virus (19).

2. *Highly purified T particles provide strong prophylaxis in mice against intracerebral infection by low challenge doses of homologous B virions.* When inoculated intracerebrally along with low lethal doses of B virions, highly purified T particles provided remarkable prophylaxis and most treated mice survived an otherwise rapidly fatal viral encephalitis as is summarized in Table 1. It was found that virus replicated to significant levels in the brains of some treated mice but not in others. In no case was the brain virus titer as high in T particle treated mice as in control mice given virus alone (19).

3. *Highly purified T particles can not protect mice from the lethal effects of large doses of B virions, but convert a rapidly lethal encephalitis to a slowly-progressing paralytic virus disease.* As Table 1 shows, high doses of infectious B virions alone kill all control animals within several days, but the presence of T particles in the inoculum greatly altered the nature of the disease process (19). In the control animals the onset of neural effects was sudden, and all animals died within a few hours to a day following the first signs of encephalitis. But the same inoculum in the presence of T particles caused a very slow onset of disease. This infection was not a rapidly fatal encephalitis but a slowly progressing disease with less virus replication in the brain. The mice exhibited gradually increasing paralysis usually appearing first in the hind limbs, then developed generalized wasting deterioration. They eventually became unable to eat or drink and most of them died slowly. Fig. 1 shows a mouse 12 days after infection. The hind limb paralysis, ruffled fur, arched back and weight loss are typical of the slower virus disease mediated by the presence of T particles. We conclude that T particles can slow down viral infections *in vivo* and profoundly alter the nature of viral disease as Huang and Baltimore suggested they might.

134

4. *Selection of B virions over T particles during* in vivo *passage of mixtures of both.* In our original study of T particles *in vivo* (18) we demonstrated that intracerebral inoculation of mixtures of large numbers of T particles plus large (or small) numbers of B virions led to the production of greatly reduced yields of B virions but T particles were either lost or were present in such small numbers that they did not cause detectable interference on first passage of brain virus yields (18). We have since repeated this observation many times and further found that T particles are not absent from the brains of these mice, they are merely present at very low levels. This could be shown by inoculating brain yields onto BHK_{21} cells then purifying the BHK_{21} yields after 24 hours. In 7 different experiments the amplifying effect of this first passage caused the production of a visible band of T particles, but there were always more B virions than T particles in these first passage yields. This explains why repeated intracerebral passage of VSV in mice does not lead to a von Magnus type accumulation of defective virus (18). A possible explanation for these results will be suggested in the discussion.

PERSISTENT NONCYTOCIDAL INFECTION OF CULTURED CELLS IS MEDIATED BY T PARTICLES

1. *Both temperature sensitive B virions and homologous T particles were required to initiate persistent noncytocidal carrier infection of BHK_{21} cells in culture.* Wagner *et al.* (10) established the first reported VSV carrier culture using a small plaque mutant of VSV. We have further studied this process to determine what is required for a virulent virus such as VSV to become persistent and non-cytocidal. We found that among all of our wild type and temperature sensitive mutant strains of VSV, only the temperature sensitive ts 31 strain of Pringle (25) readily established carrier cultures (23). Furthermore, it could do so only in the presence of the homologous short T particle (26) which it regularly produces. In the absence of T particles the cloned ts 31 B virions were cytocidal for 100% of infected cells but in the presence of homologous short T particles a small percentage of cells survived and established a carrier culture at 37°C. (23). These carrier cells underwent frequent crises of severe cytopathology at first [as did the carrier culture of Wagner *et al.* (10)]

but after 90 days in culture the carrier state became sta-
bilized. Thereafter these cells have behaved like normal
BHK_{21} cells with a doubling time of less than 24 hours even
though they are continuously producing virus at low levels
(up to several PFU/cell/day). At 170 days after carrier
establishment these cells show only scattered syncitia and
slight cytoplasmic granularity even though all cells are
infected. Fig. 2 shows carrier cells at 120 days when
cytoplasmic granularity was more prominent.

2. *All, or nearly all carrier cells are infected with B
virions and T particles, and they show strong interference
to homologous B virion challenge. Interferon is not
detectable in carrier cultures.* Several lines of evidence
suggest that the carrier cells are infected with both infectious B virions and T particle. First, nearly all carrier cells showed granular cytoplasmic inclusions during
the first 4 months in culture. Secondly, infectious center
assays demonstrate that all or nearly all cells are producing infectious B virions (23). Thirdly, each infectious
center cell producing B virions is also producing T particles as shown by first passage of every plaque picked from
carrier culture infectious centers (23). Fourthly, carrier
cells show greater than 99% yield reduction when challenged
with high multiplicities of homologous B virions, but no
reduction of yield when challenged by influenza virus or
mengovirus (23). This lack of resistance to heterologous
virus indicates that interferon is probably not the interfering agent in these carrier cells. This was confirmed
when we failed to detect interferon activity even in undiluted culture medium from carrier cells (23).

3. *A new long T particle arises during establishment of
carrier cultures, and it is this defective particle, not a
mutated B virion, which is responsible for maintaining the
persistent noncytocidal infection of the carrier cells.*
We observed (23) that shortly after initiation of the carrier cultures with ts 31 B virions and homologous short T
particles, these short T particles of 150s (26) were replaced by a new long T particle (of approximately 470s).
This newly-generated T particle has persisted throughout
the first 170 days of persistent noncytocidal carrier infection. These long T particles are continuously budded
into the culture medium along with B virions, they are

136

always produced along with B virions when carrier cells are cocultivated with normal BHK$_{21}$ cells or induced to yield virus by incubation at 33°C (23).

The following evidence shows that this long T particle is responsible for maintenance of the persistent non-cytocidal carrier state (23): Firstly, B virions isolated from carrier cells, then cloned to rid them of long T particles, are unable to re-establish persistent infections of BHK$_{21}$ cells alone (all cells are killed), but they readily do so in the presence of added purified carrier long T particles. Secondly, persistent carrier infections could be established by wild type (and other strains of B virions) when accompanied by the carrier long T particle. We conclude that this long T particle is the essential determinant of persistent noncytocidal infection in these carrier cultures.

4. *Cell-free extracts from the cytoplasm of VSV carrier cultures and rabies virus-infected BHK$_{21}$ cells exhibit little* in vitro *transcriptase activity.* Galet *et al.* (27) have shown that virulent infection by VSV leads to the appearance in cell extracts of sedimentable viral nucleo-proteins which are very active in *in vitro* transcription. We have confirmed this but have found that persistent non-cytocidal VSV carrier infection or rabies virus infection of BHK$_{21}$ cells induces only barely-detectable levels of viral RNA polymerase activity (22). Rabies virus infection is normally noncytocidal in BHK$_{21}$ cells and in most cultured cells (9). We conclude that persistent noncytocidal infection by VSV (or by rabies) induces much lower transcriptase levels than does virulent VSV infection. The long T particle must be directly or indirectly influencing the B virion-induced levels of transcriptase in carrier cultures.

5. *Wild type VSV B virions produced by cells which are also infected with carrier long T particles exhibit great-ly depressed virion transcriptase activity.* When large amounts of carrier virus were induced by cocultivation of carrier cells with normal BHK$_{21}$ cells we found that the B virions often had greatly depressed virion transcriptase activity in an *in vitro* assay. This seemed to occur when-ever there were large yields of long T particles, suggesting that B virions produced within cells which are also

replicating long T particles may be defective in virion transcriptase. We confirmed this using wild type B virions. Whenever we doubly-infected normal BHK_{21} cells with wild type B virions plus purified carrier long T particles, strong interference with B virion replication occurred. However the B virions which were produced, when purified and tested for transcriptase levels, always showed very low specific activity (10 fold or greater below the level of control B virions from singly infected cells (23). Other T particles do not show this transcription - attenuating activity. The basis for this unique regulatory effect of carrier long T particles is unknown at present. It may be of great importance in maintenance of persistent noncytocidal infection by this otherwise-virulent virus. Most T particles seem to interfere at the level of replication (28,29,30), not at the transcription level.

6. *Rabies virions lack detectable transcriptase activity* in vitro. Sokol *et al*. (31) reported that purified rabies virions lack detectable *in vitro* transcriptase activity and we have confirmed this on a number of purified HEP rabies (Flury strain) virion preparations (22).· It is possible that our reaction conditions are inadequate, but the same conditions do show small amounts of rabies virus-induced RNA polymerase activity in sedimentable complexes from infected cell cytoplasm. Cell activation of rabies virion transcriptase following infection is another possibility.

Defective interfering T particles of rabies virus have been observed and inferred in a number of laboratories, but have not yet been thoroughly studied (32-34). We have carried out serial undiluted passages of HEP rabies virus and have found an unpredictable appearance and disappearance of a distinct T particle band of about 350s (23). We have also confirmed the observation (9) of the Wistar Instutute group that the rabies B virion band is very broad (as compared to VSV). It seems likely that the broad heterogeneous B virion band includes a long T particle similar to the VSV carrier long T particle. New Jersey strains of VSV B virions behave in a similar manner, showing much greater variation and heterogeneity than VSV Indiana (29,35). We are studying rabies noncytocidal infection in greater detail but it is already clear that persistent noncytocidal carrier infections by VSV show some remarkable similarities to rabies infections of BHK_{21}

[which are normally noncytocidal (9)].

DISCUSSION

Although VSV is only a model system, these studies suggest the following general hypotheses for persistent, slow, noncytocidal infections *in vitro* and *in vivo* by enveloped negative strand RNA viruses. 1) Defective interfering particles are responsible for "slowing" virulent RNA viruses and maintaining persistent noncytocidal infection (and "slow" virus disease). 2) They probably do so by interfering at the replication level (28,29), and perhaps in some cases at the transcription level (22,23). Regulation of transcription offers considerable advantage *in vivo* where persistently infected cells may be destroyed by the immune system if they express much foreign (viral) antigen on their surface membrane. These hypotheses will be more difficult to test for measles virus and rabies virus than for VSV but we are attempting to carry out rabies virus and measles virus studies in parallel with the VSV work. However, it is clear that the original suggestion of Huang and Baltimore (1) regarding a role of defective viruses in slow virus disease is already showing considerable promise. A role for defective particles in LCM virus persistent noncytocidal infection now seems increasingly likely (36,37).

One apparent anomaly of the *in vivo* results deserves comment; that is the selection for B virions during replication of mixtures of B virions and T particles inoculated together in high dosage (18). There are two obvious explanations for this: Firstly, some cell lines promote defective particle interference whereas interference is much less in other cell lines (38,1,35), and the infected brain cells may behave in the latter manner. Secondly, B virions *in vivo* are likely to escape from T particles by being seeded to distant cells that are not simultaneously infected with T particles. Thus there would be local growth of "clones" of B virions free of T particles (until local high multiplicities generated new T particles or until T particles from a distant site were seeded into the local "clone" of B infected cells). In the body where distant seeding is a possibility, B virions (which can replicate by themselves) have an advantage over T particles (which cannot) except in local areas wherever there are high concentrations of B virion-infected cells to support T particle replication. Therefore, we propose the following evolutionary role for defective interfering particles (which are now known to be generated by nearly all animal viruses): Virulent animal viruses have a selective advantage if they can spread readily from host to host and initiate rapid growth in each before an effective immune response is mounted. However, once the virus is established, rapid cytocidal spread within tissues and organs would be fatal to the host (and to the host populations upon which these virulent viruses depend for survival). Therefore, each rapidly cytocidal virulent virus carries not only the genetic potential for rapid replication and spread, but also the genetic potential to prevent excessive damage at any local site (by generation of defective particles). Wherever local high multiplicity infection occurs in tissues and organs the possibility of organ destruction is balanced by the high probability that defective particles will be generated. This not only protects the host population from excessive virus lethality, it also provides a mechanism for long-term virus persistence in a noncytocidal intracellular state (as exemplified by the VSV carrier cultures).

The strong *in vivo* prophylactic effect of T particles against low challenge doses of infectious virus suggests that defective particles might offer unique vaccine opportunities (19), but obviously their ability to trigger slow persistent infection suggests caution with such an approach. However this point may be somewhat academic since McLaren (39) recently found that poliovirus defective particles (40) are present as a large percentage of the particles in commercially distributed polio vaccine lots and in the reference vaccine pools. Vaccine selection techniques may select not only for virus mutants, but for defective interfering particles as well. In view of the selection and production techniques for such current vaccines as measles, mumps, rubella, vaccinia etc., it would be surprising if defective particles were not present. The potential ramifications of defective particles in vaccines are intriguing at the very least.

ACKNOWLEDGMENTS

We thank E. Bussey for excellent technical assistance. The *in vivo* studies reported here were started in collaboration with Dr. M. V. Doyle. Supported by USPHS research grant No. CA10802 from the National Cancer Institute.

REFERENCES

1. A.S. Huang and D. Baltimore, Nature 226, 325 (1970).
2. A.F. Howatson, Adv. Vir. Res. 16, 195 (1970).
3. D.L. Knudson, J. Gen. Virol. 20, 105 (1973).
4. A.S. Huang, and R.R. Wagner, Virology 30, 173 (1966).
5. P. Printz, Ann. Inst. Pasteur, Paris 119, 520 (1970).
6. J.A. Mudd, R.W. Leavitt, D.T. Kingsbury, and J.J. Holland, J. Gen. Virol. 20, 341 (1973).
7. S. Matsumoto, Adv. Virus Res. 16, 257 (1970).
8. H.N. Johnson, Ann. N.Y. Acad. Sci. 48, 380 (1947).
9. F. Sokol, E. Kuwert, T.J. Wiktor, K. Hummeler, and H. Koprowski, J. Virol. 2, 836 (1968).
10. R.R. Wagner, A. Levy, R. Snyder, G. Ratcliff, and D. Hyatt, J. Immunol. 91, 112 (1963)
11. F.E. Payne, J.V. Baublis, and H.H. Itabashi, N. Engl. J. Med. 281, 585 (1969).
12. L. Horta-Barbosa, D.A. Fucillo, J.L. Sever, and W. Zeman, Nature 221, 974 (1969).
13. T.E. Henson, J.A. Brody, J.L. Sever, M.L. Dyken, and J. Cannon, J. Am. Med. Assoc. 211, 1985 (1970).
14. R. Rustigian, J. Bacteriol. 92, 1792 (1966).
15. R. Rustigian, J. Bacteriol. 92, 1805 (1966).
16. M.V. Haspell, P.R. Knight, R.G. Duff, and F. Rapp, J. Virol. 12, 690 (1973).
17. O.T. Preble, and J.S. Youngner, J. Virol. 12, 481 (1973).
18. J.J. Holland, and M.V. Doyle, Infect. Immun. 7, 526 (1973).
19. M.V. Doyle, and J.J. Holland, Proc. Natl. Acad. Sci. U.S. 70, 2105 (1973).
20. M.E. Reichmann, L.P. Villarreal, D. Kohne, J. Lesnaw, and J.J. Holland, Virology in press. (March 1974 edit.)
21. L.P. Villarreal, and J.J. Holland, Nature, new Biol.
22. L.P. Villarreal, and J.J. Holland, manuscript submitted for publication (1974).
23. L.P. Villarreal, and J.J. Holland, manuscript submitted for publication (1974).
24. P. von Magnus, Adv. Virus Res. 2, 59 (1954).
25. C.R. Pringle, J. Virol. 5, 559 (1970).

26. M.E. Reichmann, C.R. Pringle, and E.A.C. Follett J. Virol. 8, 154 (1971).

27. H. Galet, J.G. Shedlarski, Jr., and L. Prevec Can. J. Biochem. 51, 721 (1973).

28. A.S. Huang and E. Manders, J. Virol. 9, 909 (1972).

29. J. Perrault, and J.J. Holland, Virology 50, 159 (1972).

30. S. Emerson, and R.R. Wagner, J. Virol. 10, 297 (1972).

31. F. Sokol, and H.F. Clark, Virology 52, 246 (1973).

32. K. Hummeler, H. Koprowski, and T.J. Wiktor, J. Virol. 1, 152 (1967).

33. K. Yoshino, S. Taniguchi, and K. Arai, Proc. Soc.Exp. Biol. Med. 123, 387 (1966).

34. J. Crick, and F. Brown, J. Gen. Virol. 22, 147 (1974).

35. J. Perrault, and J.J. Holland, Virology 50, 148 (1972).

36. F. Lehmann-Grubbe, Virol. Monogr. 10, 1 (1971).

37. R.M. Welsh, C.M. O'Connell, and C.J. Pfau, J. Gen Virol. 17, 355 (1972).

38. P.W. Choppin, Virology 39, 130 (1969).

39. L.C. McLaren, and J.J. Holland, manuscript submitted for publication (1974).

40. C.N. Cole, D. Smoler, E. Wimmer, and D. Baltimore, J. Virol. 7, 478 (1971).

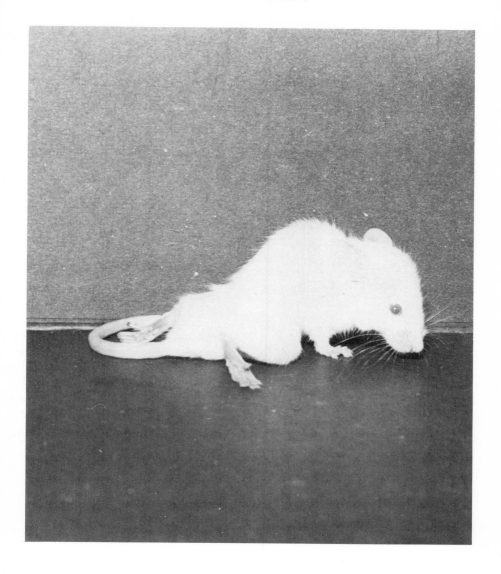

Fig. 1. Mouse exhibiting typical slow, paralytic disease caused by intracerebral inoculation of 10^5 wild type VSV B virions and 5×10^{10} homologous T particles 12 days before.

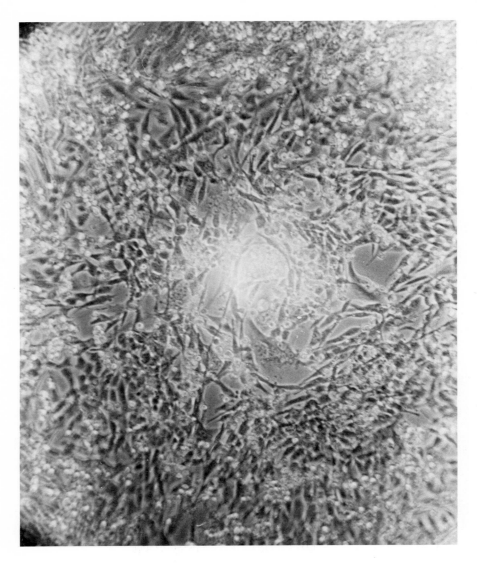

Fig. 2. Photomicrograph of BHK_{21} VSV carrier cells 120 days after initiation of persistent noncytocidal infection. Note the intracytoplasmic inclusions, granular cytoplasm and numerous syncitia at this time. After 170 days these characteristics of the carrier cultures are still present but are much less pronounced.

TABLE 1

Effect of T particles on low dosage and high dosage VSV
B virion infection of mice.

Number of mice	No. of Survivors	Aver./day of death in nonsurviving mice
small inoculum of B virions alone*		
96	8	2–3
low inoculum of B virions plus T particles*		
117	109	8–11
large inoculum of B virions alone*		
72	0	1 1/2–2
large inoculum of B virions plus T particles*		
75	12	9–14

Mice were inoculated intracerebrally with 0.02 ml volumes
of B virions alone, or mixtures of B virions plus T
particles.
*This is a summary Table from many separate experiments.
Small inocula of B virions ranged from 25 PFU to 200 PFU
inoculated per mouse. Large inocula ranged from 10^4 to
10^6 PFU inoculated per mouse. Where T particles were employed approximately 5×10^{10} physical particles were mixed
with B virions (in 0.02 ml) and inoculated as a mixture.

INCREASED PRODUCTION OF INTERFERING VIRUS PARTICLES IN CELL CULTURES FROM MICE RESISTANT TO GROUP B ARBOVIRUS INFECTION

Margo Brinton Darnell* and Hillary Koprowski

Wistar Institute
36th and Spruce Sts
Philadelphia, Pennsylvania 19104

ABSTRACT. Resistance to group B arbovirus infection in mice is inherited as a dominant autosomal allele. Comparative studies have been conducted using inbred resistant C3H/RV mice and congenic, susceptible C3H/He mice. C3H/RV mice and cell cultures derived from them produce lower virus yields after a group B arbovirus infection, then do C3H/He mice or cultures derived from them.

Serial passage of undiluted culture fluid in resistant and susceptible cultures after infection with West Nile virus (WNV), a group B arbovirus, resulted in a cyclic rise and fall in virus titer. Only viral preparations made in resistant cells contained sufficient quantities of defective interfering particles (DI) to interfere with the replication of standard WNV.

INTRODUCTION

Two instances of genetically controlled resistance to specific types of viral infections have been found among laboratory mouse populations (1-5). One is resistance to mouse hepatitis and the other, resistance to group B arbovirus infection. Resistance to group B arbovirus infection is inherited as an independent dominant allele. Mice of the inbred resistant strain, C3H/RV, possess the homozygous genotype (RR), while mice of their congenic strain, C3H/He possess the homozygous-susceptible genotype (rr).

---

*Present address: Department of Microbiology, 1060 Mayo Bldg., University of Minnesota, Minneapolis, Minnesota 55455.

The development of the resistant C3H/RV strain has allowed
comparative studies of genetically-controlled resistance to
group B arbovirus infection against a low background of other
variables (6).

The levels of neutralizing antibody, interferon, and
complement after a group B arbovirus infection have not been
found to be higher in resistant mice as compared to susceptible ones (7, 8, 9, 10). C3H/RV mice are able to survive
intracerebral injection of an undiluted preparation of the
standard 17D vaccine strain of yellow fever, whereas a 10^{-4}
dilution of this virus produces paralysis and death in all
C3H/He mice. WNV, a more virulent group B arbovirus, can
kill C3H/RV mice after intracerebral doses 10 to 100 times
greater than those required to kill susceptible mice. C3H/
RV mice are completely resistant to WNV injected intraperitoneally, whereas C3H/He are susceptible. C3H/RV mice
and cell cultures derived from them produce lower yields of
group B arboviruses, than do C3H/He mice or cultures derived
from them (7, 8, 11-14). Resistant and susceptible mice
produce equal amounts of group A arboviruses and other unrelated viruses (8, 11, 12). The reduced yield of group B
arboviruses from cultures of cells from resistant mice
(resistant cultures) was found neither to be due to an inability of these cells to be infected nor to an earlier or
greater production of interferon as compared to cultures of
cells from susceptible mice (susceptible cultures) (15).

It has been suggested that the production of DI particles, able to interfere with the production of infectious
virus, may aid in host defense and change the course of
certain viral diseases (16, 17, 18). Standard virus production remained high during serial undiluted passage of WNV
in cultures of susceptible cells, whereas viral titers dropped
rapidly during similar passage in resistant cells. Our data
indicate that DI particles are probably produced in significant numbers by resistant cells.

RESULTS

Growth of WNV in resistant and susceptible cells.
Embryofibroblasts from resistant mice produce lower yields
of WNV than cells from susceptible mice, whether or not the
cells have been transformed with SV40 (15) (Figure 1). By
36 hours after infection, the yield of WNV from susceptible
cultures was always 1 to 1 1/2 logs higher than that obtained

from resistant ones. No decrease in cell number was observed
in these cultures during the course of the experiment and
virus was continually produced by cells which showed no CPE.
Since the transformed fibroblasts showed the same differential
production of WNV as the untransformed cells, they were used
in all subsequent experiments.

Serial undiluted passage of WNV in resistant and
susceptible cells. Comparable confluent cultures of resistant and susceptible cells were infected with WNV and culture
fluids were serially passed to fresh cultures every three
days. Infectivity was assayed at each transfer. This method
allowed several cycles of virus growth to occur between
transfers (Figure 2). The yield of infectious WNV progressively decreased from both resistant and susceptible cultures
through the third passage. The fourth passage resulted in
an increased yield of WNV from the susceptible cultures,
while the yield from the resistant cultures continued to
decline. A slight increase in titer was consistently observed in resistant culture fluids after the fifth passage,
but after the sixth passage the titer decreased to an un-
detectable level.

Interferon was measured in the culture fluids from the
first six passages. The titer of interferon was low and
reflected the amount of infectious virus produced (Figure 2).

Serial undiluted passage of WNV was also conducted in
the presence of 1 ug/ml of Actinomycin D, which has been
shown to inhibit the synthesis of endogenous interferon (19)
(Table 1). The titer of WNV from resistant and susceptible
cultures decreased in a manner comparable to the control and
to the experiments shown in figure 2. It seems unlikely
that interferon is responsible for the rapid drop in virus
titer observed in culture fluids from resistant cells during
passage.

The production of DI particles is enhanced by the use
of high multiplicities of infection or multicyclic viral
growth conditions (18, 20-23), since, presumably, both procedures allow a greater chance of dual infection of a cell
by a defective particle and an infectious virion. After
infection of resistant and susceptible cultures with WNV
at multiplicities of 50, 5 and 0.5, culture fluids were
serially passaged as described previously. The results
shown in figure 3 indicate that as the multiplicity of
infection increases, there is a more rapid decrease in WNV
titer with passage.

Assay of interference. When cells are infected with
both defective and standard virus there is an inhibition of
the absolute amount of standard virus produced as compared
to that produced by cells infected with standard virus alone
(18). The ability of serially passaged culture fluids from
WNV-infected resistant and susceptible cultures to interfere
with the production of infectious WNV was assayed (Table 2).
The yield of infectious WNV from both resistant and susceptible cultures was reduced by approximately 1 log as compared
to control, when a 1:1 mixture of third passage-resistant
cell WNV and control virus (hamster brain-produced WNV) was
used for infection. Third passage-susceptible cell WNV
caused no detectable decrease in yield when it was mixed with
control virus and then this 1:1 mixture was used to infect
cells. The titer of infectious WNV in the third passage-
susceptible cell sample was 2 logs higher than that in the
comparable resistant cell sample. Since the ratio of defective to infectious particles determines the extent of interference, the lack of an observable interference by the
susceptible cell sample was most likely due to an insufficient
number of DI particles to cause a detectable interference in
the presence of the increased amount of standard virus con-
tributed by the control WNV.

Preliminary study of WNV progeny from resistant and
susceptible cultures. Virus, grown in the presence of
^{14}C-amino acids and ^{3}H-uridine was harvested from resistant
and susceptible cells 24 or 96 hours after infection. Virus
preparations were partially purified and then centrifuged on
a 5-25 % (W/V) sucrose gradient. A symmetrical peak of
infectivity was found in the same position in all gradients.
Table 3 depicts the amount of acid-insoluble radioactivity
and infectivity in the peak viral fraction from each gradient.
The CMP/ml of radioactivity in viral protein and RNA increase
during the four day labeling period and are comparable in
samples from resistant and susceptible cultures. The amount
of infectious virus produced does not, however, continue to
increase in resistant cultures.

DISCUSSION

To date DI particles have not been separated and
characterized from any of the group B arboviruses. DI particles of viruses with icosahedral symmetry appear to have

the same shape and size as the standard virion (26). Recently, DI particles from a group A arbovirus, sindbis, have been identified (24, 25). Shenk and Stollar were able to separate a sindbis particle differing in density from the infectious virus by 0.02 g/cm^3 under the special condition of a D_2O sucrose density gradient. They were unable to show a difference between the size of the RNA from this particle and that from the infectious virion.

Although we have not as yet separated or positively identified WNV DI particles, the preliminary indirect evidence presented here is consistent with the hypothesis that WNV DI particles are produced rapidly and in significant quantities in resistant cells. Some DI particles may also be produced in susceptible cells, but in much smaller quantities.

The differential production of DI particles was not observed when VSV, a rhabdovirus, was serially passaged in resistant and susceptible cells (18, A.S. Huang, personal communication). The data obtained with VSV is consistent with the hypothesis that the enhanced production of group B arbovirus DI particles in resistant cells during passage is corrolated with the group B arbovirus genetically-controlled resistance.

This report and a few others (15, 21, 27) indicate that host cells probably can affect the enrichment of DI particles and possibly also the ability of these particles to interfere with the production of standard virus. Further studies on the intracellular steps involved in the production of DI particles and in the interference of defective virus particles with standard virus production may also shed light on the mechanism of group B arbovirus resistance.

In mice ,group B arboviruses characteristically produce a slowly progressing paralytic and wasting disease with death occuring between 5 and 14 days after infection. A reduced yield of infectious virus from individual cells at the site of inoculation, possibly due to the production of DI particles, could slow the spread of the infection and shift the balance in favor of the host.

ACKNOWLEDGEMENTS

This work was supported in part by Public Health Service grants #gM 00142 from The National Institute of General Medical Sciences and RR05540 from the Division of Research Resources.

REFERENCES

1. Kantoch, M., Warwick, A. and Bang, F.B., J. Exp. Med. 117, 781 (1963).
2. Sawyer, W.A. and Lloyd, W., J. Exp. Med. 59, 533 (1931).
3. Webster, L.T., J. Exp. Med. 65, 261 (1937).
4. Sabin, A.B., Ann. N.Y. Acad. Sci., 54, 936 (1952).
5. Theis, G.A., Billingham, R.E., Silvers, W.K. and Koprowski, H., Virology 8, 264 (1959).
6. Groschel, D. and Koprowski, H., Arch Fur ges. Forsch., 18, 379 (1965).
7. Goodman, G.T. and Koprowski, H., J. Cell. Comp. Physiol., 59, 333 (1962),
8. Hanson, B. and Koprowski, H., Microbios, 1B, 51 (1969).
9. Vainio, R., Gavatkin, R. and Koprowski, H., Virology 14, 385 (1961).
10. Darnell, M.B., Koprowski, H. and Lagerspetz, K., J. Inf. Dis. March (1974).
11. Goodman, G.T. and Koprowski, H., Proc. Natl. Acad. Sci. 48, 160 (1962).
12. Webster, L.T., Johnson, M.S., J. Exp. Med. 74, 489 (1941).
13. Vainio, T., Ann. Med. Exp. Fenn. 41: Suppl. 1, 1 (1963).
14. Vainio, T., Ann. Med. Exp. Fenn. 41: Suppl. 1, 25 (1963).
15. Darnell, M.B. and Koprowski, H., J. Inf. Dis. March (1974).
16. Schlesinger, R.W. In "The Viruses", (Burnet, F.M., and Stanley, W.M., eds.) Vol. 3, pp. 157 (1959) Academic Press, New York.
17. Huang, A.S. and Baltimore, D., Nature (London) 226, 325 (1970).
18. Huang, A.S., Ann. Rev. of Micro. 27, 101 (1973).
19. Heller, E., Virology 21, 652 (1963).
20. Von Magnus, P., Advan. Virus Res. 2, 59 (1954).
21. Kingsbury, D.W. and Portner, A., Virology 42, 872 (1970).
22. Stampfer, M., Baltimore, D. and Huang, A.S., J. Virol. 7, 409 (1971).
23. Choppin, P.W., Virology 39, 130 (1969).
24. Schlesinger, S., Schlesinger, M. and Burge, B.W., Virology 48, 615 (1972).
25. Shenk, T.E. and Stollar, V., Virology 53, 162 (1973).
26. Yoshiike, K., Virology 34, 391 (1968).
27. Perrault, J. and Holland,J.,Virology 50, 158 (1972).

TABLE 1

EFFECT OF ACTINOMYCIN D ON WNV YIELD AFTER SERIAL UNDILUTED PASSAGE IN SUSCEPTIBLE AND RESISTANT T-MEF CULTURES

Passage level	WNV yield ($\log_{10}$ PFU/ml)			
	Resistant		Susceptible	
	Control	+Act D	Control	+Act D
1	5.7	5.0	6.85	6.5
2	4.6	3.6	6.25	5.9
3	3.1	2.5	4.6	4.2
4	3.35	3.0	5.8	5.2

Serial undiluted passage of WNV was conducted as described in the legend of figure 2, except that half of the cultures were supplemented with 1 ug/ml of Actinomycin D at the time of transfer.

TABLE 2

ASSAY OF INTERFERENCE BETWEEN SERIAL UNDILUTED
PASSAGE WNV AND BRAIN-PRODUCED WNV

Cell Type	Moi of brain-produced WNV	48 hour WNV yield $(\log_{10}$ PFU/ml)		
		Brain-produced WNV + medium	Brain-produced WNV + 3rd passage susceptible cell WNV	Brain-produced WNV + 3rd passage resistant cell WNV
Resistant T-MEF	1.82	2.7	-	1.9
	0.18	2.35	2.2	0.9
	0.018	1.0	1.75	Undetectable
Susceptible T-MEF	1.42	7.3	-	6.3
	0.14	6.6	6.5	5.75
	0.014	5.5	6.25	4.35

Equal volumes of diluted (10^{-1}, 10^{-2}, 10^{-3}) hamster brain-propagated WNV and undiluted third passage tissue culture fluid from either resistant or susceptible T-MEF cultures were mixed. The third passage virus samples were the same as those shown in figure 2. Resistant and susceptible T-MEF cultures were infected with 0.2 ml of the various virus mixtures. Control cultures were infected with 0.2 ml of a mixture containing equal volumes of brain-propagated WNV and medium. Media from three replicate plates were pooled for titration 48 hr after infection. The titers of the virus preparations used for infection were as follows: hamster brain-produced WNV = $10^{8.9}$ pfu/ml, third passage-susceptible cell WNV = $10^{4.5}$ pfu/ml, and third passage-resistant cell WNV = $10^{2.5}$ pfu/ml.

TABLE 3

PROGENY WNV FROM RESISTANT AND SUSCEPTIBLE
T-MEF CULTURES 24 AND 96 HOURS AFTER INFECTION

Source of virus	Hours After Infection	Acid-insoluble ^{3}H-uridine CPM/ml	Acid insoluble ^{14}C-amino acid CPM/ml	PFU/ml
Susceptible T-MEF	24	2050	450	1.3×10^7
	96	3804	2636	5.5×10^7
Resistant T-MEF	24	1250	500	1.0×10^6
	96	3610	2600	7.5×10^4

Three confluent monolayers in 32 oz. prescription bottles
were used for each sample. Cultures were infected with WNV
at a multiplicity of infection of 25. One hour after infection cultures were incubated with MEM containing 1/4 the
normal amount of amino acids and supplemented with bovine
serum albumin (0.5%) and 0.2 μc/ml of ^{14}C-amino acids and
1 μc/ml ^{3}H-uridine for either 24 or 96 hours. At the time
of harvest media were collected, clarified by low speed
centrifugation, and the virus was then pelleted in the type
30 rotor at 78,000 x g for 3 hr at 4° C. The pellets were
resuspended in a small volume of NTE buffer (0.15 M NaCl,
0.05 M Tris-HCl, 0.001 M EDTA, pH 8.0) supplemented with
0.2% BSA and then sonicated 3 times for 1 min. After clar-
ification by low speed centrifugation, virus suspensions
were layered onto a 5-25% (W/V) sucrose gradient. Samples
were centrifuged at 63,000 x g for 3 hr in the SW25.1 rotor
at 4° C. One ml fractions were collected and assayed for
infectivity by plaque assay. An aliquot of each sample was
precipitated with cold 5% TCA, collected on Millipore filters,
dried and counted.

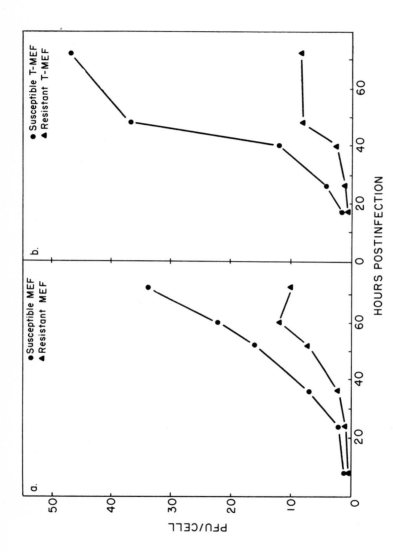

Figure 1. Growth of WNV in (a) Normal and (b) SV40-transformed resistant and susceptible mouse embryo fibroblasts (MEF) after infection with a multiplicity of infection of 20. WNV was titered by plaque assay in LLC-MK$_2$ cells.

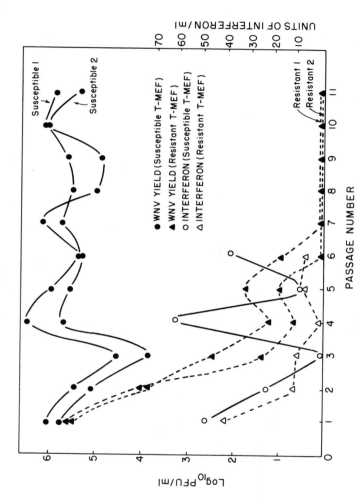

Figure 2. Serial undiluted passage of WNV in susceptible and resistant transformed-mouse embryo fibroblast cultures. Cultures were infected with hamster brain-propagated WNV (10 pfu/cell). After 3 days incubation half of the media from each flask was transferred to a fresh culture of the same type and supplemented with an equal volume of fresh media. The transfer was repeated at 3 day intervals.

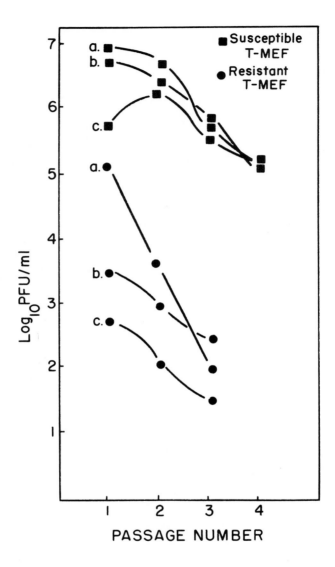

Figure 3. Effect of multiplicity on yield of WNV after serial undiluted passage in resistant and susceptible T-MEF cultures. The multiplicities used were (a) 50 pfu/cell, (b) 5 pfu/cell and (c) 0.5 pfu/cell. Passages were carried out as described in the legend of figure 2.

IV

VIRUSES IN CHRONIC
CENTRAL NERVOUS SYSTEM DISEASE

ALTERED NEUROLOGIC DISEASE INDUCED BY REOVIRUS MUTANTS

Bernard N. Fields and Cedric S. Raine

Departments of Medicine (Infectious Disease),
Cell Biology, Microbiology and Pathology
(Neuropathology) and the Rose F. Kennedy
Center for Research in Mental Retardation and
Human Development
Albert Einstein College of Medicine
Bronx, New York   10461

ABSTRACT. Temperature-sensitive mutants of reovirus type
3 have been isolated and characterized genetically and
biochemically. In contrast to the wild type virus which
produces an acute necrotizing encephalitis in rats infected by intracerebral inoculation, certain mutants
induce a slowly progressive communicating hydrocephalus.
Other mutants induce no overt disease. The biochemical
defects in those mutants which induce hydrocephalus
resides in the inability to assemble outer coat peptides.
The assembled viral outer protein shell thus appears to
be responsible for the lytic cell response and acute
encephalitis due to wild reovirus type 3.

INTRODUCTION

The availability of well characterized conditional
lethal temperature sensitive mutants of animal viruses
has opened up the possibility of studying the role of
various viral components in virus host interactions.
Thus the role of such viral components as coat or core
proteins can be examined by infecting appropriate mutants
into a suitable animal host (1). Such an approach may
also offer insight into a number of diseases that appear
to be associated with viral agents found in non-permissive
relationships to their host. The etiology of such
diseases and their relationship to defective or mutant
viruses, perhaps best typified by measles virus and

isolates of closely related viral strains from the chronic neurologic disorder subacute sclerosing panencephalitis (2) is not well understood. By utilizing viral mutants it is hoped that a better understanding of the pathogenesis of such disease states may be developed.

REOVIRUS TYPE 3. Our studies have been concerned with the replication and genetics of reovirus Type 3. The model system we have chosen for detailed analysis of viral pathogenesis is the production of encephalitis following inoculation of suckling rodents via the intracerebral route. Upon intraveneous or intraperitoneal inoculation, a variety of symptoms have been produced in such animals. Acute disease in newborn mice is characterized by an illness consisting of hepatitis, encephalitis, steatorrhea and oily skin (3). A small proportion (1 to 5 per cent) of animals survive and go on to a more chronic illness similar to a runting syndrome (4). Upon direct inoculation of appropriate doses into brains of newborn animals, an acute encephalitis ensues that is necrotic, hemorrhagic and fatal in almost 100 per cent of animals (5-7).

USE OF TEMPERATURE SENSITIVE MUTANTS. In order to evaluate the role of the outer viral coat in causing acute neuron destruction, two classes of mutants were selected for study (Table 1).

The B mutants have a defect that occurs late during the cycle; mRNA, ssRNA, dsRNA and all the major structural peptides are synthesized (8,9). However, infection leads to assembly of a virus that does not possess an outer protein coat (10). Thus, the specific defect in this mutant seems to lie in the inability of one or more of the outer-coat proteins to assemble onto the core. This mutant is also very defective in cell killing. For example, when wild-type virus infects tissue-culture cells at high temperature (39°C), lysis occurs in 90 to 95 per cent of cells by approximately 15 hours, and by 24 hours there is essentially nothing but cell debris and nuclei left. When the B mutant is used to infect cells at the higher temperature, and the same thing can be said of the C mutant, fewer than 20 per cent of the cells are killed at comparable times.

The C mutant makes small amounts of mRNA but is incapable of replicating detectable dsRNA (9). It is blocked in the pathway taking single-stranded to double-stranded RNA. All the major cytoplasmic viral proteins are synthesized (8), but a structure is assembled that is deficient in the inner structures; an empty viral capsid is assembled without a core (10). Thus, the defect is probably in an inner peptide, which functions as a replicase - the enzyme that replicates the single-stranded to the double-stranded RNA form.

Thus mutants blocked in the assembly of outer coat proteins(s) (B mutants) and inner coat proteins (C mutant) can be compared to fully assembled virions (wild type) as to their neurovirulence.

DISEASE STUDIES. Wild-type virus, with an inoculum from 10^1 to 10^8 plaque-forming units (PFU) produces an acute necrotizing encephalitis, with death generally occurring between one and two weeks (7). Forty animals were inoculated, and only four survived at the lowest doses. Survivors were observed for as long as a year, and the animals were entirely healthy. The C mutant, at very high doses (greater than 10^7 or 10^8), kills the majority of animals, and the resultant illness resembles the acute encephalitis produced by the wild-type virus. Electron microscopy of brain sections reveals neural tissue that contains viral inclusions composed of a mixture of full and empty virions. At lower doses the majority of animals survive, with no apparent long-term residua. In a large percentage of animals inoculated with the B mutants at high doses fatal encephalitis also developed, but at doses between 10^4 and 10^7 PFU of virus only a small percentage of animals became sick or died; the majority appeared clinically well (1,11). Ultra-structural examination of the brains from acutely ill animals revealed a mixture of viral cores and incompletely assembled virions. Several weeks to months after the infection, there was illness in many of the surviving animals, manifested by smaller size and humped posture. When brains of these animals were examined, a marked thinning of the cerebral cortical mantle and a dilatation of the lateral ventricles as compared to the normal rat could be seen. This progressed over a period of eight months to a condition in which gross cavitation of the cortex was present.

Virus could be isolated consistently in both mutant infected animals for 6-8 weeks and only sporadically thereafter in a few B animals (10 weeks). Analysis of neutralizing antibody revealed no significant differences in the B or C mutant infected animals. Thus, instead of a clinically apparent acute necrotizing encephalitis characteristic of wild-type infection, a disease was produced by the B mutant that had as its features degeneration of brain parenchyma with secondary enlargement of the cerebral ventricles, most nearly resembling hydrocephalus ex vacuo. Histologic examination has confirmed the presence of a communicating hydrocephalus, absence of aqueductal stenosis, attenuation of ependymal lining and preservation of subspendymal white matter up to the perimeter of the cavitated zone.

HYPOTHESIS FOR ALTERED DISEASE. What are potential models for altered disease caused by reovirus mutants (Fig. 1)? During the normal infection viruses accumulate in the cytoplasm, eventually followed by cell lysis and release of virus that is attacked by neutralizing antibody. Newly released virus infects other cells in which the same cycle subsequently develops. Once antibody is made, new virus is neutralized, and further infection of new cells is blocked. In addition, interferon is produced, also restricting viral replication. On the other hand, a rare mutant with a defect in the outer coat would multiply inefficiently, but both, by not causing efficient cell lysis as well as by releasing particles resistant to neutralizing antibody, could persist in the presence of high titers of viral-specific antibody. This would lead to a persistent viral infection, largely cell-associated, which only in an indolent fashion would produce cell damage. Other possibilities exist, and the precise mechanism is currently being explored.

IMPORTANCE TO THE STUDY OF VIRAL PATHOGENESIS. These findings of an altered disease induced by reovirus mutants suggest that such a mechanism may exist in the pathogenesis of other viral diseases. This may be particularly relevant to the altered central-nervous-system disease associated with measles virus (SSPE) or similarly with any virus (natural or mutant) producing an indolent systemic infection. In addition to directly killing cells, such a persistent aberrant virus could act as an antigen that could exist as a circulating antigen-antibody complex and possibly induce features of auto-immune disease (12). A means is now available for direct examination of these possibilities by the isolation and analysis of mutant variants of measles and other viruses and for study of their disease-producing capablilites. Such studies are currently in progress.

ACKNOWLEDGEMENTS

This work was supported by grants from the National Institutes of Health (AI-10326, NS-08952, NS-03356, NS-06735). Bernard N. Fields is the recipient of a Faculty Research Associate Award of the American Cancer Society (PRA 63) and an Irma T. Hirschl Scholar Award. Cedric S. Raine is the recipient of a Research Career Development Award from the N.I.H. (NS-70265).

REFERENCES

1. Fields, B.N., New Eng. J. Med. 287, 1026 (1972).
2. Sever, J.L. and Zeman, W., Neurology 18(1), 1 (1968).
3. Walters, M.N., Joske, R.A., Leak, P.J., et al., Br. J. Exp. Path. 44, 427 (1963).
4. Stanley, N.F., Leak, P.J., and Walters, M.N., Br. J. Exp. Path. 45, 146 (1964).
5. Margolis, G., Kilham, L., and Gonatos, N.K., Lab. Invest. 24, 91 (1971).
6. Gonatos, N.K., Margolis, G., and Kilham, L., Lab. Invest. 24, 101 (1971).
7. Raine, C.S., Fields, B.N., J. Neuropath. Exp. Neurol. 32, 19 (1973).
8. Fields, B.N., Laskov, R. and Scharff, M.D., Virol. 50, 209 (1972)
9. Cross, R.K. and Fields, B.N., Virol. 50, 799 (1972).
10. Fields, B.N., Raine, C.S. and Baum, S.G., Virol. 43, 569 (1971).
11. Raine, C.S. and Fields, B.N., Am. J. Path. (1974). In press.
12. Sinkovics, J.G., N. Eng. J. Med. 284, 107 (1971).

Table 1

FEATURES OF TEMPERATURE-SENSITIVE MUTANTS

Test	Wild-Type Virus	Temperature-Sensitive Mutant in Cistron	
		B	C
Time of defect	-	Late	Late
Cell killing	++++	+	0
ssRNA (transcription)	++++	++	+
dsRNA (replication)	++++	++	0
Peptides	++++	++	+
Morphogenesis	Virus	"Core"	Outer capsids
Possible defect	-	Outer peptide	Inner peptide (replicase)

A MODEL FOR ALTERATION IN VIRAL PATHOGENESIS

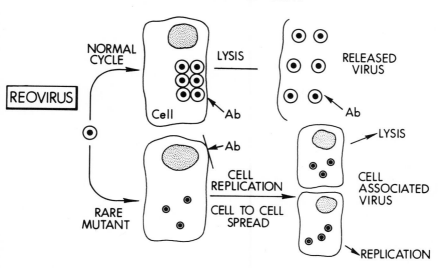

Fig. 1. A model for alteration of viral pathogenesis
(reproduced from Ref. 1 with permission of the author).

RABIES AND PARAINFLUENZA VIRUSES

Hilary Koprowski, M. D.

The Wistar Institute
Philadelphia, Pennsylvania

ABSTRACT. There are few examples of virus-host cell interactions of such contrast as that of rabies and parainfluenza type 1 infections of the cell. Rabies virus can infect and, in most cases, cause a fatal disease of the central nervous system in all warm blooded animals, and is infectious for cells in culture obtained from cold blooded animals. Ultrastructural analysis indicates that the virions are assembled either at the cell surface as budding particles, or in the intracytoplasmic matrix. Although virions of other rhabdoviruses such as vesicular stomatitus virus and Kern Canyon virus display RNA-dependent RNA polymerase activity, no such enzyme has been discovered incorporated into the virions of rabies virus. Although VSV grows in enucleated mammalian cells almost as well as in intact cells, preliminary experiments indicate that infectious rabies virus cannot be assembled in enucleated cells. The parainfluenza type 1 virus (6/94) originally isolated from cultures of brain cells obtained at autopsy of Multiple Sclerosis (MS) cases can be serially passaged in embryonated hens' eggs, preferably incubated at 32°C, but in mammalian cells it can only undergo one growth cycle. Although on examination by electron microscopy, complete virions are assembled, they are not infectious for other mammalian cells unless they are treated with diluted concentrations of trypsin. Uptake by macrophages will also make the virus infectious for mammalian cells. A chronic infection of human brain cells in culture by 6/94 virus can be established. In the course of several cell transfers, hemadsorption and immunofluorescent staining of the cells will disappear but small amounts of infectious virus can be recovered in embryonated hens' eggs.

A comparison of the properties of rabies virus and the parainfluenza type 1 virus is a study in contrasts. Except for the possibility that parainfluenza type 1,of which the hemagglutinating virus of Japan (HVJ) is the prototype, may be infectious for all warm blooded animals as is rabies, the two viruses are distinctly different (Table 1).

Infection with parainfluenza type 1 may be classified as a banal infection of the respiratory tract occurring mostly in young children. In Japan, children develop antibodies against HVJ between the first and second year of life and a majority of the population then retains these antibodies during their lifetime (1). Chronic infections of humans with HVJ have either not been encountered or have not been reported, although persistent infections of laboratory animal colonies with HVJ have been described (2). In contrast, the infectivity of rabies for humans and animals is relatively low, but once the disease develops it is very severe and often fatal. The target organ is always the brain, although the virus may replicate in vivo in cells other than those of the central nervous system (CNS) (Table 1).

Rabies spreads from the periphery via nerve trunk; if a viremia phase of rabies infection exists it plays no role in the centripetal spread of the virus. The mode of spread of parainfluenza 1 is unknown and the possible role of macrophages in the activation of the virus will be discussed below.

The target cells in CNS for rabies are neurons. Rabies antigen can be detected in the cytoplasm of neurons including brain neurons but it should be emphasized that destruction of neurons in brain tissue has rarely, if ever, been seen on histological examination. What, then, is the relationship between this virus and its host cell? Even if cultures of neurons were to become available, we still do not know enough about the mode of replication of rabies virus in the host cell to be able to undertake a study bearing directly on the problem of virus in cells of the CNS.

Ultrastructural studies of BHK cells in cultures infected with rabies (3) reveal accumulations of filamentous structures identical to the nucleocapsids of the virus in the cytoplasm five hours after the cell engulfs the infecting virus particle by pinocytosis. Progeny virus

170

particles are first seen 6 hours after infection, and
virus production through budding at the cell surface increases for up to 12 hours after infection. Nucleocapsids
are dispersed throughout the cytoplasm and do not accumulate in the vicinity of the budding particle. Virus particles can be seen budding into the cytoplasmic vacuoles 24
hours after infection; at 72 hours after infection, the
budding processes virtually cease and the development of
rod-shaped particles in the cytoplasm becomes predominant.
In contrast to the budding particles, these particles
develop a two-unit viral membrane in close proximity to
the endoplasmic reticulum (3). At that time, large matrices and dense bodies are seen in the cytoplasm. Production
of infectious virus is at its peak 18-24 hours after infection, concomitant with the presence of budding virus particles. It drops abruptly at the time when particles are
developing in the cytoplasm and when nucleocapsids are
possibly accumulating in the matrices (3). The susceptibility of the infected cell to immune lysis by antiviral
antibody is conditioned by the presence of virus particles
budding at the cell surface and there is no indication of
the interaction of antibody with cell surface antigen
other than the virus particle itself. Thus, ultrastructural observations seem to indicate a unique "double" feature of rabies "mode replication" in the cell: budding at
the cell surface as any "good" paramyxovirus should but
then developing in the cytoplasm and possibly involving
the endoplasmic reticulum. Although all these events can
be observed in the cytoplasm, the recently described site
for the transcription of the rabies virus genome (4), and
there is no indication of involvement of the nucleus in
viral replication, production of rabies virus can be
inhibited to a certain degree by DNA inhibitors such as
cytosine arabinoside (5). In addition, since no RNA transcriptase activity was detected in the virus particle, the
contribution of host cell functions to the replication of
the virus may be different in the case of rabies from that
in other rhabdoviruses.

　　　　To study this problem, we have compared the infection of enucleated TC7 (African Green Monkey Kidney
origin) cells with rabies virus to that of the Indiana
strain of vesicular stomatitis virus (VSV), another member
of the rhabdovirus group (6). As shown in Table 2, no
infectious rabies virus was recovered from cultures of
enucleated cells whereas VSV replicated almost as well in

enucleated cells as in intact cells. However, as shown
in Table 3, rabies fluorescing antigen was synthesized
almost as well in enucleated cells as in intact cells.
Rabies-infected enucleated cells also incorporated ^{3}H-
uridine whereas the non-infected cells did not.

Since synthesis of the FA antigen in intact
cells takes place concurrently with the appearance of the
nucleocapsids, it is possible that replication of virus
RNA occurs in enucleated cells, but a functioning cell
nucleus may be essential for either transcription of viral
RNA or for the assembly of the progeny virions.

A disarrangement of the production of different
viral components caused by such drastic means as enuclea-
tion of the cells was also observed in chronic rabies infection of human diploid cells maintained for a long time
in culture without cell transfer (7); these cells produced
rabies antigen without a concomitant release of infectious
virus. Whether the same condition prevails in rabies-
infected neurons, which are essentially non-dividing cells,
is not known but a search for an animal model for chronic
CNS infection has continued parallel to the tissue culture
studies.

Since street virus may persist in the organism
for months, or possibly for years, before causing signs
of sickness and since the outcome of the disease nearly
always is fatal, the question arises whether it would be
possible to cause a chronic, non-fatal disease of the CNS
in street virus-infected animals. This has been accomplished through the infection of mice by two strains of
rabies: a non-virulent attenuated HEP-Flury virus (a rabies
strain which, after its original isolation from man, has
never been carried except in an avian host), given intracerebrally, and street virus, injected intramuscularly. As
shown in Table 4, HEP inoculation had a marked sparing
effect on mice exposed to street virus (8). Depending on
the time interval between exposures to the two viruses,
many of the street virus-infected animals did not die but
became partially paralyzed. The paralysis was usually in
the street virus injected limb and lasted for an observation period that extended over one year. At that time,
the observed degeneration of a portion of the peripheral
nerves in the affected limb and the proliferation of
Schwann cells may indicate that an active infectious process caused by this supposedly lethal virus may have still

been operating in the animal. It is doubtful that the
sparing effect in street virus-injected mice was antibody
mediated since irradiation of the experimental animals did
not affect the results. It is possible, however, that
rapid induction of interferon in the blood and brain 7-14
hours after inoculation with the non-virulent HEP virus
may have been instrumental in arresting the spread of the
street virus; the mechanisms underlying the persistent
paralysis remain, however, unknown.

To further inquire into the nature of this
phenomenon, the pathogenicity of several ts mutants were
investigated. One of these mutants, the ts-2, derived
from a fixed CVS strain (9) in contrast to parenteral virus was incapable of causing plaque formation at a non-
permissive temperature of 40.5°C but retained the virulence of the parenteral strain when injected intracerebrally in three-day-old mice. When injected by the same
route into 4-6-week-old mice, however, with four lower
dilutions of the virus stock, it failed to induce signs of
illness (Table 5). Only when diluted 10^4 to 10^5, did the
injections cause sickness of animals 23-31 days after infection (10). What was most surprising, however, was the
paradoxical behavior of the same strain injected intra-
plantary into mice of the same age. The dilution containing large amounts of virus that caused no disease after intracerebral inoculation produced disease in animals
injected into the foot pad. The incubation period was 14-
20 days and the disease lasted for a week to ten days. In
brain tissue of asymptomatic, intracerebrally inoculated
mice, the virus was present for up to 7 days after infection (Table 6). From the brain tissue of paralyzed mice,
either after intracerebral or intraplantar inoculation,
the virus could be recovered both at the onset and during
the course of illness. Resistance could not be attributed
to mediation by an immune response since antibody levels
could not be correlated with the expected outcome of the
infection. Serum interferon levels were high from ten
hours after infection in asymptomatic animals infected
intracerebrally with concentrated virus, but no serum
interferon was found after inoculation with more diluted
virus in animals that were symptom-free. The presence of
brain interferon could be correlated with replication of
the virus but not with the disease itself.

Thus, we are left with the puzzling situation

in which a virus, replicating preferentially in the neurons of the CNS, does not cause disease after direct exposure of the neuronal tissue of the animal host to the
virus but causes disease after the virus "travels" from
the periphery to the neurons of the brain. If the presence of defective interfering (DI) particles could
account for the asmyptomatic infection following intracerebral infection,then either at the site of peripheral
infection, or while the inoculum spreads to the CNS, selection of virulent virus over DI particles is favored.

Thus, in contrast to the situation with the
Arbo B viruses (11,12) where the genotype of the host may
determine the ratio of defective particles to virulent
particles, in rabies infection different tissues of the
same host may determine this ratio.

In discussing rabies infection, I have tried to
envisage possible mechanisms operative in changing a
severe type of CNS infection into a chronic infection
which either causes no signs of illness or which after
prolonged persistence of the virus in the brain tissue
ultimately leads to a paralytic disease. In discussing
parainfluenza type 1, on the other hand, I would like to
investigate possible mechanisms by which a virus, that
usually causes a banal respiratory infection, may become
more pathogenic and cause a more severe disease. I shall
limit my discussion to the parainfluenza type 1 virus
ioslated by ter Meulen and me (13)from cultures of brain
cells growing out of explants of brain tissue obtained at
autopsy from a case of multiple sclerosis (14). Table 7
shows the history of the isolation of the agent which has
been called 6/94. Out of a total of 53 brain cultures
established from four plaque-adjacent areas, cells of a
pool of three cultures from one plaque area yielded virus
after fusion with the CV-1 strain of African Green Monkey
Kidney cells using lysolecithin as a fusion agent. The
cells of the fused cultures showed hemadsorption and the
presence of cytoplasmic antigen staining with parainfluenza type 1 antibody. Although these cells have been maintained for more than 100 passages in culture, positive
hemadsorption and the development of FA antigen depend
very much upon the incubation temperature of these cells,
and both were markedly suppressed immediately after fusion
if the cultures were incubated at 37°C instead of 33°C
(14). Minimal amounts of infectious virus were produced

by the chronically infected cultures but when the agent
was finally isolated in embryonated eggs, higher yields were
obtained when the eggs were incubated at 33°C than at
37°C. When chronically infected, fused cell cultures were
cloned, progeny cultures of six out of seven clones were
found to be infected, and HAD and immunofluorescence were
expressed in a much larger proportion of cells incubated
at 33°C rather than 37°C. Unfortunately, since no data on
optimal propagation temperatures are available for parainfluenza type 1 viruses isolated from either acute or
chronic infections of man and animals, it is difficult to
compare the properties of 6/94 virus with other isolates
from human subjects. Apart from temperature sensitivity,
6/94 shares other characteristics with the HVJ group of
viruses, which may be instrumental in the establishment
of chronic infections of cells and tissues. Similarly
to the Sendai virus (15,16) 6/94 virus can be propagated
for an indefinite number of passages in embryonated eggs.
However, following one growth cycle in mammalian cells,
the progeny virus cannot infect other mammalian cells but
it will be infectious for embryonated eggs. When, similarly to the treatment of Sendai virus (15), 6/94 virus
is exposed to diluted concentrations of trypsin, it becomes infectious for mammalian cells in second passages
(17, Table 8). In addition to restoring infectivity,
trypsin treatment also restores viral hemolysis. Hemagglutinin   titers are not affected by passage through
mammalian cells. Treatment with proteolytic enzymes or
exposure to chick embryo tissue apparently leads to the
digestion of "precursor" (16) glycoprotein which inhibits
infectivity of the virus for mammalian cells. Reactivation
of the virus by trypsin treatment may be extended to a virus grown in any mammalian cell system including human
brain cells maintained in culture. If, however, instead
of exposure to trypsin, a virus passaged in human brain
tissue is picked up by macrophages, its infectivity is
also restored (17, Table 9). Thus, through intervening
passages in macrophages, either mouse or human, it is
possible to transfer infectivity of this parainfluenza
type 1 agent from one group of human brain cells to
another (Table 10).

     Can this mechanism operate <u>in vivo</u>? Obviously,
experiments in animals may show whether macrophages are
the cells that not only restore viral infectivity but

also serve as a vehicle for the transportation of virus to target organs other than bronchial or lung tissue. If this were the case, a call for macrophages by mediators at the site of infection would not be very beneficial to the host. The evidence for possible involvement of macrophages as virus carriers in multiple sclerosis is highly circumstantial. There are six reports on the presence of nucleocapsids resembling filamentous or tubular structures in either the nucleus or the cytoplasm of cells adjacent to MS plaque areas (18). The structures, free in the cytoplasm, are located in cells identified as astrocytes. Nuclei containing the intranuclear structures can be classified into two types: one type of nucleus contains structures of an electron density similar to that of the chromatin, with a diameter of 200-300 Å, and of regular contour. This type of nuclei has also been described in cases of lupus erythematosis and possibly in other diseases. The other type of nuclei contains filaments of irregular contour, that are less electron dense than the chromatin and surrounded by an amorphous material (18). Cross striation is visible and the basic structure of the filament (a hollow core surrounded by an amorphous material) is similar to the rough or fuzzy nucleocapsids of paramyxoviruses. What is also interesting is the fact that such filaments are found only in macrophages (18) adjacent to the plaque area and are not seen in the nuclei of cells of neural origin. We are a long way from the time when we will be able to tie all the experimental data together and relate it to the pathogenesis of multiple sclerosis. It is quite possible, however, that the techniques of virus isolation, including the origin of cells that are searched for the presence of the virus, will have to undergo modifications and revisions.

Finally, we have directed our efforts to the problem of whether the parainfluenza 1 virus could trigger a disease in experimental animals which would progress to a chronic disease of the CNS. When 6-week-old mice were injected intracerebrally with 6/94 virus they remained symptom-free for many months of observation (19, Table 11). When they were sacrificed 3 and 7 days after inoculation, histologic examination of their brain tissue showed acute disseminated meningoencephalitis and ependymitis. The same changes were noted in mice injected with the Edmonston strain of measles virus. From the 14th day on, the inflammatory changes subsided in both groups of mice. In those inoculated with parainfluenza 1, however, destruction of paraventricular tissue, subcortical white matter and myelin was observed from the 14th day on. These lesions increased progressively throughout the 67 days observation while infectious parainfluenza 1 could be detected only through the first four days of infection (19). Measles injected animals showed no such changes. Thus, in mice, it is possible for a virus infection of brain tissue to trigger progressive asymptomatic lesions of the CNS which apparently run their course in the absence of detectable virus. This does not preclude the possibility that products or "byproducts" of parainfluenza type 1 infection may still be detected after termination of the acute infectious process. From this point of view, this system provides a useful model for the study of chronic CNS lesions triggered by virus infection.

ACKNOWLEDGEMENTS

This work was supported in part by funds from the National Multiple Sclerosis Society and the World Health Organization; and USPHS grants NS11036 from the National Institute of Neurological Diseases and Stroke and AI09706 from the National Institute of Allergy and Infectious Diseases.

REFERENCES

1. Okuna, Y., (personal communication).
2. Fujiwari, K.,(personal communication).
3. Iwasaki, Y., Koprowski, H., Müller, D., ter Meulen, V., and Käckell, Y.M., Lab. Invest.<u>28</u>, 494-500 (1973).
4. Bishop, D.L. (personal communication).
5. Campbell, J.B., Maes, R.F., Wiktor, T.J. and Koprowski, H., Virology <u>34</u>, 701-708 (1968).
6. Wiktor, T.J., and Koprowski, H., J. Virol. (submitted for publication).
7. Wiktor, T.J. and Clark, H F., Infect. Immun. <u>6</u>, 988-995 (1972).
8. Wiktor, T.J., Koprowski,H. and Rorke, L.B., Proc. Soc. Exp. Biol. & Med., <u>140</u>, 759-764 (1972).
9. Clark, H F., and Koprowski, H., J. Virol., <u>7</u>, 295-300 (1971).
10. Wiktor, J. T., Ohtani, S., Clark, H F., and Koprowski, H., (to be published).
11. Darnell, M. B., Koprowski. H., and Lagerspetz, K., J. Infect. Dis.<u>129</u>, 240-247 (1974).
12. Darnell, M.B. and Koprowski, H., J. Infect. Dis.<u>129</u>, 248-256 (1974).
13. ter Meulen, V., Koprowski, H., Iwasaki, Y., Käckell, Y.M. and Müller, D., Lancet II, 1-5, (1972).
14. Koprowski, H. and ter Meulen, V., New England J. Med. (submitted for publication).
15. Homma, M. and Ohuchi, M., J. Virol. <u>12</u>, 1457-1467 (1973).
16. Sheid, A. and Choppin, P.W., Virol. <u>57</u>, 475-490 (1974).
17. Waters, D., Koprowski, H., and Lewandowski, L.J., in Proceedings of Workshop on Measles Virus, Biochemical Society, Belfast, Ireland (1974).
18. Cited in: Tanaka, R., Iwasaki, Y., Koprowski, H., New England J. Med. (submitted for publication).
19. Iwasaki, Y., and Koprowski, H., Lancet (submitted for publication).

TABLE 1

Properties of Rabies and Parainfluenza type 1 viruses
on the level of the whole organism

Properties	Rabies	Parainfluenza 1
Host range	All homothermic species	Possibly all homothermic species (many not tested)
Host genotype	Not investigated	Not investigated
Natural mode of infection	Broken skin, intact mucosa,respiratory route	Respiratory route
Mode of spread	Via nerve trunks no viremia	Macrophage?
Replication of the virus	Muscle cells, neurons, salivary gland cells	Epithelial lining of respiratory tract, endothelium of large veins, peritoneal macrophages, ependyma and chorioid plexus epithelium
Immunopathological component	Suppression of T cells, exacerbates otherwise asymptomatic infection of mice	Immunosuppression with cyclophosphamide,but apparently not with ATS,exacerbates the disease

TABLE 2

Inability of enucleated cells to produce
progeny rabies virions

Number of cells	Intact or Enucleated	pfu/culture of produced virus	
		Rabies	VSV
10^5	Enucleated	$< 10^{1.0}$	$10^{7.8}$
	Intact	$10^{6.1}$	$10^{8.7}$
10^4	Intact	$10^{3.3}$	$10^{5.0}$

TABLE 3

Development of rabies FA antigen in enucleated cells

Rabies strain	Treatment of cells	% of cells showing positive fluorescence (48 hr.after infection)
ERA	None CB CB + centrif.	100 100 80
HEP	None CB CB + centrif.	100 100 90

CB = Cytochalasin B, 10 μg/ml
centrif = centrifugation

TABLE 4

Sparing effect of HEP Flury on Street virus
infections of mice

Conditions of Street virus infected mice which received
HEP Flury intracerebrally at times before or after street
virus (hours)

-2	+2	+6	+24	None
1/3/8	1/5/6	0/4/8	6/5/1	12/0/0

Dead/Paralyzed surviving/Surviving without signs of
illness

TABLE 5

Disease of mice infected with ts-2 strain of rabies

Route of Inoculation	Paralysis ratio after infection with virus						
	Undiluted*	10^{-1}	10^{-2}	10^{-3}	10^{-4}	10^{-5}	10^{-6}
Intracerebral	0/14	0/14	0/14	0/14	0/14	8/14 (28-30)	2/14 (28-31)
Intraplantar	10/14 (14-20)	7/14 (14-20)	1/14	0/14			

*Contains $10^{6.5}$ pfu/ml
(   ) = incubation period

TABLE 6

Isolation of infectious rabies virus from brain tissue of ts-2 infected mice

Dilution of virus	Route of inoculation	Paralysis ratio	Isolation of virus after infection								
			hours					days			
			4	10	24	48	96	7	11	14	20
Undiluted	i.c.	None*	+	+	-	+	+	-†		+†	-
	i.pl.	10/14*				-	-	-	-	+†	
10^{-1}	i.c.	None*	-	-	-	+	+	-			-
	i.pl.	7/14**				-	-	-	-	-†	-
10^{-2}	i.c.	None*	-	-	-	+	+	-			-
	i.pl.	None**				-	-	-	-	-	-
10^{-3}	i.c.	None*					+	+			-
	i.pl.	None						-	-	-	-
10^{-4}	i.c.	1/14*	None								
10^{-5}	i.c.	8/14**	None							+†	
10^{-6}	i.c.	2/14	None							+†	

*All survivors resistant to challenge inoculation
**Some survivors resistant to challenge inoculation
†Fluorescing antigen detected in brain tissue of sick animals
i.c.=intracerebral
i.pl.=intraplantar

Table 7

HISTORY OF ISOLATION OF VIRUS FROM BRAIN TISSUE OF EZ

Origin of Cell Cultures	MS Brain Tissue												Indicator Cells
	White Matter								Grey Matter Areas				CV-1
	Plaque Adjacent Area						Plaque Distant Area						
	1	2	3	4	5	6	I	II	a	b	c	d	
Morphological Changes	-	-	-	NG	+	NG	-	NG	-	-	-	-	-
Nucleocapsids / HAD	- / -	- / -	- / -		+ / -		- / -		- / -	- / -	- / -	- / -	- / -
Fusion Cultures with CV-1 Cells — No. of Pooled Cultures / Fusion Factor	S LL	LL	S	S LL			LL		S LL				S LL
Morphological Changes After Fusion	- -	-	-	- -		+①ˣ	- -		- -				- -
HAD	- -	-	-	- -		+③ˣ	- -		- -				- -
Nucleocapsid	- -	-	-	- -		+③ˣ	- -		- -				- -

Arrow indicates number of cultures pooled together for fusion experiment.

LL= Lysolecithin

S= Beta-propiolactone inactivated Sendai virus.

NG= No Growth

$\bigcirc^{x}$ Denotes passage number after fusion at which changes were observed.

HAD= Hemadsorption of guinea pig RBC

183

TABLE 8

Effect of trypsin treatment on 6/94 virus
passaged in mammalian cells

Origin of virus		Before trypsin	After trypsin*
Fertile** Hens'eggs	HA HE INF	2048 0.295 6×10^7	2048 0.294 6×10^7
MDBK** cells	HA HE INF	2048 0.123 0	2048 0.230 2×10^6

*0.0005% of trypsin for 10 min. at 37°C with occasional
  shaking
**Purified virus of 1.20 gm/cc. density
  HA = hemagglutination (1% chick RBC)
  HE = hemolysis (determined by lysis of 2% guinea pig RBC
       and measured by O.D. at 575 nm)
  INF = Infectivity determined by titration in KC (human
        glioma) cells.

TABLE 9

Infectivity of 6/94 virus grown in human brain

Trypsin treatment	Infectivity of brain passaged virus for:		
	Temperature of Incubation °C	MDBK cells	Mouse macrophages
No	32 37	6×10^1 0	3×10^4 3×10^3
Yes	32 37	3×10^5 3×10^4	3×10^5 3×10^4

Table 10

Restoration of infectivity of 6/94 virus for human brain cells after passage through either human or mouse macrophages

Passage number of virus through cells			Infectivity for cells*			
1	2	3	Human brain	Human macrophages	Mouse macrophages	Embryonated eggs
Human brain			None	3×10^3	2×10^4	6×10^4
	Mouse macrophage		2×10^3	-	6×10^5	-
	Human macrophage	Mouse macrophage	3×10^1	-	6×10^1	-
		Human brain	3×10^2	-	-	-
	macrophage	Human brain	None	-	-	-

*as determined by hemadsorption of guinea pig RBC on infected cells

TABLE 11

Progressive lesions of brain tissue of mice infected
with 6/94 strain of parainfluenza

Brain tissue examined days after inoculation	VIRUS INOCULA						
	Parainfluenza 1				Measles		
	Virus		Lesions			Lesions	
	Isolation	EM	Acute	Chronic		Acute	Chronic
3	+*	+**	Disseminated meningoence-phalitis and ependymitis	None		Disseminated meningoence-phalitis and ependymitis	None
7	-	-	Disseminated meningoence-phalitis and ependymitis	None		Disseminated meningoence-phalitis and ependymitis	None
14, 45, 67	-	-	None	Progressive destruction of paraventricular tissue, subcortical white matter and myelin		None	None

* from tissue culture explants
** in ependymal cells only

THE RELATIONSHIP OF SV40-RELATED VIRUSES TO PROGRESSIVE MULTIFOCAL LEUKOENCEPHALOPATHY

Richard T. Johnson, Opendra Narayan, and Leslie P. Weiner

Departments of Neurology and Laboratory Animal Medicine
The Johns Hopkins University School of Medicine
Baltimore, Maryland, 21205

ABSTRACT. The papovaviruses of the SV40-polyoma group recently isolated from man can be serologically divided into three types. All are morphologically indistinguishable, are oncogenic for hamsters, and have capsid and tumor antigens which cross-react to greater or lesser extents with SV40 but not mouse polyoma virus. Viruses of two types, JC and SV40-PML viruses, have been isolated only from brains of patients with progressive multifocal leukoencephalopathy, a rare subacute demyelinating disease. There is substantial evidence relating these viruses etiologically to this disease. The third serotype, BK virus, has been isolated from human urine following renal allografts but has not been related to any human disease.

INTRODUCTION

The recent recovery of viruses from progressive multi-focal leukoencephalopathy (PML) has been of greater biological than public health interest, since PML is a rare brain infection usually complicating grave, underlying systemic disease. The biological interest, however, is manifold. First, it is the first consistent isolation of viruses from a chronic human demyelinating disease and, therefore, has implications in the studies of multiple sclerosis, the most common human demyelinating disease. Second, the disease appears to represent an opportunistic infection complicating immunosuppression, due either to underlying disease or to immunosuppressive drugs given to sustain human organ transplants or to treat other illnesses. Third, the agents themselves are of interest, since these are the first papovaviruses of the SV40-polyoma subgroup which have been

187

related to human disease and since both serotypes isolated from PML have proven oncogenic in hamsters. We will first describe the disease, briefly summarize the known biological properties of the viruses, and finally discuss how these viruses can be related to the pathogenesis of human demyelination and possibly neoplasia.

PROGRESSIVE MULTIFOCAL LEUKOENCEPHALOPATHY

In 1958 Astrom, Mancall, and Richardson (1) described this chronic human demyelinating disease under the title "Progressive multifocal leukoencephalopathy, a heretofore unrecognized complication of chronic lymphocytic leukemia and Hodgkin's disease". They described three patients with progressive neurological disease that proved pathologically to have widely disseminated foci of myelin sheath destruction with relative sparing of axons. In many areas, these foci appeared to become confluent forming plaque-like lesions. Associated with the myelin destruction were unique cellular reactions. Oligodendrocytes were absent within the foci, and surrounding the foci they were enlarged and contained intranuclear inclusion bodies. On the other hand, within the lesions the astrocytes were enlarged "into bizarre gigantic forms, with unequivocal mitoses...suggesting neoplastic cells".

In 1961 Richardson (2) reviewed 10 cases of PML studied personally as well as 12 others reported in the literature. Not all were associated with lymphomas and leukemias, but cases were also found in association with sarcoidosis, tuberculosis, carcinomatosis, and, in one case, simply advanced age without associated disease. The neurological disease, however, followed a stereotyped pattern with the development of multifocal neurological signs such as paralysis, mental deterioration, visual loss, sensory abnormalities, and ataxia, which followed an ingravescent course leading to death in less than one year. The patients remained afebrile, and headaches were infrequent. The cerebrospinal fluid was usually normal. The pathological findings were highly stereotyped resembling the original three cases. Since the common feature of the underlying diseases was that all illnesses were, at times, associated with immunological hypoactivity and since the nuclear inclusions were consistent with a viral cytopathology, Richardson postulated a viral cause. A similar suggestion that the inclusion bodies might be related to viral infection have been made by Cavanagh, et al. (3).

There are now over 100 reported cases of PML, and over half of these have been associated with malignant lympho-proliferative diseases including lymphosarcoma. Chronic and acute myelogenous leukemia, carcinomatosis, tuberculo-sis, and sarcoidosis account for the majority of the remaining cases, but recently cases have been reported in patients who received immunosuppressive therapy following renal transplantation (4) and who had been treated with large doses of immunosuppressive agents for systemic lupus erythematosus (5). Several patients have not been found to have underlying disease, but in those in whom clinical immunological studies have been carried out, a consistent finding has been abnormalities of cell-mediated immune responses (6). Most of the patients have died within six months after the onset of their disease, but there have now been several cases who lived for more than a year. One patient described by Hedley-White, et al. (7) survived for five years with two periods of apparent remission. We observed a patient, who after an initial rapid deteriora-tion, survived in a stable condition for almost two years, and this period of survival was associated with an extra-ordinary rise in antibody against the papovavirus isolated from the brain (5).

In 1964 ZuRhein and Chou (8) examined the oligodendro-cyte inclusions electron microscopically and found large numbers of particles, sometimes in pseudocrystalline arrays, resembling papovaviruses. Extraction and negative stain-ing of these particles indicated a size and capsid struc-ture suggestive of papovaviruses of the SV40-polyoma sub-group (9). This initial observation was rapidly confirmed, and in 1969 ZuRhein (10) reviewed 8 cases studied person-ally as well as 19 cases studied by others, all of which contained virions ranging in size from 32 to 45 mm. These virions appeared to be located primarily, and in most cases exclusively, in the oligodendrocytes surrounding the areas of demyelination. Virions were concentrated in the nucleus but also were seen along membranes within the cyto-plasm. The particles appeared to be present in each case of PML in which there was adequate tissue available for study.

Initial attempts to isolate virus from cerebral tissue of patients with PML by inoculation of cell cultures, small laboratory rodents, and embryonated eggs and primates with long term observations were all unsuccessful (10-13).

189

During the past three years, three serologically distinct types of papovaviruses, all cross-reacting to greater or lesser extent with SV40, have been isolated from man. Two of these viruses have been isolated only from brain tissue of patients with PML. Initial isolation of an apparently new human papovavirus by Padgett, et al. (14) was accomplished by the inoculation of a homogenate of brain from a patient dying of PML onto cultures derived from human fetal brain. This virus, termed JC, has now been isolated from four cases of PML in that lab (15) as well as cases in three other laboratories (16-18). A virus anti-genically indistinguishable from SV40 was isolated from two patients with PML in our laboratory, initially by the fusion of cultured cells derived from the brain of the patient with primary cultures of African green monkey kidney cells (5), but subsequently from one case this agent has been re-isolated from homogenates of brain inoculated on cultures of human fetal brain (19). The third papovavirus was isolated by Gardner, et al. (20) from the urine of a patient follow-ing a renal allograft. Although this virus, BK, has now been recovered from urine of a number of patients (21), it has not been related to any disease in man. Since it must be regarded as a candidate virus in PML, it will be dis-cussed briefly in the following section.

BIOLOGICAL PROPERTIES OF THE NEW HUMAN PAPOVAVIRUSES

JC, SV40-PML, and BK viruses resemble SV40 and polyoma viruses, since they are non-enveloped, icosahedral virions between 30-45 nm in size and contain a circular DNA duplex with a molecular weight of 3×10^6 daltons (22, 23). Digestion with Hemophilus influenzae restriction endonu-clease preparations has shown that the SV40-PML DNAs yield 11 fragments similar to classical SV40. Nine co-migrate with fragments of SV40-DNA, and two do not (22). The two different SV40-like viruses isolated from PML differ from each other in the same two fragments that they differ from classic SV40 (24). Therefore, they appear to be strains of SV40. The DNA of JC and BK viruses show entirely different patterns when digested and electrophoretically analyzed, and they are significantly different from each other (23). Therefore, these two agents appear to be two distinct, new papovaviruses rather than SV40 variants.

Different cell cultures which have been shown to support permissive infection with these viruses. JC virus

has been shown to have cytopathic effects only in cultures
of human fetal brain cells (15), but this cytopathology may
be subtle necessitating electron microscopic monitoring of
cultures (16). JC virus multiplies to reasonable titers in
human fetal brain cells, but no replication has been demonstrated in a number of human cells, African green monkey
kidney cells, rabbit kidney cells, or mouse cells (15). In
contrast, the SV40-PML and BK viruses replicate and cause
cytopathic changes in a variety of human and primate cell
cultures (25-27). All three viruses produce tumors in
hamsters (25, 28, 29). However, JC virus is unique in
being more oncogenic when inoculated intracerebrally than
extraneurally and in producing cerebral and cerebellar
tumors resembling gliomas (28). The SV40 strains from PML
are similar to classic SV40 in producing undifferentiated
sarcomas when injected subcutaneously and choroid plexus
papillomas after intracerebral inoculation (25). Cerebral
tumors have not been induced by BK virus.

Intranuclear tumor (T) antigens produced by all three
serotypes appear to cross react by fluorescent antibody
staining with antibodies to SV40 T antigen (25, 26, 28).
In electron microscopic agglutination studies, the agents
appear to have cross-reacting capsid antigens. Sera from
rabbits obtained 10 days after a single, intravenous inoculation of virus react solely with the inoculated agent.
Therefore, these sera can be used for typing JC, SV40-PML,
or BK viruses. However, these sera do not differentiate
SV40-PML variants from classic SV40 virus. Hyperimmune
sera show varying degrees of cross-reaction between JC, BK,
and SV40 viruses indicating that they share minor capsid
antigens, but no cross-reaction is found with mouse polyoma
virus (30). Slight to moderate degrees of cross-reactivity
has also been demonstrated in hyperimmune serum assaying
for hemagglutination inhibiting, fluorescing, and neutralizing antibodies (16, 18, 20, 25, 26). Both JC and BK
viruses possess particle-associated hemagglutinin similar
to polyoma virus but the strains of SV40 isolated from PML
do not (20, 31, 32).

Serologic studies have shown that both JC and BK
viruses are ubiquitous in human populations. Sero-conversion of a majority of persons to BK virus occurs in early
childhood (33, 34), and sero-conversion to JC virus appears
to occur in later childhood or adolescence (32). In contrast, serological surveys show that neutralizing antibody
to SV40 virus is variable, running as high as 27% in

191

monkey handlers and 20% in children of an age group having a high risk of exposure to contaminated killed poliovirus vaccines. Non-monkey sources of infection have been suggested by the finding of antibody in 2 to 4% of individuals who have had little or no contact with rhesus monkeys and who were bled either prior to the introduction of contaminated vaccines or were born after vaccines were cleared of SV40 (35).

RELATIONSHIP OF PAPOVAVIRUSES TO PML

Isolation of viruses from tissues of patients with PML has proven to be a tedious and time-consuming procedure. Furthermore, the necessity of maintaining inoculated cultures for long periods of time and the use, in some studies, of cultures of simian origin have raised the spector that some isolates might represent laboratory contaminants or even recombinants with simian viruses latent in cell cultures (36). However, monospecific sera have made it possible to identify these viruses directly by fluorescent antibody staining of viral antigens in the brain tissue and by electron microscopic agglutination to differentiate virions extracted directly from the brain (37). Utilizing these methods we have studied brain tissue of 13 patients with PML, identified JC virus in 11, and SV40 viruses in two (6). BK virus was not implicated in the disease within this series nor were cases encountered, where adequate material was available, in which there was a failure to identify a papovavirus.

In contrast to these findings, no papovavirus has ever been isolated from or serologically identified in normal brains or in brain tissue of other diseases. Papovavirus-like particles have been reported in electron microscopic studies of cell cultures derived from human brain tissues (38), and particles the size of papovaviruses have been reported in human brain biopsies (39) and in a human choroid plexus papilloma (40). However, a subsequent study of similar particles in choroid plexus tumors indicated histochemically that these were glycogen granules (41). Therefore, it appears that papovaviruses are not found in other diseases or normal brain, can be consistently identified in the brain in PML, and are present in such extraordinary quantity that virions can be extracted from brain and examined serologically, in most cases, without concentration (42).

Since PML is associated with defects in cell-mediated immunity (6), it probably results from activation of virus latent in the brain or other tissue since childhood infection. On the other hand, the rare patient who succumbs to PML might be one who failed to acquire immunity during childhood and has a first encounter with the virus after an illness has interferred with cell-mediated immune responses. As yet, neither SV40 or JC viruses have been demonstrated in human tissues other than the brain.

The mechanism by which these viruses produce unique cytopathological changes in the brain is suggested both by studies in cell cultures of human fetal glial cells as well as histological studies of the diseased brains. In cultures of human fetal glial cells, there appear to be two predominant types of cells. The large, translucent vesicular cells with prominent nuclei, abundant cytoplasm, and multiple processes have been thought to represent astrocytes; the small bipolar, dark, refractile cells have been called spongioblasts and are thought to represent the germinal cells giving rise to neurons and/or oligodendrocytes. Inoculation of these cultures with either JC or SV40 virus produces lysis of the spongioblasts (14, 43). Inoculation with classic SV40 or SV40 strains isolated from PML also causes later lysis of most astrocytes, but surviving astrocytes contain intranuclear T antigen on immunofluorescent staining and, although no virus replication is evident as tested by inoculation of freeze-thawed cells onto African green monkey cells, virus can be rescued by co-cultivation of these cells with BSC-1 or primary African green monkey cells (25). Thus, within the cultures of human fetal glial cells, there appear to be two cell populations, one permissive and one non-permissive for these agents.

In the human brain, neurons show no evidence of disease in PML. In the white matter of the brain which contains the axons of these neurons there are two glial cell populations (Fig. 1). The oligodendrocytes are the glial cells whose cytoplasmic extensions form the myelin sheath which wrap the axons. The astrocytes make up the other major glial population but are not associated with myelin. Oligodendrocytes are depleted within the foci of myelin loss, and the oligodendrocytes around the periphery of the demyelination are distorted and their enlarged nuclei packed with virions. Fluorescent staining confirms the presence of viral antigen in the enlarged cells surrounding the areas of demyelination. It would appear, therefore, that in PML a permissive infection of oligodendrocytes with these opportunistic viruses causes their lysis and demyelination.

Within the areas of demyelination, the astrocytes are large and distorted, often contain multiple nuclei, hyperchromatic distorted nuclei, and many mitotic figures (Fig. 1). In the original description of PML, these were likened to malignant cells (1). They rarely contain virions by electron microscopic examination. In sections of brain T antigen has not been demonstrated within these cells. The cells grown from brains of patients with PML yielding SV40 viruses appear to be largely astrocytes. These cells had been shown not to contain virions by electron microscopy (5), to contain T antigen by fluorescent antibody staining, and to yield virus when fused to permissive cells (25).

In summary, of the three major cell types in the brain, neurons appear unaffected by these papovaviruses while both glial cell populations are involved. The oligodendrocytes appear to be involved in a permissive infection resulting in demyelination, and the astrocytes in a nonpermissive infection resulting in some features of transformation. For this reason, studies are currently in progress to determine whether these agents might be related, in some cases, to the induction of astrocytic tumors, the most common brain tumors of man.

ACKNOWLEDGMENTS

This work was supported by a grant from the National Institute of Neurological Diseases and Stroke (NS 08838) and a contract from the National Cancer Institute (NO1-CP-43266). Leslie P. Weiner is the recipient of a research career development award (NS 50274).

REFERENCES

1. Astrom, K.-E., Mancall, E.L., and Richardson, E.P., Brain 81, 93 (1958).
2. Richardson, E.P., New Engl. J. Med. 265, 815 (1961).
3. Cavanagh, J.B., Greenbaum, D., Marshall, A.H.E., and Rubinstein, L.J., Lancet 2, 524 (1959).
4. Manz, H.J., Dinsdale, H.B., and Morrin, P.A.F., Ann. Int. Med. 75, 77 (1971).

5. Weiner, L.P., Herndon, R.M., Narayan, O., Johnson, R.T., Shah, K., Rubinstein, L.J., Preziosi, T.J., and Conley, F.K., New Engl. J. Med. 286, 385 (1972).
6. Narayan, O., Penney, J.B., Jr., Johnson, R.T., Herndon, R.M., and Weiner, L.P., New Engl. J. Med. 289, 1278 (1973).
7. Hedley-Whyte, E.T., Smith, B.P., Tyler, H.R., and Peterson, W.P., J. Neuropath. Exp. Neurol. 25, 107 (1966).
8. ZuRhein, G.M., and Chou, S.M., Science 148, 1477 (1965).
9. Howatson, A.F., Nagai, M., and ZuRhein, G.M., Canad. Med. Ass. J. 93, 379 (1965).
10. ZuRhein, G.M., Progr. Med. Virol. 11, 185 (1969).
11. Schwerdt, P.R., Schwerdt, C.E., Silverman, L., and Rubinstein, L.J., Virology 29, 511 (1966).
12. Dolman, C.L., Furesz, J., and Mackay, B., Canad. Med. Ass. J. 97, 8 (1967).
13. Gibbs, C.J., Gajdusek, D.C., and Alpers, M.P., In Pathogenesis and Etiology of Demyelinating Diseases. Add. ad Int. Arch. Allergy 36, 519 (1969).
14. Padgett, B.L., Walker, D.L., ZuRhein, G.M., Eckroade, R.J., and Dessel, B.H., Lancet 1, 1257 (1971).
15. Walker, D.L., Padgett, B.L., ZuRhein, G.M., Albert, A.E., and Marsh, R.F., In Slow Virus Diseases (Ed. Zeman, W., and Lennette, E.). Williams and Wilkins, Baltimore, p. 49 (1973).
16. Weiner, L.P., Narayan, O., Penney, J.B., Jr., Herndon, R.M., Feringa, E.R., Tourtellotte, W.W., and Johnson, R.T., Arch. Neurol. 29, 1 (1973).
17. Cathala, F., Hauw, J.-J., and Escourolle, R., C.R., Acad. Sc. Paris 276, 1081 (1973).
18. Field, A.M., Gardner, S.D., Goodbody, R.A., and Wood-house, M.A., J. Clin. Path., In press.
19. Weiner, L.P., Herndon, R.M., Narayan, O., and Johnson, R.T., J. Virol. 10, 147 (1972).
20. Gardner, S.D., Field, A.M., Coleman, D.V., and Hulme, B., Lancet 1, 1253 (1971).
21. Coleman, D.V., Gardner, S.D., and Field, A.M., Brit. Med. J. 3, 371 (1973).
22. Sack, G.H., Narayan, O., Danna, K.S., Weiner, L.P., and Nathans, D., Virology 51, 345 (1973).
23. Osborn, J.E., Robertson, S.M., Padgett, B.L., ZuRhein, G.M., Walker, D.L., and Weisblum, B., J. Virol. 13, 614 (1974).
24. Narayan, O., and Nathans, D., Unpublished data.

25. Narayan, O., Unpublished data.
26. Takemoto, K.K., and Mullarkey, M.F., J. Virol. 12, 625 (1973).
27. Major, E.O., and DiMayorca, G., Proc. Natl. Acad. Sci., 70, 3210 (1973).
28. Walker, D.L., Padgett, B.L., ZuRhein, G.M., Albert, A.E., and Marsh, R.F., Science 181, 674 (1973).
29. Shah, K.V., Daniel, R.W., and Warszawski, R., Fed. Proc. 33, 753 (1974).
30. Penney, J.B., Jr., and Narayan, O., Infect. Immun. 8, 299 (1973).
31. Mantyjarvi, R.A., Arstila, P.P., and Meurman, O.H., Infect. Immun. 6, 824 (1972).
32. Padgett, B.L., and Walker, D.L., J. Infect. Dis. 127, 467 (1973).
33. Gardner, S.D., Brit. Med. J. 1, 77 (1973).
34. Shah, K.V., Daniel, R.W., and Warszawski, R.M., J. Infect. Dis. 128, 784 (1973).
35. Shah, K.V., Am. J. Epidemiol. 95, 199 (1972).
36. Black, P.H., and Hirsh, M.S., New Engl. J. Med. 286, 429 (1972).
37. Penney, J.B., Jr., Weiner, L.P., Herndon, R.M., Narayan, O., and Johnson, R.T., Science 178, 60 (1972).
38. Oyanagi, S., terMeulen, V., Muller, D., Katz, M., and Koprowski, H., J. Virol. 6, 370 (1970).
39. Vernon, M.L., Horta-Barbosa, L., Fuccillo, D.A., Sever, J.L., Baringer, J.R., and Birnbaum, G., Lancet 1, 964 (1970).
40. Bastian, F.O., Lab. Invest. 25, 169 (1971).
41. Carter, L.P., Beggs, J., and Waggener, J.D., Cancer 30, 1130 (1972).
42. Johnson, R.T., and Gibbs, C.J., Jr., Arch. Neurol. 30, 36 (1974).
43. Shein, H.M., J. Neuropath. Exp. Neurol. 26, 60 (1967).

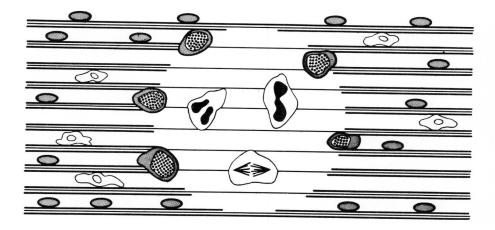

Fig. 1. Schematic diagram of the demyelinated lesion of
PML showing the varied cytopathic reactions in the white
matter. The axons from the neurons (shown as fine horizontal lines) are generally intact, but the myelin sheaths
(heavy horizontal lines) are disrupted within the lesion.
The myelin sheaths are extensions of the cytoplasmic membranes of oligodendrocytes (shaded cells) which are lost
within the demyelinated area. In the periphery the oligodendrocytes are enlarged and have intranuclear inclusions
containing many virions (shown as dots). The astrocytes
(clear cells) are normal distant from the lesion, but
within the lesion they are greatly enlarged and often
contain multiple nuclei, hyperchromatic distorted nuclei,
and mitotic figures.

MEASLES VIRUS LATENCY AND NEUROVIRULENCE

Fred Rapp, Martin V. Haspel, Ronald Duff and Paul Knight

Department of Microbiology
The Milton S. Hershey Medical Center
The Pennsylvania State University
Hershey, Pennsylvania 17033

ABSTRACT. Measles virus can enter an in vitro latent
state in hamster embryo fibroblasts. Infectious measles
virus can be rescued from the latently infected cells by
co-cultivation with susceptible cells, incubation at 33.5°,
or by treatment with chemicals able to induce cells to
produce virus. Studies with inhibitors reveal that little
or no RNA or protein synthesis is required for the isolation of infectious virus following the procedures enabling
virus rescue. Interferon is not responsible for the latent infection. Autointerference between a temperature-
sensitive (ts) mutant and another virus variant is probably
the mechanism of latency. Newborn hamsters can be protected from acute encephalitis by maternally derived measles
neutralizing antibody. Measles virus can establish latent
infection of the central nervous system in the maternal
antibody protected animals. Cyclophosphamide treatment
causes activation of the latent infection resulting in the
development of neurological symptoms. Selection for ts
mutants is accompanied by attenuation of measles virus
neurovirulence.

INTRODUCTION

Measles virus induces both acute encephalitis (1) and
chronic neurological disorders such as subacute sclerosing
panencephalitis (SSPE) and possibly multiple sclerosis
(2,3). Transient EEG changes as well as cerebrospinal
fluid pleocytosis associated with "uncomplicated" measles
(4-6), suggests that neurological involvement by measles
virus is relatively common. Lifelong immunity to measles
virus has been demonstrated even in the absence of booster
immunization by natural re-exposure to the virus (7).
Measles virus may therefore enter a latent state as a
consequence of the normal disease process. Measles virus,

as well as other paramyxoviruses such as mumps and New-castle disease virus (NDV), can also enter a latent state in cell culture (8-14). In vitro latency is a useful model for the elucidation of the molecular mechanisms of measles virus latency. This paper reviews work carried out concerning in vitro and in vivo latent infections with measles virus.

DEVELOPMENT OF IN VITRO LATENT INFECTION

A latent infection with Schwarz measles vaccine derived virus was obtained when the infected hamster embryo fibro-blast (HEF) cells were maintained in a non-proliferative state (8). Upon subsequent cell passage, the latently infected cells (S cells) were demonstrated by immunofluor-escence techniques to contain measles virus antigens, but they did not release infectious virus. Infectious measles virus could be rescued from the S cells by co-cultivation with BSC-1 cells. The co-cultivation technique has been successful in recovering infectious measles virus from non-producer cells such as those obtained from the brains of SSPE patients (15).

ALTERATION OF THE CELL-VIRUS RELATIONSHIP

DURING CELL PASSAGE

After about 20 cell passages, small amounts of virus were spontaneously released from the S cells at 37°. Virus leakage could be eliminated by incubation at 39° or enhanced by incubation at 33.5° (Table 1). The virus obtained from the S cells by incubation at 33.5° (TR), un-like the virus obtained by co-cultivation (CC), replicated as a temperature-sensitive (ts) mutant at 39° (Figure 1). The CC and TR viruses demonstrated similar thermal stabil-ity (9). The viruses isolated by these different methods also differed in plaque size and the ability to replicate in Vero cells without adaption (Table 2). The CC and TR viruses therefore represented distinct variants of measles virus.

During continued cell passage, the cell-virus relation-ship was further altered. After cell passage 45, virus began to be spontaneously released at 39° (Table 1).

Although a 100-fold increase in virus release still occurred at 33.5°, the TR virus was no longer temperature-sensitive (9), nor was it distinguishable in any way from the CC virus (Table 2).

OTHER METHODS OF VIRUS INDUCTION

A 100-fold increase in infectious virus released at 37° occurred following chemical induction (16). Treatment of the S cells with BUdR (50 µg/ml), IUdR (50 µg/ml) or mitomycin C (1 µg/ml) for 72 hours resulted in virus induction. Cytosine arabinoside, actinomycin D and cycloheximide were ineffective.

THE STATE OF THE LATENT VIRUS IN THE S CELLS

The peak titers of infectious virus obtained by co-cultivation, unlike a primary infection of BSC-1 cells, occur within 20 hours. This finding suggested that some of the components of the virus obtained by co-cultivation were probably pre-formed.

5-Azacytidine (50 µg/ml) inhibits the production of infectious measles virus during primary infection by incorporation into virus RNA. The early release of infectious measles virus by co-cultivation is not inhibited by 5-azacytidine (Figure 2). RNA synthesis is therefore not required for the early release of virus. After 16 hours, an inhibition, probably due to exhaustion of pre-formed measles RNA, was observed. It has been reported that in another measles in vitro latency system, there are no qualitative differences between RNA synthesis in lytically and latently infected cells (17).

It has been demonstrated that little or no protein synthesis is required for the release of infectious mumps virus from latently infected cells (18). Cycloheximide (10 µg/ml) inhibits the appearance of infectious virus in lytically infected cells but does not alter the early release of virus by co-cultivation (Figure 2). A decrease in virus release was observed 8 hours after the addition of the BSC-1 cells. Little or no protein synthesis is therefore required for the early virus release; inhibition by cycloheximide probably occurs after the pool of pre-formed virus proteins is depleted.

Studies by indirect immunofluorescence methods reveal that measles virus antigens are present in the perinuclear region of the cell (8). Electron microscopy also demonstrated myxovirus-like nucleocapsids in the perinuclear region (16). During virus induction, the antigens were observed to spread outward throughout the cytoplasm from the perinuclear region. The measles virus therefore appears to be pre-formed in the S cell, and is probably blocked at a late maturational step.

A POSSIBLE MECHANISM FOR THE LATENT

INFECTION AND ITS ACTIVATION

The S cells are resistant to superinfection by Edmonston measles virus. Although this measles virus strain reaches titers of 10^5 plaque-forming units per ml in HEF cells, no virus is detectable above the background of spontaneously released virus when S cells are superinfected with Edmonston measles virus (16). Interferon does not appear to be responsible for either the resistence to superinfection or the maintenance of virus latency. Vesicular stomatitis virus, which is very sensitive to the effects of interferon, replicates equally well in both HEF and S cells. In addition, interferon does not inhibit the release of measles virus by co-cultivation (Figure 2). Work done in two other laboratories has also demonstrated that human cells persistently infected with measles virus were resistant to superinfection by measles but not by other viruses (10,11). Interferon did not appear to be involved in these other systems.

Temperature-sensitive (ts) mutants are intimately involved in the establishment and maintenance of in vitro latent infections of NDV (12,13). We have isolated a ts mutant by incubation of the S cells at 33.5°. In another measles virus latent system (11), an increase in virus release occurred when the cells were incubated at 33°; there is no information available as to whether or not a ts mutant could be isolated from these cells at the lower temperature. It is evident however, that ts mutants are somehow involved in virus latency in vitro. Resistance of cells to superinfection in the absence of detectable interferon suggests an interference phenomenon. The replication of the ts mutant is inhibited at the higher temperature. It is possible that the mutant further inhibits the non-temperature sensitive variant isolated by co-cultivation. During the course of frequent cell passage, the ts mutant was lost from the S cells. Concomitant with the loss of the ts mutant was the spontaneous release of virus at 39°.

The transition from a latent to a persistent infection is most probably due to the continued passage of the cells. Frequent cell passage at 37° would select against a slowly replicating virus and result in the loss of the ts mutant. In addition, measles virus replicates most efficiently in rapidly proliferating cells (9). There is a direct relationship between the proliferative activity of the S cells and the amount of infectious virus in each cell (Figure 3). The latent infection was developed by maintaining the cells in a non-proliferative state. The breakdown of the latent infection may have occurred by the maintenance of the S cells in a highly proliferative state by frequent cell passage. It should be noted that there is at least one reported instance of the isolation of measles virus from SSPE cells without the requirement of co-cultivation, after these cells had been passaged extensively in cell culture (19). Cell passage therefore appears to be involved in the activation of another measles virus latent infection.

MEASLES VIRUS NEUROVIRULENCE: IMMUNOLOGICAL FACTORS

Measles virus induces encephalitis in newborn hamsters following intracranial injection (20,21). Hamsters born to mothers hyperimmune to measles virus, have high levels of measles neutralizing antibody (22). Newborn hamsters were injected (intracranial route) with 10^4 PFU of brain adapted Schwarz measles virus. All of the unprotected animals developed acute encephalitis while only 17% of the animals possessing maternal antibody developed encephalitis within 16 days of inoculation (22). As the protected animals matured, they developed active immunity suppressing the measles infection. Only a few of these animals later developed neurological symptoms (between 26 and 70 days after inoculation). Immunosuppression by cyclophosphamide (200 mg/Kg body weight) activated the latent infection resulting in the development of neurological symptoms in 30% of the animals previously protected by maternal antibody.

Maternal antibody was thus able to protect newborn hamsters from acute encephalitis. The measles virus was, however, latent in the central nervous system. It is interesting to note that about 50% of the patients with SSPE had measles virus infections prior to age 2 (23). It is possible that the presence of maternal antibody to measles virus may influence virus latency. The activation of the latent infection may then result in the pathogenesis of SSPE.

MEASLES VIRUS NEUROVIRULENCE: VIROLOGICAL FACTORS

Non-neurotropic polioviruses replicate as ts mutants (24). In addition, ts mutants of reovirus exhibit decreased neurovirulence (25). Six ts mutants of measles virus have been isolated in our laboratory. Newborn hamsters were injected intracranially with 3×10^4 PFU of either the parental strain or one of the ts mutants. All of the ts mutants were less neurovirulent than the parental strain (Table 3). Some mutants, however, were more attenuated than others. The neurovirulence is not due to reversion, as virus could be isolated from mutant infected brains, and was found to still be mutant. All of the mutants were capable of replicating at the hamster body temperature (37°). The degree of attenuation may depend upon the nature of the temperature-sensitive block; studies are now being carried out to evaluate this possibility.

The attenuation of the properties of measles virus responsible for the induction of acute neurological diseases may permit the development of chronic neuropathies. Ts mutants should prove as useful in experimental pathology as they have in the study of the genetics and other biological properties of viruses.

ACKNOWLEDGEMENTS

This study was conducted under Contract No. 70-2024 within the Virus Cancer Program of the National Cancer Institute, National Institutes of Health, U.S. Public Health Service and Public Health Service Grant No. 5 R01 CA11647-05.

REFERENCES

1. La Boccetta, A.C. and Tornay, A.S., Amer. J. Dis. Child. 107,247 (1964).
2. Ter Meulen, V., Katz, M. and Müller, D., Curr. Topics Microbiol. 57,1 (1972).
3. Weiner, L.P., Johnson, R.T. and Herndon, R.M., New Eng. J. Med. 288,1103 (1973).
4. Gibbs, F.A., Gibbs, E.L., Carpenter, P.R. and Spies, H.W., J.A.M.A. 171,1050 (1959).
5. Pampiglione, G., Griffith, A.H. and Bramwell, E.C., Lancet 2,5 (1971).
6. Ojala, A., Ann. Med. Intern. (Fenn.) 36,321 (1947).
7. Dekking, F., Arch Ges. Virusforsch. 16,208 (1965).
8. Knight, P., Duff, R. and Rapp, F., J. Virol. 10,995 (1972).
9. Haspel, M.V., Knight, P.R., Duff, R.G. and Rapp, F., J. Virol. 12,690 (1973).
10. Rustigian, R., J. Bact. 92,1792 (1966).
11. Norrby, E., Arch. Ges. Virusforsch. 20,215 (1967).
12. Preble, O.T. and Youngner, J.S., J. Virol. 9,200 (1972).
13. Preble, O.T. and Youngner, J.S., J. Virol. 12,481 (1973).
14. Walker, D.L. and Hinze, H.C., J. Exp. Med. 116,739 (1962).
15. Horta-Barbosa, L., Fuccillo, D.A., Sever, J.L. and Zeman, W., Nature (London) 221,974 (1969).
16. Knight, P., Doctoral Dissertation, Pennsylvania State University (1973).
17. Winston, S.H., Rustigian, R. and Bratt, M.A., J. Virol. 11,926 (1973).
18. Northrop, R.L., J. Virol. 4,133 (1969).
19. Payne, F.E. and Baublis, J.V., Perspectives in Virology, VII, M. Pollard (Ed.), Academic Press, New York, 1971, p.179.

20. Burnstein, T., Jensen, J.H. and Waksman, B.H., J. Infec. Dis. 114,265 (1964).
21. Wear, D.J. and Rapp, F., Nature (London) 227,1347 (1970).
22. Wear, D.J. and Rapp, F., J. Immunol. 107,1593 (1971).
23. Jabbour, J.T., Duenas, D.A., Sever, S.L., Krebs, H.M. and Horta-Barbosa, L., J.A.M.A. 220,959 (1972).
24. Sabin, A.B. and Lwoff, A., Science 129,1287 (1959).
25. Fields, B.N., New Eng. J. Med. 287,1026 (1972).

Table 1

THE INDUCTION OF INFECTIOUS MEASLES VIRUS FROM
DIFFERENT PASSAGE LEVEL S CELLS.

Method of virus release	T^a	$P< 20^b$	$P\ 20-45^c$	$P>45^d$
Co-cultivation	$33.5°$	ND^e	2.5×10^4 f	1.8×10^5
	$37°$	5.0×10^5	2.4×10^4	1.4×10^6
	$39°$	ND	1.4×10^5	1.6×10^6
Temperature-Release	$33.5°$	ND	3.0×10^4	8.0×10^2
	$37°$	$<1.0 \times 10$	4.0×10^2	9.5×10^2
	$39°$	ND	$<1.0 \times 10$	6.2×10^2

[a] Temperature of cultivation.

[b] S cell passage <20.

[c] S cell passages 20-45.

[d] S cell passage >45.

[e] Not Done

[f] PFU/ml assayed in BSC-1 cells.

Table 2

PROPERTIES OF VIRUSES RELEASED BY CO-CULTIVATION OR TEMPERATURE

Property	P 20-45[a]		P>45[b]	
	CC[c]	TR[d]	CC[c]	TR[d]
Replication at 39°	Normal	Temperature sensitive	Normal	Normal
Plaque Size at 37°	$\geq$ 1 mm	$\leq$ 0.5 mm	$\geq$ 1 mm	$\geq$ 1 mm
Growth in Vero cells without adaptation	virus detectable 24 hours after inoculation	No virus detectable at 36 hr.	Virus detectable 24 hours after inoculation	Virus detectable 24 hours after inoculation

[a] S cell passages 20-45.

[b] S cell passages >45.

[c] CC= Co-cultivation released virus

[d] TR= Temperature released virus.

Table 3

NEUROVIRULENCE OF TEMPERATURE SENSITIVE MUTANTS OF
MEASLES VIRUS IN THE NEWBORN HAMSTER

Virus[a]	SI[b]	NU[c]
Parental	0	5
Ts Mutant A	106	1
Ts Mutant B	103	1
Ts Mutant C	16	4
Ts Mutant E	84	1
Ts Mutant F	55	2
Ts Mutant G	24	3

[a]Approximately 60 hamsters were inoculated with 3 X 10^{4}PFU of each virus within 24 hr. of birth.

[b]Survival Index.

$$\frac{\% \text{ animals surviving 45 days after intracranial injection of virus}}{\% \text{ animals surviving 45 days after intracranial injection of uninfected cells}} \times 100$$

[c]Degree of neurovirulence.

1= little or no neurovirulent potential

The rating is dependent upon: 1. Length of time until onset of neurological symptoms (if exhibited): 2. Severity of symptoms: 3. Slope of the mortality curve.

209

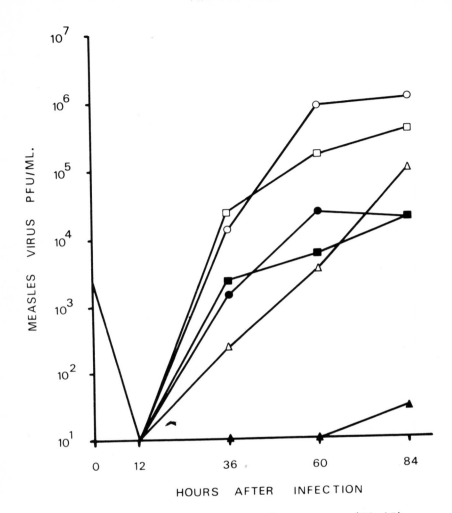

Fig. 1. Growth of early passage (20–45) co-cultivation (CC)-released viruses, temperature-released (TR) viruses, and Schwarz measles virus in BSC-1 cells at 33.5° and 39° C. Symbols: ▲ , TR 39°C; △ , TR 33.5°C; ● , CC 39°C; ○ , CC 33.5°C; ■ , Schwarz 39° C; and □ , Schwartz 33.5°C. Measles virus was assayed in BSC-1 cells by the plaque technique. From Haspel <u>et al</u>. (9) reprinted by permission of the American Society for Microbiology.

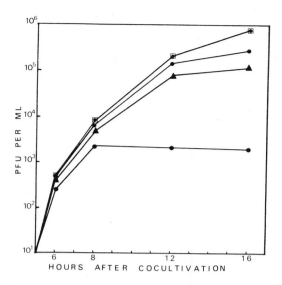

Fig. 2. Effect of 50 μg or 5-azacytidine per ml (-▲-), 10 μg of cycloheximide per ml (-●-), or 90 units of interferon per ml (-◉-) on the release of measles virus after co-cultivation of BSC-1 cells with hamster embryo fibroblast cells latently carrying measles virus. Co-cultivation involved 5 X 10^6 BSC-1 cells and 10^5 infectious units of latently infected hamster embryo fibroblast cells. Number of cellular infectious units was determined by infectious center assay. Cycloheximide or 5-azacytidine were added at the time of co-cultivation and remained in culture medium until samples were collected for infectious virus assay. BSC-1 cells were pretreated 18 hours before co-cultivation as well as during co-cultivation with interferon. Results obtained were compared to normal release of infectious measles virus after co-cultivation (-⬛-). From Knight et al. (8) reprinted by permission of the American Society for Microbiology.

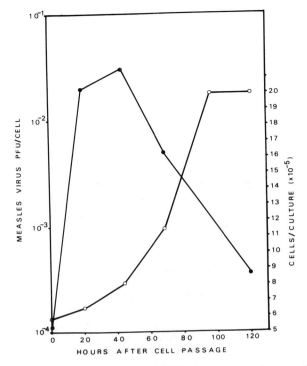

Fig. 3. Increased production of measles
virus in late system cultures after cell passage.
Latently infected cultures were passed by trypsin dispersion of cell monolayers and multiple
replicate cultures were grown in 60-mm plastic
petri dishes. Three cultures were harvested
at 0, 20, 44, 68, and 120 h after cell passage
and assayed for infectious measles virus by
the plaque method in BSC-1 cells. Three additional replicate cultures were also trypsinized
at 0, 20, 44, 68, 96, and 120 h after cell passage, and the total number of cells on each plate
was determined. Results are presented as the
average number of infectious measles virus particles per cell (●) and as the average number
of cells per 60-mm petri dish (○). From Haspel
et al. (9) reprinted by permission of the American
Society for Microbiology.

V

WHERE IS THE VIRUS OF HUMAN HEPATITIS?

STRUCTURE OF HEPATITIS B ANTIGEN (HB Ag)

John L. Gerin

Molecular Anatomy (MAN) Program
Oak Ridge National Laboratory
Rockville, Maryland 20852

ABSTRACT. HB Ag occurs in the serum of chronic carriers in a variety of particulate forms: a small 22 nm spherical particle, the predominant form; filaments of 22 nm diameter and of various lengths; and a larger 43 spherical particle with a complex morphology, the Dane particle. The various forms of each subtype of HB Ag were purified from human serum by multistep zonal centrifugation procedures. Characterization of the 22 nm form by electrophoresis on SDS-acrylamide gels revealed 7 proteins, two of which appear to be glycoproteins based on PAS staining. Antibodies to the isolated polypeptides reacted with the native particulate antigen by radioimmunoprecipitin and passive hemagglutination assays. The individual polypeptides stimulated both group (a) and subtype (d or y) specific antibodies in guinea pigs. The Dane particle occurs in the serum of most HB Ag carriers and contains a 27 nm core particle as a distinctive characteristic. The core was purified by isopycnic banding in CsCl after removal of the coat with 1% NP-40. While the coat of the Dane particle possesses the antigenic determinants of the 22 nm form, the core represents a quite separate antigenic system. The available evidence suggests that the Dane particle is the virus of hepatitis B and contains at least 6 native protein antigens; a, d or y, w or r on its surface, a "matrix" protein, the core antigen (s), and a DNA polymerase enzyme located within the core particle.

INTRODUCTION

Hepatitis B antigen (HB Ag) occurs in the serum of chronic carriers in a number of particulate forms. The

predominant form is an approximately 22 nm spherical
particle, however, filamentous forms of the same 22 nm
diameter but of varying lengths are usually observed often
in high concentration. A third form is the Dane particle,
a 43 nm spherical particle with a complex morphology
consisting of an outer coat and an internal 27 nm core.
All three particulate forms share common surface antigens
(HB$_S$Ag) as demonstrated by techniques such as immune
electron microscopy (IEM) while the core of the Dane
particle represents a distinct antigenic system (HB$_C$Ag).
The surface antigens of a given particle consists of a
group-specific determinant (a) and two subtype-specific
antigens d or y and w or r which behave in an allelic
manner and appear to be specified by the hepatitis B viral
genome (1, 2).

I will attempt to summarize results obtained in our
laboratory over the last several years from studies of the
physical, chemical and immunological properties of the
HB Ag particulate forms. Obviously, the data represents
the combined efforts of many colleagues and individual
credit will be appropriately indicated in the text.

PURIFICATION OF THE PARTICULATE ANTIGEN

The various forms of HB Ag are purified from human
serum by multiple-step zonal centrifuge procedures (5)
Usually, 500 ml of serum obtained by plasmapheresis of
a chronic carrier of HB Ag is used as starting sample in a
CsCl isopycnic banding step using a batch-type rotor.
The HB Ag with a buoyant density of 1.20 g/cm^3 is
recovered from the gradient and rebanded in the same rotor
by a flotation procedure which results in good purification
of the HB Ag from the higher density and lower molecular
weight serum proteins. Rate zonal centrifugation of the
1.20 g/cm^3 HB Ag using a continuous "isokinetic" sucrose
gradient separates the 22 nm from the remaining soluble
serum contaminants, and from the various filamentous
forms which have a higher sedimentation coefficient.

Under the conditions used to purify the 22 nm particle, the larger 1.20 g/cm^3 Dane particle is recovered on the sucrose cushion together with the longer filamentous forms. Rebanding of the appropriate fractions from the rate-zonal step in CsCl represents the final purification step for the preparation of HB$_S$Ag. Various analyses of the final preparations have failed to reveal the presence of contaminating serum proteins and such preparations were used for the further biochemical studies.

BIOCHEMICAL PROPERTIES OF HB$_S$Ag

The ultraviolet absorption spectra for the 22 nm and filamentous particles are similar and quite typical of protein with a maximum at 280 nm and a OD$_{260}$/OD$_{280}$ ratio of about 0.7. Analysis of the filamentous and 22 nm spherical forms of HB$_S$Ag after solubilization under reducing conditions and electrophoresis on SDS-acrylamide gels revealed no differences between them in either the number or apparent molecular weights of their constituent polypeptides. We have concentrated our efforts on the anaylsis of the predominant 22 nm spherical form and this work represents mainly the efforts of Dr. James Shih of our laboratory.

Amino acid analysis of purified preparations of both the adw and ayw subtypes of HB$_S$Ag showed them to have a very similar amino acid composition with a difference index (3) of 5.7. The numbers of tyrosine and tryptophane residues were not sufficient to account for the high extinction coefficients reported for the antigen (4 , 5). The analyses also showed the absence of amino sugars.

Many different preparations of purified HB$_S$Ag, including adw, ayw and adr subtypes, have been analyzed by acrylamide gel electrophoresis in SDS gels after solubilization under reducing conditions, and based on Coomassie Blue staining of fixed gels six polypeptides with molecular weights ranging from 23,000 to 97,000 daltons were consistently observed. A seventh protein of 54,000 daltons was present in some preparations but not in association with a particular antigenic subtype. The proteins designated P-1 through P-7 (Table I) in order of their increasing molecular weights (5).

PAS staining of gels for carbohydrate (6) after electrophoresis of chloroform-methanol (2:1) extracted $HB_S Ag$ revealed two bands at positions identical the major (P-2) and minor (P-5) polypeptide and we consider these polypeptides to be glycoproteins although amino acid analysis of the major P-2 polypeptide (see below) failed to reveal the presence of amino sugars.

The individual polypeptides of both an $HB_S Ag/\underline{adw}$ and $HB_S Ag/\underline{ayw}$ were isolated from the acrylamide gels, removed from reducing conditions, and used to immunize guinea pigs using Freund's complete adjuvant. Each of the polypeptide preparations stimulated group-specific antibody to native $HB_S Ag$ (anti-$HB_S/\underline{a}$) as evaluated by passive hemagglutination (4) and radioimmunoprecipitation (7) assays. Using a modification of the passive hemagglutination assay for the detection of subtype antibody (8), Dr. Jon Gold (NIAID) also found either anti-$HB_S/\underline{d}$ or anti-$HB_S/\underline{y}$ antibody in most of these sera. Importantly, polypeptides from the $HB_S Ag/\underline{adw}$ subtype stimulated only anti-$HB_S/\underline{ad}$ antibodies and not anti-$HB_S/\underline{y}$ antibodies, while those prepared from an $HB_S Ag/\underline{ayw}$ particle stimulated only anti-$HB_S/\underline{ay}$ and not anti-$HB_S/\underline{d}$ (Table I). Since the P-1 and P-2 proteins represent the major polypeptides of $HB_S Ag$ we obtained larger quantities of these proteins from gels for further analysis. The proteins were extracted from gels under renaturing conditions and analyzed in the following manner. One aliquot was used to immunize guinea pigs as before, another was hydrolyzed for amino acid analysis, and another was electrophoresed on SDS gels for an analysis of purity. The individual polypeptides migrated to their

previous positions on electrophoresis when compared with
a gel containing all of the polypeptides and run in the same
experiment. An optical scan of the stained gels showed
that P-1 was free of detectable P-2 contamination while
P-2 contained about 5% P-1. The polypeptide preparations
were free of the larger $HB_S Ag$ proteins, P-3 through P-7.
As before, each polypeptide stimulated both group-specific
and subtype-specific antibodies. Amino acid analyses of
the P-1 and P-2 preparations showed them to have an
essentially identical amino acid composition with a difference index of less than 2.0.

These data have some important implications. First,
the individual polypeptides contained both the group-specific and subtype-specific determinants of $HB_S Ag$. Since P-1
and P-2 each stimulate both antibodies, the antigenic
determinants are protein in nature and are not due to the
carbohydrate moiety. Secondly, the similarities in their
immunochemical and compositional properties suggest
that the various polypeptides are not separate primary
products of the viral genome and has interesting implications for the mechanisms of replication of the hepatitis
B virus in vivo.

THE DANE PARTICLE

The Dane particle is a very minor HB Ag component
in most serum of chronic carriers. When we first became
interested in the Dane particle as a potential candidate
for the virion of hepatitis B, we screened sera from a
number of chronic HB Ag carriers by IEM and found that
greater than 80% contained detectable Dane particles
irregardless of the $HB_S Ag$ subtype (d or y). The electron
microscopy was performed by Mrs. Eugenie Ford of our
laboratory. From our initial screening of some 60 sera
we selected eight which were relatively rich in Dane
particles and did not have circulating immune complexes
(about 70% of the antigen carriers circulate immune
complexes in their sera as detected by electron micro-

scopy). The Dane particles from these sera were concentrated 20X by volume and partially purified from the 22 nm form by pelleting at moderate centrifugal speeds.

The Dane particle-rich preparations were examined in thin section after staining with uranyl acetate and the Dane particle cores were scored morphologically as to whether they were empty, full or partially full. Analysis of several preparations showed, very approximately, that 10% of the cores were full, 10% empty, and 80% partially full. On the assumption that full cores represented hepatitis virions which contained nucleic acid, we speculated that they could be separated on the basis of their buoyant density in CsCl. In fact, isopycnic banding of the Dane-rich preparations in CsCl resulted in the separation of two density populations of morphological Dane particles, one at 1.20 g/cm^3 and another at $1.24-1.25$ g/cm^3.

The Dane particle preparations were also used by Dr. Robert Purcell (NIAID) to develop a sensitive radio-immunoassay for the core antigen (9). We found that treatment of the Dane particles with 1% NP-40 effectively removed the outer coat of the Dane and that the core could then be recovered both antigenically and morphologically at a density of 1.31 g/cm^3 in CsCl gradients. This value may not represent the true buoyant density of the core particle however, since it appears to be aggregated by a small protein inter-connecting the particles. This protein could represent anti-core antibody (anti-HB$_c$) which we now know to exist in high titers in the sera of chronic carriers, or an internal "matrix" protein not removed by the NP-40 treatment. No data are yet available to distinguish between these postulated alternatives.

The eight Dane-rich preparations were also found to contain a DNA polymerase activity by Dr. William Robinson and his colleagues at Stanford (10), as he will describe in detail in the following paper. An evaluation of the Dane

220

rich preparations on the basis of the three parameters just discussed (Table 2)revealed a close correlation between the level of DNA polymerase activity and the presence of a heavy subpopulation of Dane particles, and an approximate correlation with the core antigen concentration. Since we can assume that the polymerase requires a nucleic acid template within the core, the data suggest that the enzyme activity is restricted to the heavy subpopulation of Dane particles, and that the higher buoyant density is indeed due to the presence of nucleic acid, possibly the genome of the hepatitis B virus.

From the considerations mentioned above, it is clear that the Dane particle possesses a number of separate antigenic determinants which can be structurally assigned to this complex particle. The outer coat contains a group-specific antigen (a) and two subtype-specific determinants (d or y; w or r). The particle may contain a "matrix" protein located internally between the outer coat and the core, but this possibility is only an hypothesis at this time. The surface of the core represents another antigenic system (HB$_c$Ag) and should be considered an internal structural antigen of the Dane particle. Finally, the DNA polymerase enzyme located within the core is surely an antigenic protein, but direct assays for its antibody must await the successful isolation of the active enzyme from the core particle.

ACKNOWLEDGEMENTS

The Rockville Laboratory of the MAN Program is supported by the NIAID under Union Carbide's contract with the U.S. AEC.

REFERENCES

1. G. L. LeBouvier, et al, J. Amer. Med. Ass. 222, 928 (1972).

2. W. H. Bancroft, F. K. Mundon, and P. K. Russell, J. Immunol. <u>109</u>, 842 (1972).
3. H. Metzger, <u>et al</u>, Nature <u>219</u>, 1166 (1968).
4. G. Vyas and N. Shulman, <u>Science</u> <u>170</u>, 332 (1970).
5. J. L. Gerin, In: Hepatitis and Blood Transfusion (Eds., G. Vyas, H. Perkins, and R. Schmidt). New York: Grune and Stratton, Inc. (1972).
6. D. P. Bolognesi and H. Bauer, <u>Virology</u> <u>42</u>, 1097 (1970).
7. J. J. Lander, H. J. Alter, and R. H. Purcell, J. Immunol. <u>106</u>, 1166 (1971).
8. J. W. Gold, <u>et al</u>, J. Immunol. <u>112</u>, 1100 (1974).
9. R. H. Purcell, <u>et al</u>, <u>Intervirology</u> (In Press).
10. P. M. Kaplan, et al, J. <u>Virology</u> <u>12</u>, 995 (1973)

TABLE 1

POLYPEPTIDES OF HB_sAg

Protein	MW	GP*	Stimulated Ab to:		
			a	d**	y***
P1	23–26	–	+	+	±
P2	30–32	+	+	+	+
P3	36	–	+	+	+
P4	42	–	+	+	+
P5	54	+	+	+	+
P6	68–72	–	+	±	+
P7	97	–	N.T.	N.T.	N.T.

*   PAS positive in gels
**   Proteins from HB_sAg/adw
*** Proteins from HB_sAg/ayw
N.T. = not tested

TABLE 2

ANALYSIS OF DANE PARTICLE CONCENTRATES FOR
POLYMERASE, CORE ANTIGEN, AND
HIGH DENSITY DANE PARTICLES.

SAMPLE	^{3}H-CPM ENZYME*	^{125}I-CPM CORE**	HEAVY DANES***
1	7,330	4,297	4+
2	6,625	10,811	3+
3	3,961	6,722	3+
4	1,628	993	1+
5	1,151	1,501	1+
6	1,087	554	1+
7	1,085	1,224	1+
8	1,047	1,201	1+
NHS	30	230	–

*   Endogenous DNA polymerase activity
**   Micro SP–RIA assay for core antigen
***   Based on isopycnic banding in CsCl
NHS= Normal human serum

A HUMAN HEPATITIS B VIRUS CANDIDATE

William S. Robinson

Department of Medicine
Stanford University School of Medicine
Stanford, California 94305

ABSTRACT. One of the particulate forms bearing hepatitis B antigen in human blood, the 42 nm Dane particle, has been shown to contain a small circular double stranded DNA with a molecular weight around 1.6×10^6 daltons and a DNA polymerase. The circular DNA functions as a primer-template for the DNA polymerase. The circular DNA, the DNA polymerase and the DNA product of the enzyme reaction appear to be internal components of the 28 nm core of the Dane particle.

INTRODUCTION

The infectious form of hepatitis B virus has not been identified, although the hepatitis B surface antigen (HB_sAg) found in large amounts in the plasma of infected patients is undoubtedly viral antigen. HB_sAg is present on the surface of several particulate structures found in plasma, the most common by far being 16 to 25 nm spherical particles (1). The heterogeneity of the particles (2) and the failure to find nucleic acid in purified preparations of them (3) suggest that they are not complete virions, but more likely incomplete virus coat particles. A second and larger form which bears HB_sAg on its surface is a 42 nm particle with more complex structure first described by Dane et al. (4). Detergent was used by Almeida et al. (5) to prepare 28 nm inner core structures from Dane particles. Cores were shown by immune-electron microscopy to be specifically aggregated by a human convalescent serum free of antibody to HB_sAg (anti-HB_s). Thus the core antigen (HB_cAg) is clearly distinct from HB_sAg. Here I will review recent work done in my laboratory for the most part show-

225

ing that Dane particles have features of a complete virus: a unique nucleic acid and a DNA polymerase. A schematic representation of the structural forms containing HB_sAg, HB_cAg, DNA polymerase and DNA is shown in Fig. 1.

DNA POLYMERASE ASSOCIATED WITH HB_sAg

Hirschman et al. (6) first described DNA polymerase activity in crude pellets obtained by high speed centrifugation of three HB_sAg positive sera. The reaction was thought to be dependent on an endogenous RNA template or primer since treatment of the preparations with high concentrations of RNase appeared to reduce their activity. The reaction, however, appeared to be stimulated by the addition of poly dAT and not by poly rA-oligo dT as are known RNA dependent DNA polymerases (7). Subsequently several laboratories (e.g. ref. 3) failed to find DNA polymerase activity in highly purified preparations of 16 to 25 nm HB_sAg bearing particles. Dr. John Gerin and I then decided to examine crude high speed pellets prepared from plasma of chronic HB_sAg carriers for DNA polymerase to attempt to confirm the findings of Hirschman et al. Instead of examining plasmas from random chronic HB_sAg carriers, plasmas which were relatively rich in Dane particles were selected for study with the idea that Dane particles might contain DNA polymerase. Concentrated particulate preparations from such plasmas were then shown to incorporate ^{3}H-TTP into acid precipitable radioactivity in a reaction dependent on 4 deoxynucleoside triphosphates and $MgCl_2$. The enzyme activity was increased two-fold by addition of the detergent NP40 and the reaction rate was not affected by the addition of DNA or RNA to the reaction mixture. Subsequently 8 of 8 preparations from Dane particle rich plasmas (8), none of 6 similar preparations from HB_sAg negative controls (8) and 40 of 80 unconcentrated serum samples from random chronic HB_sAg carriers (9) were found to contain this enzyme activity. As will be subsequently shown the enzyme described here has significantly different properties from the one reported by Hirschman et al. (6) suggesting that the two are different enzymes.

IDENTIFICATION OF THE DNA POLYMERASE CONTAINING PARTICLE

Several lines of evidence now strongly indicate that

the DNA polymerase found in Dane particle rich HB_SAg preparations is a component of Dane particles and antigenically distinct cores prepared from Dane particles by NP40 detergent treatment.

1. Before detergent treatment the DNA polymerase containing particles were precipitated by serum containing antibody to HB_SAg (anti-HB_S) and not by serum containing antibody to the Dane particle core antigen (anti-HB_C) (10). The reaction with anti-HB_S containing serum was blocked by highly purified 16 to 25 nm particles which have HB_SAg on their surface.

2. After treatment with detergent NP40, which disrupts Dane particles, the enzyme activity was precipitated by anti-HB_C containing serum and not by anti-HB_S (10). The reaction with anti-HB_C was not blocked by purified 16 to 25 nm HB_SAg bearing particles.

3. After sucrose gradient sedimentation of concentrated Dane particle rich HB_SAg preparations, the enzyme activity was found in the same position in the gradient as 42 nm Dane particles detected by electron microscopy (8).

4. After NP40 treatment, the DNA polymerase activity was found at the same position in a sucrose gradient as 28 nm Dane particle core structures detected by electron microscopy and radioimmunoassay (8). Although the DNA polymerase activity sedimented within the density range of HB_CAg, the average density for enzyme was slightly greater than the average for HB_CAg suggesting that the enzyme was associated with a subpopulation of cores.

5. No enzyme activity has been found in purified 16 to 25 nm HB_SAg bearing particles (3,8).

DANE PARTICLE DNA

The observation that the DNA polymerase reaction carried out by Dane particle core structures did not require added DNA or RNA suggested that the Dane particle core contained nucleic acid which served as a primer-template for the reaction. Experiments were thus done to examine Dane particle cores for the presence of nucleic acid (11). Enzyme containing particles from 1 liter amounts of Dane particle rich plasma were concentrated by centrifugation and then purified by repeated equilibrium centrifugation in sucrose density gradients. The preparations were treated with DNase 1 to eliminate free DNA not within a structure such as Dane particles. After NP40 treatment Dane particle cores were isolated by rate zonal sedimentation in a sucrose density gradient. Cores were retreated with DNase and pelleted by centrifugation to concentrate and remove DNase. The core pellet was resuspended in SDS containing buffer to disrupt cores and release nucleic acid. The resulting solution was then layered over a sucrose density gradient and centrifuged at high speed to pellet any nucleic acid with sedimentation coefficient greater than about 10S. Examination of the pellet by electron microscopy revealed circular DNA molecules exclusively (Fig. 2). Incubation with DNase 1 before examination eliminated all of the circular molecules. The smooth, open configuration of the molecules indicates that they are double stranded and spreading in formamide to demonstrate single stranded DNA or RNA revealed no additional molecules of any kind. The open appearance of the molecules on the electron microscope grids and absence of superhelical forms suggest an open circular conformation. Whether this appearance is due to a true open circular conformation with a nicked strand or to a closed circular structure with a low superhelix density is not clear from the results here. The same circular DNA molecules were found in Dane particle core preparations from 3 out of 3 chronic HB_sAg carriers. No circular DNA was found in the plasmas of 4 HB_sAg negative control subjects processed in the same way.

The combination of equilibrium centrifugation to par--tially purify Dane particles followed by rate zonal sedimentation to further purify cores, resulted in elimination of all HB_sAg and other particulate material. The finding of a single species of DNA molecules after DNase treatment of core preparations purified this way suggests that the DNA is a component of the core. When DNase treatment of cores was omitted, some linear DNA molecules with a wide distribution of lengths (0.5 to 12 microns) in addition to the circular molecules were observed. The elimination of the linear DNAs by DNase treatment of core preparations indicates that they were not in a protected position within

the cores as were the circular molecules. Length measurements on 225 circular molecules revealed a mean length of
0.78 $\pm$ 0.09 microns (11). This is more heterogeneity than
found for circular DNAs of known viruses such as SV-40
after infection at low multiplicity (12) or PM-2 (13).
After infection with SV-40 at high multiplicity, the viral
DNA exhibits a wider length distribution similar to that of
Dane particle DNA (12).

In other experiments, preparations of Dane particles
purified as described above were incubated with 7 m lithium
thiocyanate to dissociate particulate structures and then
directly spread on grids for electron microscopy (14).
Again small circular molecules were the only recognizable
nucleic acid molecules present (Fig. 3).

THE DNA POLYMERASE REACTION PRODUCT

After a DNA polymerase reaction with NP40 treated
Dane particle preparations, radioactive DNA product remains
associated with a 110S structure (8). This structure has
been identified as Dane particle core by its cosedimentation with core-associated DNA polymerase activity (8) and
by its precipitation with serum containing anti-HB_c but not
with serum containing anti-HB_s (10). Incubation of the
core with SDS and ME results in release of the radioactive
enzyme reaction product from cores. The resulting radioactive DNA in 0.11 m NaCl has a sedimentation coefficient
of 15S (8) and it is made completely acid soluble by incubation with DNase 1 and is not affected by RNase A (8 and
Table 1) as expected for DNA. Examination of the 15S
radioactive band by electron microscopy after rate zonal
sedimentation in a CsCl density gradient revealed exclusively circular double stranded DNA molecules indistinguishable from those recovered from Dane particle cores
without a DNA polymerase reaction (11). This suggests that
the circular DNA molecules recovered from Dane particle
cores serve as primer-template for the DNA polymerase
reaction.

Several findings indicate that the radioactive DNA
product of the enzyme reaction is in a double stranded or
base paired form. 1) In 0.16 m salt the DNA sediments only
about 10% faster than in 0.002 m salt (Fig. 4), unlike
single stranded nucleic acid, the sedimentation coefficient
of which can change as much as 9 fold with a similar change

in ionic strength (15). 2) The complete resistance of the ^{3}H-DNA to S_1 nuclease before heating (Table 1) indicates that none of the radioactive DNA is single stranded. 3) The sharp temperature transition from S_1 nuclease resistant to susceptible (Fig. 5) confirms that it is in a highly ordered form before heating.

The base composition of Dane particle DNA can be calculated from thermal transition and buoyant density measurements using circular DNA molecules made radioactive in a DNA polymerase reaction. Fig. 5 shows that the midpoint temperature for the thermal transition curve of the ^{3}H-DNA in 0.01 m sodium phosphate and 0.001 m EDTA buffer was 72°, and for PM-2 C^{14}-DNA 69°. These values correspond to G+C contents of 49% and 42% respectively (16). The latter is in agreement with the published G+C content for PM-2 DNA (13). Fig. 6 shows the results of equilibrium centrifugation of SV-40 ^{32}P-DNA and Dane particle ^{3}H-DNA in a CsCl density gradient. The mean buoyant density of the ^{3}H-DNA was approximately 0.007 gms per ml higher than that for the ^{32}P-DNA. Using 41% for the G+C content of SV-40 DNA (17), the ^{3}H-DNA can be calculated (18) to have a G+C content of 48%, in close agreement with the value calculated from the thermal denaturation experiment above.

EVIDENCE FOR AN INTERNAL LOCATION OF THE DNA POLYMERASE, DNA PRIMER-TEMPLATE AND DNA REACTION PRODUCT WITHIN THE DANE PARTICLE CORE

As described above the DNA polymerase, circular DNA molecules and the DNA product of the DNA polymerase reaction are all associated with the core of the Dane particle. Further evidence indicates that each of these components is probably an internal component of the core which appears to be impermeable to large molecules such as protein and nucleic acid but permeable to small molecules. This is suggested by the observations that the DNA polymerase utilizes the endogenous circular DNA as primer-template (11) and cannot be stimulated by added DNA or RNA (8), indicating that such macromolecules fail to reach the enzyme within the intact core. Human convalescent sera with anti-HB$_s$ and anti-HB$_c$ in high titer (10) do not inhibit the core associated DNA polymerase activity. Either such sera do not also contain antibody to the enzyme or antibody present cannot reach the enzyme within the core. Similarly

the small circular DNA molecule found in cores is not
attacked or altered by treatment of cores with DNase although following extraction from cores with SDS it is completely DNase susceptible (11). Similarly the primer-
template activity of this DNA is not affected by pretreatment of cores with DNase before an enzyme reaction (8).
Thus the core DNA is not available as substrate for DNase
when in intact cores. Finally, ^{3}H-DNA newly synthesized
in DNA polymerase reactions remains associated with 110S
cores and is not digested by DNase until after disruption
of cores with SDS (8), indicating that it is in a protected
position within the core before SDS treatment.

Small molecules such as $MgCl_2$ and deoxynucleoside
triphosphates on the other hand appear to readily enter
cores and reach the enzyme during a DNA polymerase reaction, and inhibitors of the reaction such as actinomycin D
and daunomycin can reach the DNA primer-template (8).

The observations that natural DNAs and RNAs as well
as synthetic polyribo and polydeoxyribonucleosides when
added to the reaction mixture do not stimulate the reaction
and high concentrations of RNase do not inhibit the reaction carried out by the Dane particle associated DNA polymerase (8) is different from the results reported by
Hirschman et al. (6) for enzyme activity in concentrated
preparations from plasma. RNase inhibited and poly dAT
stimulated that reaction. This suggests that the enzyme
described by Hirschman et al. and the Dane particle enzyme
described here are not the same. We have found DNA polymerase activity in plasma samples from occasional normal or
HBAg carriers that is not in a particulate form and is
stimulated by adding DNA to the reaction. This activity
does not appear to be related to the Dane particle associated DNA polymerase described here.

DISCUSSION

Our experiments indicate that DNA polymerase and circular double stranded DNA molecules are components of the
Dane particle and are localized in a protected position
within the core of the Dane particle. The circular DNA
molecules in cores appear to function as primer-template
for the DNA polymerase reaction carried out by Dane particle cores. The presence of DNA in Dane particle cores is
consistent with the hypothesis that the Dane particle is a

hepatitis B virion. If that hypothesis is correct, the
Dane particle core would represent viral nucleocapsid. The
morphological appearance of the Dane particle, and the
presence of a uniquely small circular double stranded DNA
and DNA polymerase in the particle indicate that the Dane
particle does not belong to any known group of viruses.
The function of the DNA polymerase and its possible utility
for virus infection and replication is not clear.

The circular DNAs described here average about 0.78
microns in length which would correspond to a molecular
weight around 1.6×10^6 daltons. This is smaller than
double stranded DNA found in any known virus and is similar
in molecular weight to single stranded DNAs found in minute
virus of mice (19), adenoassociated virus (19,20) and
latent rat virus (21). The genetic information carried by
double stranded DNA of molecular weight 1.6×10^6 daltons
must be very limited. Three viral functions, each of which
is probably associated with one or more different virus
coded proteins, have been identified in Dane particles:
the hepatitis B surface or envelope antigen (HB_sAg), the
hepatitis B or Dane particle core (nucleocapsid) antigen
(HB_cAg) and the Dane particle associated DNA polymerase.
The circular DNA found in these experiments could probably
code for no more than the proteins associated with these 3
viral functions. Gerin (3) has described 2 major and 4 or
5 minor peptides in highly purified preparations of 20 nm
HB_sAg bearing particles which were probably free of Dane
particles and cores. If these proteins in addition to Dane
particle core proteins are all virus coded, more genetic
information would be needed than that probably available in
DNA molecules the sizes of the small circular molecules
described here. This suggests the possibility that the
circular DNAs come from defective viruses containing DNAs
with large deletions. The heterogeneity of DNA lengths
(0.78 ± 0.09 microns) would be consistent with such a
possibility. The relatively wide distribution of molecular
lengths found here is much greater than for circular DNA
isolated from SV-40 virus after low multiplicity infection,
although similar to DNA from SV-40 passed at a high multiplicity (12). If the circular DNAs do come from defective
forms of virus, infectious particles with larger DNA molecules might be present in these preparations but in numbers
too small to be detected by these experiments. Alternatively, a second virus or helper virus not yet identified

might be required for their replication as for example adenoviruses are required for replication of small DNA containing adenoassociated viruses (22,23).

The origin of the linear DNA molecules found in these preparations is not clear but their heterogeneity in length and susceptibility to DNase digestion in Dane particle core preparations suggests that they may represent molecules of the DNA thought to be present in a soluble form in all human sera (24).

ACKNOWLEDGMENTS

I gratefully acknowledge the collaboration and helpful discussions with Drs. John L. Gerin, Richard L. Greenman, Paul M. Kaplan, David A. Clayton, Jack Griffith, Robert Purcell and Thomas Edgington on different parts of the work reviewed here and the technical assistance of Ms. Nona Stone. This work was supported by U.S. Public Health Service grants CA-10467 and CA-23487.

REFERENCES

1. Bayer, M. E., Blumberg, B. S., and Werner, B., Nature (London) 218, 1057 (1968).
2. Almeida, J. D., Postgrad. Med. J. 47, 484 (1971).
3. Gerin, J. L., Hepatitis and Blood Transfusion, G. N. Vyas, H. A. Perkins, and R. Schmidt (eds.), Grune and Stratton, New York, 1972, p. 205.
4. Dane, D. S., Cameron, C. H., and Briggs, M., Lancet 1, 695 (1970).
5. Almeida, J. D., Rubenstein, D., and Stott, E. J., Lancet 2, 1225 (1971).
6. Hirschman, S. Z., Vernace, S. J., and Schaffner, F., Lancet 1, 1099, (1971).
7. Temin, H. M., and Baltimore, D., Adv. Virus Res. 17, 129 (1972).
8. Kaplan, P. M., Greenman, R. L., Gerin, J. L., Purcell, R. H., and Robinson, W. S., J. Virol. 12, 995 (1973).
9. Greenman, R. L., Kaplan, P. M., and Robinson, W. S., Clin. Res. 22, 125A (1974).
10. Greenman, R. L., and Robinson, W. S., J. Virol., in press, 1974.
11. Robinson, W. S., Clayton, D. A., and Greenman, R. L., submitted for publication, 1974.

12. Tai, H. T., Smith, C. A., Sharp, P. A., and Vinograd, J., J. Virol. 9, 317 (1972).
13. Espejo, R. T., Canelo, E. S., and Suisheimer, R., Proc. Nat. Acad. Sci. USA 63, 1164 (1969).
14. Griffith, J., and Robinson, W. S., unpublished experiments.
15. Boedtker, H., J. Mol. Biol. 2, 171 (1960).
16. Marmur, J., and Doty, P., J. Mol. Biol. 5, 109 (1962).
17. Crawford, L. V., and Black, P. H., Virol. 24, 388 (1964).
18. Sueoka, N., Marmur, J., and Doty, P., Nature 183, 1429, (1959).
19. Crawford, L. V., Follet, E. A. C., Burdon, M. G., and McGeoh, P. J., J. Gen. Virol. 4, 37 (1969).
20. Rose, J. A., Berus, K. I., Hoggan, M. D., and Koczot, F. J., Proc. Nat. Acad. Sci. USA 64, 863 (1969).
21. Salzman, L. A., White, W. L., and Kakafuda, T., J. Virol. 7, 830 (1971).
22. Atchison, R. W., Caste, G. C., and Hammon, W. M., Science 149, 754 (1965).
23. Hoggan, M. D., Blacklow, N. R., and Rowe, W. P., Proc. Nat. Acad. Sci. USA 55, 1467 (1966).
24. Kamm, R. C., and Smith, A. G., Clin. Chem. 18, 519 (1972).

THE HEPATITIS B CANDIDATE VIRUS

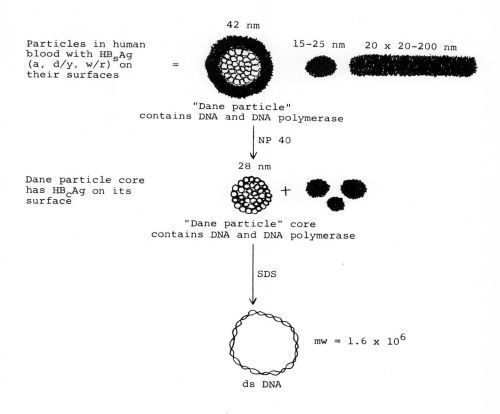

Fig. 1.   Schematic drawing of the particulate forms bearing hepatitis B antigens in human blood.

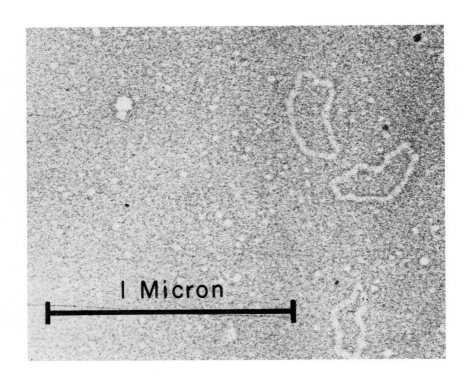

Fig. 2.   Electron micrograph of circular viral DNA
mounted by the aqueous technique (experiment by D. Clayton
and W. Robinson).

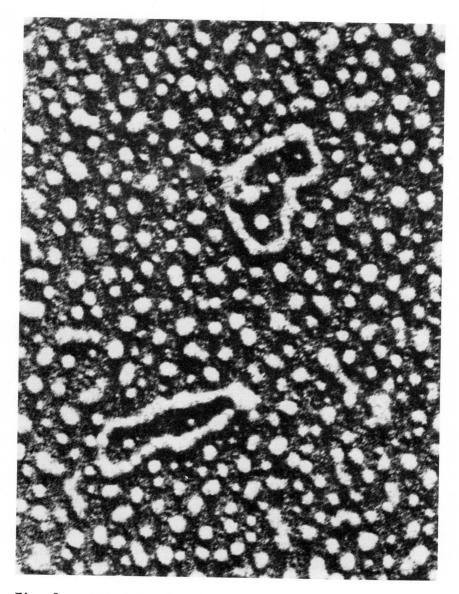

Fig. 3.   DNA molecules from a Dane particle preparation after incubation with 7 m Li SCN and mounted by the formamide technique.   X560,000.   (Experiment by J. Griffith and W. Robinson).

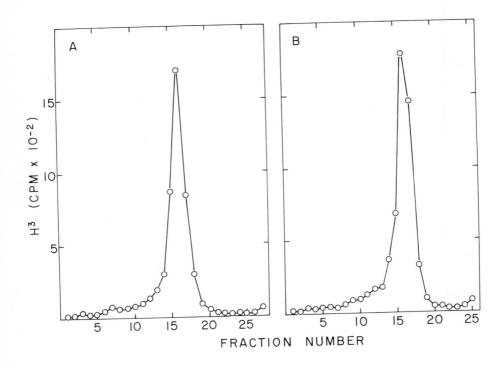

Fig. 4. Rate zonal sedimentation of Dane particle ^{3}H–DNA in solutions with high and low ionic strength. ^{3}H–DNA was prepared in a DNA polymerase reaction containing purified Dane particles and ^{3}H–TTP, and the ^{3}H–DNA was isolated by SDS treatment and sucrose gradient sedimentation as previously described (8). Samples of ^{3}H–DNA in either 0.15 m NaCl, 0.01 m Tris–HCl pH 7.4 and 0.001 m EDTA (A) or 0.001 m Tris–HCl pH 7.5 and 0.001 m EDTA (B) were layered over 5 to 20% sucrose density gradients containing the same respective buffers and centrifuged at 50,000 RPM, 4 for 5 hours in a Spinco SW 65 rotor. Acid precipitable ^{3}H was determined on fractions collected from the bottom of each tube.

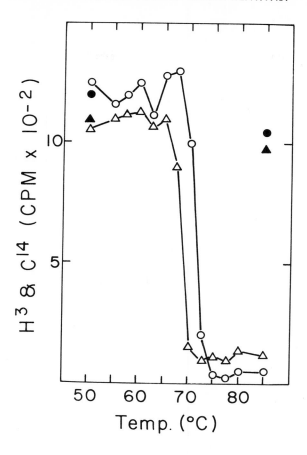

Fig. 5.   Thermal denaturation of Dane particle ^{3}H-DNA.
A solution containing ^{3}H-DNA prepared as for the experiment in Fig. 4 and calf thymus DNA at 10 ug per ml in
0.01 m Na phosphate pH 7.2 and 0.001 m EDTA was placed in
a water bath and heated sequentially to the temperatures
designated.   After 10 min at each temperature, 50 ul aliquots were removed, rapidly cooled in an ice-water bath and
diluted to 1 ml with S_1 buffer containing 10 ug per ml calf
thymus DNA.   After aliquots were obtained at all temperatures, TCA precipitable [3]H (circles) was determined either
before (solid symbols) or after (open symbols) incubation
with S_1 nuclease.   ^{14}C-DNA (triangles) from PM-2 virus was
used in a parallel experiment.

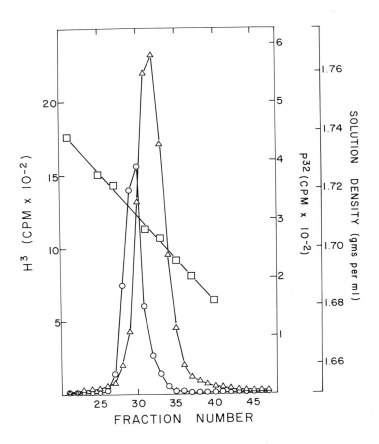

Fig. 6. Equilibrium sedimentation of Dane particle
[3]H-DNA and SV-40 virus P[32]-DNA in a CsCl density gradient.
A 4 ml solution containing ^{3}H-DNA prepared as for the experiment in Fig. 4, P[32]-DNA from SV-40 virus, 100 ug calf
thymus DNA, 0.1 m Tris-HCl pH 7.4 and 0.005 m EDTA was
added to 5.0 gms solid CsCl in a polyallomer tube, overlaid
with mineral oil and centrifuged at 45,000 RPM and 20 for
64 hours in a Spinco 50 Ti rotor. Solution density
(squares) by refractometry (12) and TCA precipitable [3]H
(circles) and P[32] (triangles) were determined on 0.1 ml
fractions collected from the bottom of the tube.

Table 1   Nuclease Digestion of Dane Particle ^{3}H-DNA[a]

Nuclease (37°,1 hour)	Unheated DNA	Heated DNA
none	2,268[b]	2,170
DNase 1 (20 μg per ml)	85	96
S$_i$ (20 u per ml)	2,210	35
RNase A (20 μg per ml)	2,315	2,395

[a]Data taken from Robinson et al. (11).

[b]TCA precipitable radioactivity in cpm.

PATTERNS OF HEPATITIS B VIRUS GENOME EXPRESSION *IN VIVO*

Thomas S. Edgington

Department of Molecular Immunology
Scripps Clinic and Research Foundation
La Jolla, California 92037

ABSTRACT. The Hepatitis B virus (HBV) appears not to be an obligate cytopathic agent *in vivo*; however, intrahepatic cytopathology and extrahepatic tissue injury are observed in certain forms of HBV infection. The pathogenesis of HBV disease involves complex interrelationships between host and agent and appears to be associated with both: 1) qualitative and quantitative patterns of HBV genome expression and/or integration in the host cell; and 2) quantitative and qualitative aspects of the host immune response. Intrahepatocellular HBV genome expression has been characterized by immunohistochemical means employing reagents specific for antigenic markers of the HBV coat and the HBV core. Patterns of intracellular synthesis of viral products and cytologic atypism differ in various forms of HBV hepatic disease. Data is consistent with differing patterns of HBV genome expression included within: a) productive, and b) hypothetically postulated non-productive patterns of virus:cell interaction. Current observations suggest that HBV is an elective cytopathogenic agent and that complex HBV:Host interactions must determine the character of disease.

INTRODUCTION

The Hepatitis B virus (HBV) has been characterized in respect to the various morphological forms isolated from plasma (1-7); and the properties of the HBV-associated coat antigen (HB Ag) proteins and the internal core (HB$_{core}$) have been described (8). The presence of a DNA transcriptase has recently been recognized which appears to be a DNA instructed enzyme (9). Further evidence now indicates the presence of a DNA, recoverable from HB_{cores}, which has a size of approximately 1.5 x 10^6 daltons (10). This elusive agent is not readily classifiable within current taxonomic groups and may represent a unique class of viruses. This agent is highly restrictive in species distribution and is usually transmissible only in man (11-13) and chimpanzees (14,15). Recent work by Purcell has indicated the possibility of transmission in the Rhesus (16,17).

HBV infection may be transient, prolonged, or persistent; and it may be associated with a variety of clinical manifestations of significant disease or with no apparent disease (18). HBV infection frequently may be silent and probably transient as attested to by the relatively high frequency of low levels of specific antibody in the population. HBV-associated disease is considered within two generic groups which probably differ in their pathogenesis. First, there is primary hepatic disease which includes a variety of forms. Quite independently, a variety of extra-hepatic diseases are occasionally observed in association with HBV infection and include acute arthritis, arthralgia, fever, vasculitic purpura, periarteritis nodosum, glomerulonephritis and enteritis (19-22). These appear to be attributable to secondary immune complex disease. There is also an inordinately high incidence of HB Ag positivity in patients with hepatoma (23).

With this background I would like to address myself to one topic possibly related to the pathogenesis of HBV infection. First, I would like to consider the expression of HBV genome *in vivo* through analysis of the tissue distribution of structural components of the agent. Second, I will provide some evidence that the pattern of viral genome expression may vary considerably in different individuals and in association with different forms of hepatic disease attributable to this agent. The possible role of the host immune response in the pathogenesis of HBV-associated disease remains an important additional factor.

Late immune or hyperimmune human antisera to HB Ag is directed to group specific and subtype antigens (24), present on the surface of 22 nm spherical particles, filamentous particles, and 43 nm Dane particles (26)(Table 1). These appear to be specified by the virus. A possible host component x has been suggested by LeBouvier (24). The existence of HB$_{core}$ antigens not expressed on the surface but present on the internal 27 nm core of Dane particles was described by Almeida *et al.* (25) and has been further characterized (8).

In vivo distribution of HBV gene products has been analyzed immunochemically utilizing antisera to the structural components of the virus. A number of potent human antisera to HB Ag, as well as guinea pig antisera produced by immunization with purified HB Ag 22 nm particles, have been employed in immunofluorescence techniques to demonstrate the presence of these coat antigens in the cytoplasm of hepatocytes from humans (26) and chimpanzees (14) during HBV infection. The reactions are completely blocked by neutralization of the reagents with purified HB Ag 22 nm particles possessing appropriate antigenic type and subtype determinants. This cytoplasmic localization is observed for both the group specific "a" antigens as well as for the "d" and "y" subtype antigens. In the majority of cases there is conspicuous concentration of HB Ag in the cytoplasms in the vicinity of the hepatocyte surface. Although most commonly found in a diffuse distribution involving most or all hepatocytes in early acute hepatitis and the chronic carrier state, focal distribution of HB Ag positive hepatocytes suggestive of focal infection is also seen on occasion and may involve small islands of only 10-50 contiguous cells. In still other cases one may observe only very local synthesis by a small proportion of isolated hepatocytes.

Quite independent localization of HB$_{core}$ Ag to hepatocyte nuclei is observed (14). This is observed as minute granules in the nucleoplasm but usually not the nucleolus. The reactions employ the same human antiserum originally used by Almeida *et al.* (25) to delineate the HB$_{core}$ Ag system by immune electron microscopy; however, identical nuclear localization of HB$_{core}$ can be demonstrated using antiserum produced by immunization of rabbits with purified HB$_{core}$ provided by Dr. W.S. Robinson (9,10). These reactions are not inhibited by absorption of the anti-HB$_{core}$ Ag antiserum with purified HB Ag 22 nm, but specific neutralization is observed using HB$_{core}$ Ag rich particulate fractions of serum from individuals during acute

245

Hepatitis B infection. Further evidence for independence of HB Ag and HB_{core} Ag is gathered from experiments where each reaction is blocked only by antisera of homologous specificity (Table 2).

HB Ag is quite resistant to proteolytic enzymes, whereas HB_{core} Ag *in situ* is destroyed by trypsin and chymotrypsin. These cytologic observations, suggested from study of Hepatitis B in chimpanzees (27) support the morphologic structure and organization for HBV suggested by Gerin (8), in this symposium. The antigenic expression of HBV gene products can be morphologically and cytologically assigned as outlined in Table 3. It is suggested that the core of the virion is synthesized within the nucleus and invested with a virus coded protein expressing HB_{core} Ag. This particle then moves to the cytoplasm where it is invested with an envelope containing polypeptides also coded for by HBV. This expresses coat antigens, or HB Ags. Envelope synthesis may be in marked excess in order to account for the surplus of incomplete 22 nm particles and filaments found in plasma.

Immunologic analysis of genome expression by immunofluorescence and in conjunction with cytologic analysis of hepatocytes in our laboratory has led to the following observations.

1) During early acute hepatitis associated with hepatocellular injury both HB Ag and HB_{core} Ag are present. HB Ag is typically distributed in a diffuse fashion in the cytoplasm of hepatocytes throughout the tissue.

2) In the healthy carrier state a diffuse distribution of HB Ag antigen is found, in the absence of HB_{core} Ag or with only rare cells showing slight expression of HB_{core} Ag in their nuclei. The latter cases more frequently exhibit greater evidence of hepatic disease. Cytologic atypism of hepatocytes is not usual.

3) In some forms of persistent hepatitis following HBV infection it is difficult to demonstrate either HB Ag or HB_{core} Ag in cells, and when observed it usually appears restricted in a local fashion to a minor proportion of hepatocytes. Cytologic localization of HB Ag may appear

restricted not only to few cells but even to minute intracytoplasmic loci. Although few cells are positive for
HB Ag, most cells show cytologic aberrations including
cell enlargement, morphologic pleomorphism and irregular
histological organization within the hepatocellular plate.
The possibility of persistent but nonproductive infection
by HBV is speculated. The cells may contain viral genome
and reflect a non-productive viral infection; however, in
the absence of suitable methods of viral rescue this is
not currently susceptible to direct experimentation.

These observations suggest that expression of HBV
genome by infected hepatocytes may be divisible into
recognizable patterns that may bear some relationship to
hepatic injury (Table 4). The complete pattern with demonstrable synthesis of structural components of both coat
and core by virtually every cell has been observed only in
the very early phase of acute transient hepatitis. The defective patterns associated with persistent and chronic
infection may be responsible at least in part for the
limited cytopathology with these forms of disease.

In evaluation of possible factors associated with
the pathogenesis of hepatocellular injury in association
with HBV infection it is relatively apparent that a
requisite cytopathic effect of HBV infection independent
of the type of genome expression can be effectively ruled
out in view of the silent carrier state (Table 5).
Variable cytopathology may be influenced by: 1) the
genetic constitution of the host; 2) presence of complete
or partial viral genome; or 3) variable patterns of viral
genome transcription. The possibility that there is
virtually no cytopathology associated with HBV infection
of hepatocytes remains an alternate and highly tenable
hypothesis. The pathogenesis of the varied hepatic
diseases induced by this agent may be associated with
differing patterns of genome expression included within
experimentally demonstrable productive and hypothetically
postulated non-productive biological cycles. Though firmly
established pathogenetic factors responsible for disease
associated with HBV infection remain to be established,
current progress suggests that such data may be rapidly
and effectively developed.

THOMAS EDGINGTON

ACKNOWLEDGMENTS

This work has been supported by Contract 73-2509 from the National Institutes of Allergy and Infectious Diseases. This is publication EP-838.

REFERENCES

1. Boyer, M.L., Blumberg, B.S., and Werner, B., *Nature* 218, 1057 (1968).

2. Dane, D.S., Cameron, C.H., and Briggs, M., *Lancet* 1, 695 (1970).

3. Jokelainin, P.T., Krohn, K., Prince, A.M., and Finlayson, N.D.C., *J. Virol.* 6, 685 (1970).

4. Almeida, J.D., Waterson, A.P., Trowell, J.M., and Neale, O., *Microbios.* 2, 145 (1970).

5. Bond, H.E. and Hall, W.T., *J. Infect. Dis.* 125, 263 (1972).

6. Gerin, J.L., Purcell, R.H., Hoggan, M.D., Holland,P.V. and Chanock, R.M., *J. Virol.* 4, 763 (1969).

7. Gerin, J.L., Holland, P.V., and Purcell, R.H., *J. Virol.* 7, 569 (1971).

8. Gerin, J.L., this publication.

9. Kaplan, P.M., Greenman, R.L., Gerin, J.L., Purcell, R.H., and Robinson, W.S., *J. Virol.* 12, 995 (1973).

10. Robinson, W.S., Greenman, R.L., Kaplan, P.M., Gerin, J.L., and Purcell, R.H., this publication.

11. Prince, A.M., *Proc. Nat. Acad. Sci.* 60, 814 (1968).

12. Krugman, S., Giles, J.P., and Hammond, J., *J. Am. Med. Assoc.* 200, 365 (1967).

13. Barker, L.F., Shulman, N.R., Murray, R., Hirschman, R.J., Ratner, F., Diefenbach, W.C.L., and Geller, H.M., *J. Am. Med. Assoc.* 211, 1509 (1970).

14. Barker, L.F., Chisari, F.V., McGrath, P.P., Dalgard, D.W., Kirschstein, R.L., Almeida, J.D., Edgington, T.S., Sharp, D.G., and Peterson, M.R., *J. Infect. Dis.* 127, 648 (1973).

15. Maynard, J.E., Hartwell, W.V., and Berquist, K.R., *J. Infect. Dis.* 123, 660 (1971).

16. Purcell, R.H., London, W.T., Alter, H.J., and Edgington, T.S., *J. Infect. Dis.* - Submitted.

17. Purcell, R.H., this publication.

18. Iwarson, S., Lindholm, A., Lundin, P., and Hermodsson, S., *Vox Sang.* 22, 501 (1972).

19. Alpert, E., Isselbacher, K.J., and Schur, P.H., *New Engl. J. Med.* 285, 185 (1971).

20. Onion, D.K., Crumpacker, C.S., and Gilliland, B.C., *Ann. Int. Med.* 75, 29 (1971).

21. Gocke, D.J., Hsu, K., Morgan, C., Bombardieri, S., Lockshin, M., and Christian, C.L., *J. Exp. Med.* 134, 330S (1971).

22. Nowaslawski, A., Krawczynski, K., Brzosko, W.J., and Madalinski, K., *Am. J. Path.* 68, 31 (1972).

23. Prince, A.M., LeBlanc, L., Krohn, K., *et al.* *Lancet* 2, 711 (1970).

24. LeBouvier, G.L., *J. Infect. Dis.* 123, 671 (1971).

25. Almeida, J.D., Rubenstein, D., and Stott, E.J., *Lancet* 2, 1225 (1971).

26. Edgington, T.S. and Ritt, D.J., *J. Exp. Med.* 134, 871 (1971).

27. Purcell, R.H., *et al.*, In progress.

TABLE 1

HEPATITIS B VIRUS ASSOCIATED ANTIGENIC EXPRESSIONS

Type	Antigenic Determinants	Origin
I. Coat (HB Ag)		
Group specific	a	virus specified
Group specific	x	host specified
Subtype specific	d/y	virus specified (allelic)
Subtype specific	r/w	virus specified (allelic)
II. Core (HBcore Ag)		
Capsid protein	"core"	virus specified

TABLE 2

ANTIGENIC INDEPENDENCE OF HB AG AND HB CORE

Blocking Antibody	F–Anti–HB Ag Cytoplasmic Fluorescence	F–Anti–HB Core Nuclear Fluorescence
None	+	+
Anti–HB Ag	0	+
Anti–HB Core	+	0

TABLE 3

STRUCTURAL AND ANTIGENIC FORMS
OF THE HEPATITIS B VIRUS

Particle	Morphology	Antigens	Tissue Location
Dane (complete HBV)	43 nm spheres	HB Ags HB core Ag	Hepatocyte nucleus, cytoplasm, plasma
HB core	27 nm spheres	HB core Ag	Hepatocyte nucleus
HB coat	20–22 nm spheres and filamentous forms	HB Ags a, d/y, r/w	Hepatocyte cytoplasm, plasma

TABLE 4

PATTERNS OF HBV GENOME EXPRESSION BY HEPATOCYTES

Cycle	HB Core	HB Coat	Cytologic Atypism
Complete	+	+	0
Defective Core	0	+	0
Defective Coat	+	0	0
Non-Productive	0	0	+

TABLE 5

POSSIBLE RELATIONSHIPS BETWEEN HBV INFECTION
AND HEPATOCELLULAR INJURY

I. Primary Cellular Cytopathology

    Requisite

    Variable - genetically dependent

             - state of viral genome

             - pattern of viral gene expression

    None

VI

MECHANISMS OF CELL TRANSFORMATION
BY DNA TUMOR VIRUSES

GENE FUNCTIONS OF POLYOMA VIRUS AND SIMIAN VIRUS 40

Walter Eckhart

The Armand Hammer Center for Cancer Biology
The Salk Institute
Post Office Box 1809
San Diego, California 92112

ABSTRACT.   Temperature-sensitive mutants of polyoma virus
and Simian Virus 40 (SV40) fall into at least four classes.
Two classes are blocked early after infection at the restrictive temperature. The function of one of these
classes is required for viral DNA synthesis, probably for
the initiation of each round of viral DNA replication.
Mutants of the other class are blocked in both induction
of cellular DNA synthesis and viral DNA synthesis at the
restrictive temperature. Two classes of mutants are
blocked at later stages of infection, after the synthesis
of viral DNA. Some of these mutants appear to contain
altered virion proteins. It is likely that an early viral
function is involved in regulatory alterations in the infected cell.

INTRODUCTION

This session of the 1974 ICN-UCLA Conference on
Mechanisms of Virus Disease is devoted to a discussion of
the mechanism of cell transformation by DNA tumor viruses.
Transformation refers to the hereditary acquisition of new
growth properties by cells. DNA tumor viruses are able to
cause cancer in animals and produce transformation of infected cells in culture. Polyoma and Simian Virus 40
(SV40) are the most thoroughly studied DNA tumor viruses,
primarily because of the small size of their genomes
(approximately 3.4×10^6 daltons molecular weight).

In the last several years a number of general features
of transformation by polyoma and SV40 have been established
(for review see Sambrook (1)). Viral DNA persists in the
transformed cell, and can be detected by molecular hybridization, or by the rescue of infectious virus by fusion of
transformed and susceptible cells. Viral genetic information is expressed in the transformed cell, as judged by the
presence of virus-specific messenger RNA, but apparently

255

only part of the viral information is expressed, because
"late" functions, such as virion antigens, are not detected
in the transformed cell. An important mechanism of regulation of viral gene expression, both during lytic infection
and in the transformed cell, is exerted at the level of
transcription of viral DNA into stable messenger RNA (mRNA).
During lytic infection viral information is expressed in a
coordinated way, so that only "early" species of mRNA corresponding to approximately one-third of the viral genome,
are present prior to viral DNA replication, whereas "late"
species corresponding to the entire viral genome appear
after viral DNA replication. In the transformed cell viral
gene expression also appears to be regulated by a mechanism
involving transcription, because the major species of
functional mRNA correspond to the "early" region of the
viral genome. Regulation of transcription will be discussed in detail by Dr. Malcolm Martin during this session.

The presence and regulated expression of viral genetic
information in transformed cells suggests that viral gene
functions may be important in transformation. It seems
clear that cell growth control is a very complex phenomenon
and that most of the properties of transformed cells will
be determined by cellular genes and selection during the
growth of transformed cells in culture. Therefore, in addition to searching for the role of viral genes in transformation it is important to consider the ways in which
cellular genes influence the phenotype of the transformed
cell. This subject will be discussed by Dr. Robert
Pollack in this session.

In recent years several lines of evidence have pointed
to the role of viral genes in establishing and maintaining
cell transformation by polyoma and SV40 (for review see
Eckhart (2)). I shall review briefly what is known about
the gene functions of polyoma and SV40.

MUTANTS OF POLYOMA AND SV40

Several kinds of mutants of polyoma and SV40 have been
selected for the purpose of identifying the viral genes
(2). These mutants include temperature-sensitive mutants,
host range mutants, and various kinds of defective mutants
containing deletions or insertions in their genetic material. Analysis of temperature-sensitive mutants of polyoma
and SV40 has shown that they fall into at least four

classes: two classes are defective early, prior to viral
DNA synthesis at the restrictive temperature, whereas two
classes are defective late, after viral DNA synthesis but
before the formation of infectious progeny virus.

At least some of the late mutants appear to be defective in structural genes coding for virion proteins, because some of the late mutant virions are more heat labile
than wild-type or SV40 (3,4). Polyoma virions contain
three proteins that might be virus coded, having molecular
weights of approximately 47,000, 35,000 and 23,000 daltons
(for review see Crawford (5)). Recently Friedmann has
suggested that all three proteins may be derived from a
common precursor (6). Identification of the genes coding
for the virion proteins by genetic complementation analysis
may be complicated if the virion proteins are derived by
cleavage from a common precursor. Peptide analysis of the
virion proteins derived from wild-type virus and several
mutants appears to be a good approach to this problem.

The early mutants are the most interesting from the
point of view of trying to understand transformation, because it was established some time ago that one of the
early viral genes (the tsA gene) is required for transformation (7), and the early region of the viral genome is
the one transcribed into functional mRNA in the transformed cell. The properties of some mutants blocked early
after infection at the restrictive temperature are described below.

THE TSA GENE OF POLYOMA AND SV40

Both polyoma and SV40 have an early gene required for
viral DNA synthesis, referred to as the tsA gene. Mutants
in this gene carry out certain early events of lytic infection (such as induction of cellular DNA synthesis)
normally at the restrictive temperature, but are blocked
in viral DNA synthesis (8). The tsA function appears to
be required for the initiation of each round of viral DNA
replication, but not for the completion of a round of
replication once it has begun (9,10). Because both
polyoma and SV40 have a fixed origin of replication on
the viral DNA molecule (11,12,13), the tsA gene function
may promote a site specific association of the viral DNA
with elements of the replicative apparatus.

The tsA gene function is required transiently for the initiation or fixation of transformation, but not for the maintenance of the characteristics of transformed cells (7). The properties of polyoma tsA mutant transformed mouse 3T3 cells, which can be induced to produce virus by a shift from the restrictive to the permissive temperature, suggest that the tsA function may be involved in integration or excision of the viral DNA from the cellular DNA (14,15). It is attractive to speculate that integration of viral DNA into the cellular genome may be the step in transformation for which the tsA function is transiently required.

Both polyoma and SV40 tsA mutants show reduced ability to synthesize T antigen at the restrictive temperature (16,17), but it is not clear whether the tsA gene actually codes for the T antigen protein.

Host range mutants of polyoma have been isolated and have been shown to be defective in transformation and in causing cell surface alterations (18,19). The relationship between these mutants and the temperature-sensitive mutants of polyoma has not been established.

OTHER MUTANTS BLOCKED IN EARLY FUNCTIONS

It is likely that there is at least one other early gene function of polyoma and SV40 besides the tsA function, because induction of cellular DNA synthesis requires a viral gene function, and this induction is carried out normally by the tsA mutants at the restrictive temperature (8). The ts3 mutant of polyoma and the ts*101 mutant of SV40 both are blocked early after infection at the restrictive temperature, before the induction of cellular DNA synthesis (20,21). These mutants share two unusual properties: they are not complemented during mixed infection by other temperature-sensitive mutants, and infection by purified viral DNA is not temperature-sensitive (20,21). It has been suggested that these properties may result from an alteration in a virion protein of the virus, so that early viral gene expression is blocked (20). The properties could also be explained in other ways, such as by a cis-acting early viral function and leakiness of the mutant because of the high input multiplicity involved in viral DNA infection.

There is evidence that the ts3 and ts*101 functions may be involved in maintaining some of the properties of transformed cells. BHK cells transformed by ts3 show temperature-dependent expression of cell surface properties and growth properties (22). BALB/3T3 cells transformed by ts*101 show temperature-dependent expression of T antigen (23). It is attractive to speculate that an early viral gene function leads to regulatory alterations during lytic infection that are also important in transformation.

REGULATORY EFFECTS DURING LYTIC INFECTION

The clearest example of a regulatory effect resulting from polyoma or SV40 infection is the "helper effect" of SV40 for adenovirus growth in monkey cells. When adenoviruses infect monkey cells all species of viral mRNA are synthesized, but some capsid proteins are made in reduced amounts, and virus growth is defective (24,25). Co-infection by SV40 overcomes this defect, presumably because of the influence of an early SV40 gene function, because tsA mutants of SV40 exhibit helper activity normally at the restrictive temperature (26). Recently it has been suggested that the SV40 helper activity operates by allowing the attachment of certain species of adenovirus mRNA's to polysomes (27). SV40-transformed monkey cells are permissive for adenovirus growth (28). Therefore the SV40 helper activity is expressed in transformed cells as well as in lytically infected cells. Such an activity could influence the expression of cellular genes if it affected post transcriptional regulation of cellular mRNA as well as viral mRNA. It will be important to determine how such regulatory alterations might affect the properties of transformed cells.

ACKNOWLEDGMENT

Some of the work described in this presentation was supported by Grant No. CA-13884 from the National Cancer Institute.

REFERENCES

1. Sambrook, J., Adv. in Canc. Res. 16, 141 (1972).
2. Eckhart, W., Ann. Rev. Genetics (in press)(1974).

3. Eckhart, W., Virology 38, 120 (1969).
4. Kimura, G. and Dulbecco, R., Virology 49, 394 (1972).
5. Crawford, L. V., Brit. Med. Bull. 29, 253 (1973).
6. Friedmann, T., Proc. Nat. Acad. Sci. USA (in press) (1974).
7. Fried, M., Proc. Nat. Acad. Sci. USA 53, 486 (1965).
8. Fried, M., Virology 40, 605 (1970).
9. Francke, B. and Eckhart, W., Virology 55, 127 (1973).
10. Tegtmeyer, P., J. Virol. 10, 591 (1972).
11. Nathans, D. and Danna, K., Nature New Biol. 236, 200 (1972).
12. Fareed, G. C., Garon, C. F., Salzman, N. P., J. Virol. 10, 484 (1972).
13. Crawford, L. V., Syrett, C. and Wilde, A., J. Gen. Virol. 21, 515 (1973).
14. Vogt, M., J. Mol. Biol. 47, 307 (1970).
15. Cuzin, F., Vogt, M., Dieckmann, M. and Berg, P., J. Mol. Biol. 47, 317 (1970).
16. Oxman, M. N., Takemoto, K. K. and Eckhart, W., Virology 49, 675 (1972).
17. Robb, J. A., Tegtmeyer, P., Ishikawa, A. and Ozer, H. L., J. Virol. 13 (in press)(1974).
18. Benjamin, T. L., Proc. Nat. Acad. Sci. USA 67, 394 (1970).
19. Benjamin, T. L. and Burger, M. M., Proc. Nat. Acad. Sci. USA 67, 929 (1970).
20. Robb, J. A. and Martin, R. G., J. Virol. 9, 956 (1972).
21. Eckhart, W. and Dulbecco, R., Virology (in press)(1974).
22. Eckhart, W., Dulbecco, R. and Burger, M. M., Proc. Nat. Acad. Sci. USA 68, 283 (1971).
23. Robb, J. A., J. Virol. 12, 1187 (1973).
24. Fox, R. and Baum, S., J. Virol. 10, 220 (1972).
25. Lucas, J. J. and Ginsberg, H. W., J. Virol. 10, 1109 (1972).
26. Jerkofsky, M. and Rapp, F., Virology 51, 466 (1973).
27. Hashimoto, K., Nakajima, K., Oda, K. and Shimojo, H. J. Mol. Biol. 81, 207 (1973).
28. Rapp, F. T. and Trulock, S. C., Virology 40, 961 (1970).

THE DIFFERENT STABLE PATTERNS OF GROWTH CONTROL
INDUCED BY SV40 INFECTION OF NORMAL CELLS

Robert Pollack and Rex Risser

Cold Spring Harbor Laboratory
Cold Spring Harbor, New York 11724, USA

ABSTRACT. When different assays of growth control are
used, SV40 is found to induce more than one type of transformed cell.

INTRODUCTION

By definition, transformed cells must be able to grow
where normal cells do not. Conditions which severely
restrict the in vitro growth of normal cells while per-
mitting the growth of transformed cells are presented in
Table 1. A fully transformed cell line is one that can
grow in all of these restrictive conditions.

Previous work on in vitro transformation has focused
on cells which show unrestricted growth in all of these
assays. We demonstrate here the existence of virus
infected cells which show unrestricted growth in only one
or a few of these assays and discuss their significance for
the mechanism of virally induced transformation. In studying the process of in vitro transformation, we have used
the small DNA-containing tumor virus SV40 (1,2,3) and two
different types of "normal" cells.

The first cell type is the mouse fibroblast line 3T3,
a post-crisis, established, heteroploid, clonable line
derived from Swiss mouse embryo culture (4). The second
cell type is a diploid culture of rat embryo cells called
REF. REF cells are prepared directly from 14 day rat
embryos by mincing and trypsinization (Risser and Pollack,
unpublished observations).

Both REF and 3T3 cells are unable to grow in three
of the four selective conditions (Table 1). However, they
differ in their ability to grow when plated very sparsely,

261

a characteristic referred to as cellular autonomy. Like
most cells taken directly from an animal, REF cells are not
autonomous, i.e. they cannot form separate colonies when
innoculated at less than 10 cell/cm^2. 3T3 cells, on the
other hand, can form colonies at any initial density with
an efficiency of about 50%.
  We demonstrate here that SV40 induces a variety of new
patterns in cellular behavior, not simply the fully transformed pattern. The most common alteration by SV40 of 3T3,
which is already capable of forming colonies, is the
acquisition of a reduced serum requirement for growth
(Table 1). The most common alteration of REF by SV40 is
simply the acquisition of the ability to form a colony.
Furthermore, we have found that these two changes always
occur in any REF or 3T3 cells which show the other changes
more commonly thought of as transformation (Table 1).

SV40 TRANSFORMATION OF 3T3

  Historically, transformed cell lines have been
isolated from post-crisis "normal" cell lines by their
ability to grow under conditions which prevent the growth
of the normal cell lines. Since post-crisis lines are
already able to form colonies with a high efficiency, such
lines cannot be used to assay the acquisition of autonomy
induced by SV40 infection. However, the three other
selective assays (Table 1) do permit isolation of transformants. While cell lines recovered from any of these
assays after SV40-infection of 3T3 are clearly different
from uninfected 3T3 clones, no selective assay can provide
information on the sum of possible physiological states
that SV40 can induce in 3T3 cells. In particular, clones
transformed by one selective assay do not always show
transformed behavior in the other selective assays (5).

CONTINUUM OF STABLE ALTERATIONS IN 3T3 AFTER SV40-INFECTION

  To isolate all possible types of SV40 transformants, a
sparse culture of 3T3 was infected with purified SV40 at a
high multiplicity. After adsorption of virus, the culture
was trypsinized and cells were plated at very high dilution,
to give 10-20 colonies per dish. At the same time, mock-
infected 3T3 cultures were plated at the same high dilution.
After two weeks, 40 well-isolated colonies from dishes of

infected cells and four colonies each from dishes of mock-infected cells were picked by the cloning-ring technique.

The standard assay for density transformation (Table 1) was also carried out at the same time. Here, transformants are defined as densely growing foci. In the non-selective assay 15% of clones picked were judged to be density-transformed, indicating that our cloning procedure did not accidentally favor density-transformants. Four dense foci from lower dilutions were also picked as standard trans-formants.

All clones were grown up for about one month, then frozen. The frozen clones were thawed a few at a time and their phenotypes systematically characterized. At no time was any culture subjected to low serum or high cell density. Thus, this assay yielded clones representative of all cell types arising after SV40 infection (6).

PROPERTIES OF CLONES

The clones isolated here were divisable into four classes (Table 2). The first class consists of clones identical to 3T3 in all of the selective assays (Table 1). The second class consists of clones identical to standard transformants. The third and fourth classes are composed of clones that are not identical to 3T3, but that would probably be indistinguishable from 3T3 in the standard transformation assay. Class III clones are able to grow well in 1% calf serum and are about two-fold denser than 3T3. Otherwise, they are indistinguishable from 3T3. Class IV clones are intermediate transformants. They contain SV101-like and 3T3-like cells.

The minimal and most common alteration in 3T3 after SV40 infection is the acquisition of the ability to grow in reduced serum (Table 2). Fully 88 percent of the experimental clones were able to grow in 1% calf serum, while none of the four mock-infected clones could do so (Table 2). Furthermore, the 12 percent of experimental clones that grew poorly in 1% calf serum were also untransformed in any other assay (6).

PERSISTENCE OF VIRAL Tag IN 3T3-CLONES TRANSFORMED BY SV40

Mock-infected clones, of course, were free of T-antigen by both assays (Table 2). The presence and amount of T-antigen correlated well with the degree of anchorage-transformation and with the degree of density transformation. The intermediate clones, in particular, had low levels of T-antigen and a mosaic distribution of positive and negative cells. Clones in the largest class of transformants, the minimal-transformants (Table 2), did not contain T-antigen. Thus, the most common new clone is one with the ability to grow in restrictive serum, while lacking T-antigen and lacking the transformed properties which correlate with T-antigen--high density and growth in methocel.

EFFECTS OF SV40 ON RAT EMBRYO FIBROBLASTS

To isolate all possible types of SV40 transformants that form colonies, the following selective protocol was used. A confluent culture of REF cells (Figure 1A) was infected with purified SV40 at an input multiplicity of about 100 PFU/cell. After adsorption of virus, the culture was trypsinized and the cells were also plated at very high dilution, to give 1000 cells per dish. At the same time, mock-infected REF cultures were plated at the same high dilutions. While more than 100 colonies were seen on infected plates, less than one was seen on mock-infected plates (Figure 1B,C). All colonies of infected REF cells must have been altered in some way by SV40 in order to grow; we define this alteration as the acquisition of autonomy by normal fibroblastic cells. The colonies induced by SV40 did not all resemble each other. In particular, most colonies resembled the rare colony arising on a dish of mock-infected cells (Figure 2A,B). Other colonies of infected cells were slightly denser than the majority (Figure 2C). A small minority were very dense (Figure 2D).

PERSISTENCE OF VIRAL Tag IN REF COLONIES

To determine whether infected colonies contained Tag, SV40-infected and mock-infected REF cells were plated on glass coverslips at 10^2 cell/cm^2 and examined by immunofluorescent stain. To our surprise, many of the colonies did not contain T-antigen. We conclude that the minimal effect SV40 can have on a normal cell is to confer autonomy on that cell in the absence of persistent T-antigen and in the absence of any apparent transformation to high density.

PROPERTIES OF REF COLONIES

We cloned 12 colonies from an infected plate resembling Figure 1C. Each of these clones was grown up, recloned, and assayed for the retention or loss of growth control (Table 1). Since even uninfected REF cells grow to high densities in 10% serum, we were not surprised to find that all 12 clones also grew to high densities. However, the colonies differed markedly from one another and from uninfected REF cells in their ability to grow in low serum or in suspension in methocel. All clones grew in 1% serum, while REF cells did not. Fewer than one REF cell in 10^5 can form a colony in methocel. Each REF clone had a stable plating efficiency in methocel, which ranged from one cell in 10 to one cell in 10^5. Preliminary results suggest that, for these SV40-transformed REF clones, growth in methocel and production of a cellular activator of plasminogen (7; Rifkin, this volume) are well correlated (Pollack, Risser, Arelt, and Rifkin, unpublished observations).

IMPLICATION FOR VIRAL GENETICS

SV40 apparently has many different effects on a transformable cell, but these fall into two distinct classes. The first is detected by the assays of autonomy and serum-transformation. The second is detected by the assays of density and anchorage. The second class seems to be dependent on the first: All transformants of the second class so far examined are also transformed in autonomy or serum. However, transformants of the first class need not be transformed in density or anchorage.

The role of viral genes in either class is unproven, but the presence of the one known viral gene product, T-antigen, correlates with the second class, and not the first. Most, if not all, attempts to assay variant SV40 strains for effects on transformation have been assays on the final steps in transformation, and thus have actually been attempts to isolate viruses that are simultaneously defective in their ability to cause both classes of transformation. We believe it unlikely that such mutants will be picked up. Rather, we suggest that new virus selective systems be constructed, in which viruses can be detected even if they are only ts or defective in one of the two classes.

IMPLICATION FOR DIFFERENTIATION

When any embryo is minced and its cells placed in culture, only a small minority of the cells survive the initial few days and divide (8). Of these, the fibroblasts are the most common (9). Other differentiated cells normally do not divide for long, even in dense culture. No normal cell can be expected to grow into a clone in sparse culture. We have shown that SV40 can confer the ability to plate on rat embryo fibroblasts with high efficiency. Many of these colonies lack T-antigen and appear normal. Other normal embryonic tissues should be infected with SV40, to determine whether SV40 can be used as a reagent for production of clonable, normal differentiated cell lines.

ACKNOWLEDGMENTS

We thank Sue Arelt and Carole Thomason for excellent, reliable technical assistance. Robert Goldman suggested the possible use of SV40 to establish differentiated normal lines. This research was supported by funds from the National Cancer Institute, NIH. R.R. was supported by NIH predoctoral fellowship 4-501-GM-49503-04.

REFERENCES

1. Black, P. and Rowe, W., Virology 19, 107 (1963).
2. Shein, H. and Enders, J., Proc. Nat. Acad. Sci. 48, 1164 (1962).
3. Todaro, G. and Green, H., Virology 23, 117 (1964).
4. Todaro, G. and Green, H., J. Cell. Biol. 17, 299 (1963).
5. Smith, H., Scher, C., and Todaro, G., Virology 44, 359 (1971).
6. Risser, R. and Pollack, R., Virology, in press (1974).
7. Unkeless, J.C., Tobia, A., Ossowski, L., Quigley, J.P., Rifkin, D.B., and Reich, E., J. Experimental Medicine 137, 85 (1973).
8. Sato, G., Zaroff, L., and Mills, S., Proc. Nat. Acad. Sci. 46, 963 (1960).
9. Dulbecco, R., Proc. Nat. Acad. Sci. 38, 747 (1952).

Table 1. Selective Assays Yielding Transformed Cell Lines

System		Assay	Typical Value	
Virus	Cell		Normal	Transformed
SV40	REF	Autonomy: Ability to form a colony	<0.1 colony per 10^2 cells	>10 colonies per 10^2 cells
SV40	3T3,REF	Serum: Ability to grow in limiting serum	Doubling time >75 hr	Doubling time <30 hr
SV40	3T3,REF	Density: Ability to form a dense colony	5×10^4 cell/cm^2	10^6 cell/cm^2
Py SV40	BHK 3T3,REF	Anchorage: Ability to form a colony suspended in gel	<0.001 colony per 10^2 cells	>10 colonies per 10^2 cells

Table 2. Classes of 3T3 Clones Induced by SV40

Class	Percent of Clones	T-antigen	Density(a)	Doubling Time in 1% CS(b)	Anchorage(c)
I Normal	12	-	8.5 (7.6-9.5)	78 (55-100)	$\leq$.001
II Transformed	25	+	47 (35-60)	34 (24-45)	32 (11-58)
III Minimal-transformed	38	-	15 (9.5-16.5)	34 (26-49)	$\leq$.001
IV Intermediate-transformed	25	$\pm$	25 (15-45)	32 (29-41)	4 (.5-14.6)
Control					
Normal		-	7.8 (7-9)	70 (60-86)	$\leq$.001
Transformed		+	53 (47-60)	37 (26-43)	25 (16-30)

(a) cells/cm^{2}x10^{-4}

(b) hrs

(c) percent cells forming visible colonies (>0.3mm diameter) in 21 days in methocel

268

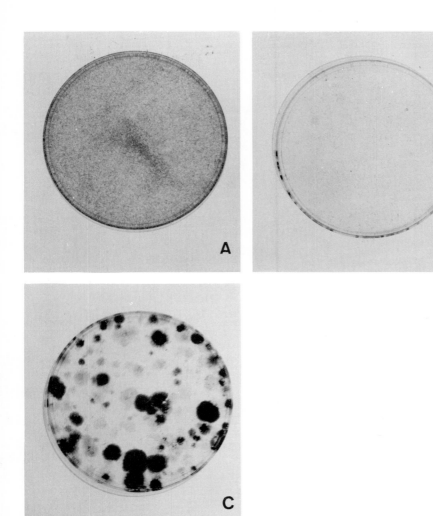

Fig. 1. Transformation of rat embryo fibroblasts by SV40. Fixed and stained plates: (A) confluent plate of REF cells at time of infection, (B) uninfected confluent plate was trypsinized and replated at 10^3 cells per plate (cells were cultured for 14 days), (C) infected confluent plate was trypsinized and replated at 10^3 cells per plate (cells were cultured for 14 days).

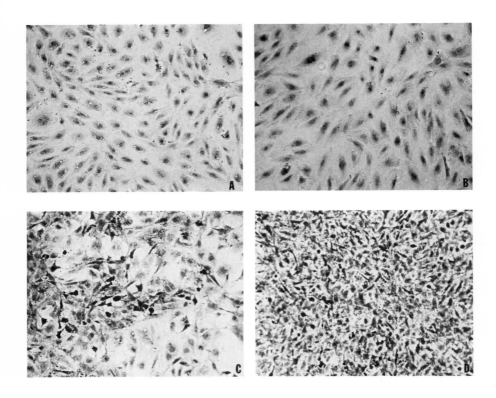

Fig. 2. SV40 transformed REF colonies. (A) Colony from mock-infected plate (PE~10^{-3}), (B-D) colonies from infected plate (PE~10^{-1}): (B) low density colony resembling mock-infected colony, (C) intermediate density colony, (D) high density colony. Relative frequency of different colony morphologies: B>C>D.

VII

CELL TRANSFORMATION BY RNA TUMOR VIRUSES

CONTROL OF REVERSION IN MSV TRANSFORMED CELLS AFTER SINGLE AND MULTIPLE TRANSFORMING CYCLES

Shigeko Nomura and Peter J. Fischinger

National Cancer Institute
Bethesda, Maryland 20014

ABSTRACT. The Moloney murine sarcoma virus (M–MSV)[1]–transformed mouse cells (S+L- cells) spontaneously gave rise to flat revertants from which MSV could no longer be rescued. Reversion frequency increased by exposure of S+L- cells to 5-Fluorodeoxyuridine or Colcemid. Retransformation of S+L- revertants by M–MSV resulted in a number of metastable states, and no second cycle of reversion was observed. The S+L- revertants retransformed by Kirsten MSV (Ki–MSV) demonstrated a rescuable and inducible MSV, and a second cycle of reversion occurred in these cases. Flat variants, which were negative for Ki–MSV rescue by MuLV, were also isolated from a nonproducer clone of BALB/3T3 transformed by Ki–MSV. Reversion was observed from feline cells transformed with MSV but not from human S+L- cells.

INTRODUCTION TO THE PROBLEM OF REVERSION

There have been several reports of reversion in cells transformed by both DNA tumor viruses such as polyoma and SV40 (1,2,3,4) and by the avian RNA (Rous sarcoma) tumor

---

[1] Abbreviations used: M–MSV, Moloney murine sarcoma virus; Ki–MSV, Kirsten murine sarcoma virus; MuLV, murine leukemia virus; gs, group specific; S+L-, sarcoma positive leukemia negative; FdUrd, 5-Fluorodeoxyuridine; Ki–BALB, a clonal line of BALB/3T3 transformed by Ki–MSV; IdUrd, 5-Iodo-deoxyuridine; FEF, feline embryonic fibroblasts; HEMS, human embryonic muscle-skin cells; SR, FR and CF, spontaneous, FdUrd- and Colcemid-induced revertants, respectively; FLV and GLV, Friend and Gross leukemia virus; FIU, focus-inducing unit; FFU, focus-forming unit.

virus (5). Reversion resulted apparently by the suppression of the transformed state by cellular genes. In most of these studies, however, the transforming genome was not native to the species of origin. In the mouse system, 3T3 cells could be transformed by the wild-type M-MSV in the absence of murine leukemia virus (MuLV) (6) with a loss of contact inhibition of growth and hyperrefractile appearance. The transformed cell contained the group specific (gs)-1 antigen of MuLV, an MSV genome which is rescuable by MuLV infection, C-type particles, and reverse transcriptase activity but no infectious MSV or MuLV. These cells have been termed sarcoma positive leukemia negative (S+L-) (7,8). Several sublines of S+L- cells spontaneously gave rise to flat variant cells termed revertants with some properties of nontransformed cells and from which MSV could no longer be rescued by MuLV infection (9,10). Reversion frequency increased by exposure of S+L- cells to 5-Fluorodeoxyuridine (FdUrd) or Colcemid (11). Initially it was not known whether the MSV genome was lost or phenotypically repressed, but recently some revertants derived either spontaneously or after FdUrd treatment could rarely of their own accord back-transform to the S+L- state indicating that the MSV genome must have persisted in a nonrescuable form in at least some revertant cells (11). Because most of the S+L- cell derived revertants examined were hypersensitive to retransformation by MSV, they were studied in some detail using several MSV isolates (12).

A clonal subline of Ki-MSV-transformed nonproducer BALB/3T3 (Ki-BALB) cells (13) also spontaneously produced flat variant sublines from which Ki-MSV could not be rescued by MuLV. The parental Ki-BALB cells did not contain infectious MSV or MuLV, detectable MuLV gs antigen(s), reverse transcriptase activity or C-type particles. However, superinfection of cells with MuLV resulted in the rescue of MSV (13), and MSV also could be induced by exposure of cells to 5-Iododeoxyuridine (IdUrd) (14). The behavior of Ki-BALB revertants is compatible with deletion of some, if not all, of the Ki-MSV genome. It is definite that each S+L- or Ki-BALB cell has the intrinsic ability to control the expression of tumor virus native or part native to the species after the conversion has already taken place, since revertant cells have been detected in multiply cloned S+L- and Ki-BALB cell population (9).

We now describe the isolation and characterization of S+L- and Ki-BALB revertants, the complex derivation and the properties of clones isolated from retransformed S+L- revertants by several sarcoma viruses, and some attempts to isolate revertants from M-MSV transformed human and cat cells.

GENERAL MATERIALS AND METHODS

The S+L- cells were initially isolated as two individual soft agar colonies after single-hit infection with M-MSV. The S+L- lines derived from these differed significantly in their reversion frequency (9,11). The cell which reverted frequently was termed FG10 and the other less reverting cell as 3197. The MSV genomes present in these cells have been described as m1 and m3, respectively. The 3T3FL (6), NIH 3T3 (15), BALB/3T3 (16), normal rat kidney cells (NRK) (17), FG10 (6), XC cells (18), feline embryonic fibroblasts (FEF) and human embryonic muscle-skin cells (HEMS) were used for virus assays and cocultivation where appropriate (10,11,12).

Cloning and nomenclature of variant sublines: To isolate flat variants, 0.2 ml of cell suspension, containing 1 cell/ml were delivered into multiple microtiter wells (Falcon Plastics) and 7-10 days after plating, individual colonies were isolated. Alternatively, cells were first seeded into plastic plates (60x15 mm) at a concentration of 50-100 cells per plate. After 7 days of incubation, flat colonies were recloned in microtiter wells. To isolate FdUrd- and Colcemid-induced flat variants, cells were exposed to 10 µg/ml of FdUrd (Calbiochem) for 1 hr at 37° or 0.04 µg/ml of Colcemid (Grand Island Biological Co.) for 24 hr at 37° before cloning (11). A rapid screening procedure was used to determine reversion frequency if the natural frequency was very low (19). To isolate the MSV-transformed revertant cells, DEAE-Dextran pretreated cell cultures were infected with various dilutions of filtered MSV stock.

275

About 2 weeks later, a terminal focus was isolated and cloned in microtiter wells. The following abbreviations and nomenclatures will be used (11,12). Because revertants could be obtained from S+L- cells either spontaneously (SR) or by chemical means such as after FdUrd (FR) or Colcemid treatment (CR), letters can be used to designate the mode of reversion. The first transforming MSV genome is designated by a preceding subscript; e.g., an m1-MSV(MuLV) transformed S+L- cell which spontaneously changes to a revertant cell is $_{m1}SR1$. When revertants are subjected to a second MSV transforming cycle then the transformed cell is characterized by a following superscript; e.g., if the $_{m1}SR1$ were transformed by m3-MSV(MuLV) then the resulting cell would be known as $_{m1}SR1^{m3}$. Symbols such as "mw" or "k" represent the wild strain of M-MSV or the Ki-MSV. If multiple cycles of reversion become possible then the sequence of transforming genomes can be grouped with the subscripts. If a revertant were to back-transform spontaneously then it would either exhibit rescue by MuLV infection or not, and the superscript would be bs^+ or bs^-. As an example after FdUrd treatment a revertant was derived which later transformed spontaneously but was in contrast to many previous observations, rescuable by MuLV (11). Accordingly such a transformed cell line can be accurately defined as $_{m3}FR^{bs+}$.

Viruses and antisera. The Moloney (MLV-IC), Friend (FLV) and Gross leukemia virus (GLV) isolates have all been adapted to grow in 3T3FL cells (20,21). The sources of defective MSV were M-MSV and Ki-MSV which had been rescued from S+L- (FG10 and 3197) and Ki-BALB cells by MLV-IC infection, and were designated m1-MSV(IC), m3-MSV(IC) and Ki-MSV(IC), respectively. MuLV was titrated either by the XC-plaque assay (22) and focus induction assay (23), and MSV was quantitated by a modified focus-forming assay (24). For human or feline cells the Rickard strain of feline leukemia virus or CCC virus pseudotypes of m1-MSV were prepared and appropriate helper viruses at optimal concentrations ($2x10^4$ focus-inducing units (FIU)/10^5 cells) were used to express all focus-forming units (FFU) of MSV in each cell system as previously described (25). The antisera used for neutralization were anti-MSV-IC, anti-GLV, anti-FLV and the serum from aged New Zealand black mice (12). Neutralization of

MuLV or of their respective MSV pseudotypes was carried out as described (21).

To rescue MSV from S+L- or Ki-BALB cells, cells were infected by MLV-IC at an m.o.i., $\geq$2, and culture fluids were tested for the presence of MSV (26). For MSV induction, cells were treated with 20 to 200 µg/ml of IdUrd (Calbiochem) for 20-30 hrs (27,28). The filtered culture fluids from 2 to 7 days post treatment were assayed for MSV on DEAE-Dextran pretreated NIH 3T3, 3T3FL, revertant cells, NRK, FEF, or HEMS cells. To detect MuLV induction, we used a modified XC-plaque assay (Lowy et al. (27)), which consisted of cocultivating IdUrd-treated cells with susceptible normal mouse or rat cells.

Tests for saturation density, MuLV gs antigen(s) (29), reverse transcriptase activity (30), chromosome counts, and electron microscopic studies were carried out as described elsewhere (10,11).

RESULTS IN REVIEW

Revertants derived from S+L- cell. The S+L- revertants demonstrated a high degree of contact inhibition, a low saturation density, a low cloning efficiency in soft agar, a lack of infectious MSV or MuLV and a lack of reverse transcriptase activity. However, they were agglutinable by concanavalin A and contained MuLV gs-1 antigen in a majority of sublines. MSV could no longer be rescued from these revertants by superinfection with MuLV or by cocultivation with normal mouse, rat and cat cells. After IdUrd treatment, reverse transcriptase activity and noninfectious virus particles were only rarely induced. As may be seen in Table 1, all revertants were susceptible to MSV and MuLV infection, and some degree of enhancement of sensitivity to MSV and MuLV infection was observed in most revertant cultures (9, 10). The frequency of occurrence of revertants increased after treatment with FdUrd or Colcemid. In one S+L- subline (3197-360), spontaneous reversion occurred at the rate of about 1 in 80 colonies, and after treatment with Colcemid or FdUrd, revertants were observed in 1 in 20 and 30 colonies, respectively. In another S+L- subline (3197-321), spontaneous reversion normally occurred less than 1 in 1000 colonies, and the

same treatments increased the frequency to approximately
1 in 70 and 55 colonies, respectively. Some revertant
clones spontaneously underwent back-transformation during
extended cultivation. Back-transformation with a rescuable
MSV genome was observed in 1 of 4 SR and 2 of 5 FR cells,
but in none of 4 CR. Furthermore, 1 of 5 FR cells gave
rise to a clone which was flat but which otherwise
resembled S+L- cells. In the SR and CR cells, the loss of
expression of transformation was associated with an
increase in chromosome number. However, the chromosome
number of FR was similar to or slightly less than that of
S+L- cells (10, 11) (Table 1). These studies demonstrated
that reversion of S+L- cells to flat variants probably
occurred by different mechanisms involving either the
viral or cellular genes or both, and that some flat
variant sublines had retained at least one complete MSV
genome in a totally covert form.

Revertants derived from Ki-BALB cells. In our hands,
cloned Ki-BALB cells produced SR cells at frequencies of
0.01 - 0.001. Such revertants were epithelioid, contact
inhibited, grew to low saturation density and exhibited
variable cloning efficiencies in soft agar. No MuLV gs
antigen(s), no reverse transcriptase activity, and no
infectious virus were demonstrated, yet these flat cells
were agglutinable by concanavalin A. MuLV was induced
after IdUrd treatment from revertants as well as from
parental Ki-BALB cells. However, Ki-MSV could not be
rescued from these revertants by superinfection with MuLV,
nor induced by treatment with IdUrd. No back-transformation was observed during 20-30 subcultures. The tumori-
genicity of revertants in syngeneic BALB/c mice was
markedly reduced compared to that of the Ki-BALB cells.
All revertants were susceptible to MSV and MuLV infection.
FdUrd or Colcemid had no effect on the increase in reversion frequency. The loss of the transformed phenotype in
Ki-BALB revertants was associated with a decrease in
chromosome number to a level similar to BALB/3T3 cell.
These observations suggest that a deletion of some or all
of the Ki-MSV genes may be involved in this reversion.
These studies are summarized in Table 2.

Retransformation of S+L- revertants by MSV. The S+L-
revertants were susceptible to a second cycle of single-hit
MSV transformation and the acquisition of the second transforming MSV genome resulted in a number of metastable
states (12). 1) A transformed S+L- like state with a
rescuable MSV, which in contrast to parental S+L- cells,
was also inducible by IdUrd ($_{m1}$SR^{m1} 13). 2) A transformed
S+L- clone which could give rise to a secondary flat S-L-
like clone, which when followed over several generations
could turn again into a stable S+L- type cell ($_{m1}$SR^{m3} 411).
3) A previously S+L- type MSV retransformed revertant
began to extrude infectious MSV with or without an atypical
MuLV ($_{m1}$SR^{m3} 91). 4) An S+L- type second cycle MSV
transformed cell resulted in both a stable S+L- type
subline ($_{m3}$SR^{mw} 101) and a subline releasing an excess of
MSV over atypical MuLV ($_{m3}$SR^{mw} 102).

The S+L- type retransformed revertant resembled
parental single cycle MSV transformed S+L- cells containing
MuLV gs antigen(s) and C type particles. Some but not all
second cycle MSV transformed S+L- revertants produced
infectious MSV on chemical induction. The second cycle of
reversion was a very rare event, if both the first and
the second transforming genome were M-MSV (Table 3), but
was demonstrated recently to occur at a frequency between
10^{-4} to 10^{-5} by the rapid screening technique for revertants (19).

The atypical MuLV which spontaneously appeared in
some MSV retransformed revertants was not the xenotropic
endogenous MuLV. This form of MuLV replicated in mouse
cells, less in rat cells, but not at all in human or cat
cells. Neutralization revealed that it was closely related
to the Moloney type of MuLV.

Two sublines of S+L- (3197) revertants were retransformed by single-hit Ki-MSV infection. The retransformed
sublines $_{m3}$SR^{k} 382 and 16 had the following properties:
they contained a rescuable and an inducible MSV, but did
not contain infectious MSV or MuLV (Table 3). Rescued
MSV from these sublines was characterized as the Ki-MSV
type based on its titration pattern, focus morphology on

279

3T3FL cells, and the high MuLV/MSV ratio of the rescued virus stocks from these cells. Two nonrescuable flat variants were isolated from 43 colonies of the 382 subline.

Flat variants derived from heterologous cells transformed by single-hit MSV infection. Single-hit infection by MSV of feline CCC or human amnion cells resulted in each case in S+L- type cells (25,31). A special marker feature of the transformed cell was the presence of the MuLV gs-1 antigen in good quantity. No C-type particles or reverse transcriptase activity was ever seen in human S+L- cells but in the cat cell the endogenous CCC virus was released spontaneously (25,31). A superinfection by leukemia C-type helper virus such as FeLV or the xenotropic MuLV-X resulted in the rescue of the MSV genome coated with the envelope of the infecting helper virus. The spontaneous release of the endogenous CCC virus from cat cells resulted also in the rescue of MSV(CCC) (25).

Flat clones were obtained from human cells especially after IdUrd pretreatment. These were grown to culture and the flattest clones were recloned several times. Despite their flat appearance, these cells yielded MSV after MuLV infection in all cases indicating that only cell morphology was affected. Additionally on prolonged cultivation these flatter variants segregated typical human transformed S+L- cells.

The feline MSV transformed cells could at times release the endogenous CCC virus. The CCC releasing and nonreleasing cloned, MSV transformed cell derivatives were examined for the appearance of flat variants. These occurred at a high frequency of about ∿0.1 in the 8C subline and only rarely <0.01 in the 6D subline. Six such flat variants were examined and found negative for MSV rescue by FeLV infection, susceptible to retransformation by MSV in several helper virus envelopes but not by MSV coated with the xenotropic endogenous CCC virus. These flat variants lost the MuLV gs-1 antigen which was the MSV marker in the cat cell.

DISCUSSION OF PRESENT STATUS OF REVERSION

In S+L- cells, the control of reversion from transformed state achieved by well defined genomes native to

the species is apparently a function of both the viral
genome and the cell because cloned mouse cell sublines
initially transformed by the identical MSV genome can
diverge to yield hundredfold differences in reversion
frequency (11). The state of integration of the MSV
genome may also be complicated. A lack of permanent
chromosomal attachment of the MSV genome may result in a
relatively high frequency of revertants with an MSV genome
in a temporarily disconnected state as has been seen in
bacteriophage systems (32). Occurrence of back-transformation in S+L- revertants indicates that the MSV genome
must have persisted in at least some revertants in a
nonrescuable form (11) and that cellular control leads to
phenotypic suppression of the MSV genome.

In contrast, the revertants from Ki-BALB cells
display properties which are compatible with a loss of
some or all of the MSV genome. No spontaneous back-transformation was ever observed in Ki-BALB revertants. Susceptibility of Ki-BALB revertants to Ki-MSV was not always
increased. Reversion of Ki-BALB cells to flat morphology
resulted in a decrease in chromosome number. Chemicals
which significantly increase reversion frequency from S+L-
cells have no effect on the present Ki-BALB cells.

Retransformation of S+L- revertants by M-MSV can give
rise to several complex functional states despite repet-
itive cycles of cloning. A second cycle of MSV transformation apparently destabilizes cellular control over
transforming genome, and the cell is apparently unable
to achieve further cycles of reversion.

The failure to isolate revertants from human S+L-
cells suggests that the MSV genome, which in its native
system can form a less firm association with the cell
may be, nevertheless, capable of forming a heritable and
essentially irreversible interaction in one of the heterologous systems but not in another heterologous cell
system.

The molecular information of the Ki-MSV genome
apparently does not exist in its entirety in the normal
mouse cell (33), and both human and cat cells don't seem

to harbor murine C-type virus information (unpublished). Thus all of the above systems can now be dissected to see whether reversion is in all cases a phenotypic control problem or whether an actual physical eviction of the transforming genome can take place.

REFERENCES

1. M. C. Weiss, B. Ephrussi and L. Scaletta, Proc. Nat. Acad. Sci. U.S. 59, 1132 (1968).
2. R. E. Pollack, H. Green and G. J. Todaro, Proc. Nat. Acad. Sci. U.S. 60, 126 (1968).
3. Z. Rabinowitz and L. Sachs, Nature 220, 1203 (1968).
4. G. Martin and I. Macpherson, J. Virol. 3, 146 (1969).
5. I. Macpherson, Science 148, 1731 (1965).
6. R. H. Bassin, N. Tuttle and P. J. Fischinger, Int. J. Cancer 6, 95 (1970).
7. R. H. Bassin, L. A. Phillips, M. J. Kramer, D. K. Haapala, P. T. Peebles, S. Nomura and P. J. Fischinger Proc. Nat. Acad. Sci. U.S. 68, 1520 (1971).
8. P. J. Fischinger, W. Schäfer and E. Seifert, Virology 47, 229 (1972).
9. P. J. Fischinger, S. Nomura, P. T. Peebles, D. K. Haapala and R. H. Bassin, Science 176, 1033 (1972).
10. S. Nomura, P. J. Fischinger, C. F. T. Mattern, P. T. Peebles, R. H. Bassin and G. P. Friedman, Virology 50, 51 (1972).
11. S. Nomura, P. J. Fischinger, C. F. T. Mattern, B. I. Gerwin and K. J. Dunn, Virology 56, 152 (1973).
12. P. J. Fischinger, S. Nomura, N. Tuttle-Fuller and K. J. Dunn, Virology In press (1974).
13. S. A. Aaronson and C. A. Weaver, J. Gen. Virol. 13, 245 (1971).
14. S. A. Aaronson, Proc. Nat. Acad. Sci. U.S. 68, 3069 (1971).
15. J. L. Jainchill, S. A. Aaronson and G. J. Todaro, J. Virol. 4, 549 (1969).
16. S. A. Aaronson and G. J. Todaro, J. Cell Physiol. 72, 141 (1968).
17. H. Duc-Nguyen, E. N. Rosenblum and R. F. Zeigel, J. Bacteriol. 92, 1133 (1966).
18. J. Svoboda, Nature 186, 980 (1960).
19. S. Nomura, K. J. Dunn and P. J. Fischinger, Nature 246, 213 (1973).

20. P. J. Fischinger, C. O. Moore and T. E. O'Connor, J. Nat. Cancer Inst. 42, 605 (1969).
21. W. Schäfer, P. J. Fischinger, J. Lange and L. Pister, Virology 47, 197 (1972).
22. W. P. Rowe, W. E. Pugh and J. W. Hartley, Virology 42, 1136 (1970).
23. R. H. Bassin, N. Tuttle and P. J. Fischinger, Nature 229, 564 (1971).
24. J. W. Hartley and W. P. Rowe, Proc. Nat. Acad. Sci. U.S. 55, 780 (1966).
25. P. J. Fischinger, P. T. Peebles, S. Nomura and D. K. Haapala, J. Virol. 11, 978 (1973).
26. P. T. Peebles, R. H. Bassin, D. K. Haapala, L. A. Phillips, S. Nomura and P. J. Fischinger, J. Virol. 8, 690 (1971).
27. D. R. Lowy, W. P. Rowe, N. Teich and J. W. Hartley, Science 174, 155 (1971).
28. N. Teich, D. R. Lowy, J. W. Hartley and W. P. Rowe, Virology 51, 163 (1973).
29. J. W. Hartley, P. W. Rowe, W. I. Capps and R. J. Huebner, Proc. Nat. Acad. Sci. U.S. 53, 931 (1965).
30. J. Ross, E. M. Scolnick, G. J. Todaro and S. A. Aaronson, Nature New Biol. 231, 163 (1971).
31. P. T. Peebles, P. J. Fischinger, R. H. Bassin and A. G. Papageorge, Nature New Biol. 242, 98 (1973).
32. E. A. Adelberg and P. Bergquist, Proc. Nat. Acad. Sci. U.S. 69, 206 (1972).
33. E. M. Scolnick, E. Rands, D. Williams and W. P. Parks, J. Virol. 12, 458 (1973).

Table 1

PROPERTIES OF SPONTANEOUS REVERTANTS FROM MOUSE 3T3FL DERIVED S+L- CELLS

	Normal 3T3FL cells	S+L- cells	Revertants
Morphology	Flat	Transformed	Flat
Average cell density	$6 \times 10^4/\text{cm}^2$	$2.5 \times 10^5/\text{cm}^2$	$3 \times 10^4/\text{cm}^2$
Cloning in soft agar	0.002%	11%	0.001-0.4%
"C" type particles	-	+	-
MuLV gs-1 (C.F.)	-	+	+ or -
Reverse transcriptase	-	+	-
MSV rescue by MuLV	-	$>10^5$FFU/ml	-
Inducibility by IdUrd	-	-	-
Agglutinability by Con. A	-	+	+
Susceptibility to MSV	Standard	Unknown	Increased
Susceptibility to MuLV	Standard	Normal to increased	Increased
Chromosome number	Standard	Decreased	Increased

Table 2

PROPERTIES OF SPONTANEOUS REVERTANTS FROM Ki-BALB CELLS

	Normal BALB/3T3 cells	Ki-BALB cells	Revertants
Morphology	Flat	Transformed	Flat
Average cell density	$1.3 \times 10^5/\text{cm}^2$	$5.6 \times 10^5/\text{cm}^2$	$8.5 \times 10^4/\text{cm}^2$
Cloning in soft agar	0.04%	28.8%	0.1-22.9%
"C" type particles	-	-	-
MuLV gs-1 (C.F.)	-	-	-
Reverse transcriptase	-	-	-
MSV rescue by MuLV	-	10^5 FFU/ml	-
MSV induction by IdUrd	-	10^{2-3} FFU/ml	-
MuLV induction by IdUrd	-	+	+
Agglutinability by Con. A	-	+	+
Susceptibility to MSV	Standard	Unknown	Decreased or increased
Susceptibility to MuLV	Standard	Decreased	Decreased
Chromosome number	Standard	Increased	Standard
Tumorigenicity	-	+	Markedly decreased

Table 3

PROPERTIES OF MOUSE S+L- CELL DERIVED REVERTANTS RETRANSFORMED BY M-MSV OR Ki-MSV

	S+L- type			MSV+ type		NP^a type
	$m1SR^{m1}$	$m1SR^{m3}$	$m3SR^{mw}$	$m3SR^{mw}$	$m1SR^{m3}$	$m3SR^{k}$
	"13"	"411"	"101"	"102"	"91"	"382"
MSV rescue by MuLV	+	+	+	NA^b	NA	+
Presence of MuLV	-	-	-	±	±	-
Infectious MSV	-	-	-	+	+	-
"C" type particles	NT^c	+	+	+	+	-^{d}
MSV induction by IdUrd	+	-	±	NA	NA	+
MuLV gs-1	+	+	+	+	+	+
Reversion to flat no MSV rescue	-	-	-	-	-	+

^{a}Nonproducer

^{b}Not applicable

^{c}Not tested

^{d}Searched for at least 2 hrs.

Tables 1, 2, and 3. A summary of properties displayed by representative sublines of S+L- and Ki-BALB revertants, and MSV retransformed S+L- revertants. MuLV gs antigen(s) was assayed either by complement fixation or immuno-diffusion. C-type particle presence was detected by electron microscopy. Tests for infectious MSV both after MuLV infection or IdUrd treatment was performed on mouse, rat, cat and human cells. Infectious MuLV content was generally assayed both on S+L- and XC cells. Concanavalin A was used at the contrations of 100-500 µg/ml.

RECOMBINANTS OF AVIAN TUMOR VIRUSES:
AN ANALYSIS OF THEIR RNA

Peter Duesberg, Karen Beemon, Michael Lai[*] and Peter K. Vogt[*]

Department of Molecular Biology
and Virus Laboratory
University of California
Berkeley, California 94720

and

[*]Department of Microbiology
University of Southern California
School of Medicine
Los Angeles, California 90033

ABSTRACT. The RNAs of several avian tumor virus recombinants which had inherited their focus forming ability from a sarcoma virus and the host range marker from a leukosis virus were investigated. Electrophoresis and analysis of oligonucleotide fingerprints showed that the cloned sarcoma virus recombinants contained only size class a RNA, although they had acquired a marker which resided on class b RNA in the leukosis virus parent. Class a RNA of different recombinant clones, derived from the same pair of parental viruses and selected for the same biological markers, differed slightly in electrophoretic mobility from each other and from the parental sarcoma virus. Small electrophoretic differences were also observed between the class a RNAs of various strains of avian sarcoma viruses and between class b RNAs of leukosis viruses, but these minor variations in RNA size were not related to the size of recombinant RNAs derived from these viruses.

Recombinants of the same cross and selected for the same pair of markers were also found to have different fingerprints of RNase T1-resistant oligonucleotides. The average complexity of the 60-70S RNA prepared from wild type sarcoma viruses was estimated to correspond to 2.7×10^6 daltons, suggesting that the genome of RNA tumor viruses is polyploid.

All these observations led us to propose that recombination among avian tumor viruses occurred by crossing over between homologous pieces of nucleic acid.

INTRODUCTION

Nondefective avian sarcoma viruses can undergo high frequency genetic recombination with avian leukosis viruses
(1,2,3). Since the 60-70S RNA of avian tumor viruses consists
of several pieces (4), it appeared likely that this recombination represented reassortment of markers situated on different genome subunits. However preliminary electrophoretic
analysis of the RNA from a recombinant between PR-B sarcoma
and RAV-3 leukosis virus led us to propose that recombinants
between avian tumor viruses originate from crossing over (5,6).
This proposal was based on the following argument: Cloned
nondefective sarcoma viruses contain only 30-40S RNA of size
class a. The 30-40S pieces of leukosis viruses are of the
smaller size class b. In a cross between PR-B sarcoma and
RAV-3 leukosis virus, the recombinant is selected for the
focus forming ability of the sarcoma virus linked to the host
range marker of the leukosis virus, thus combining markers
which on parental RNAs are situated on size a and b molecules
respectively. However, the RNA of the PR-B x RAV-3 recombinant contained only class a pieces, and thus the leukosis-
derived marker must have become incorporated into class a RNA.
To distinguish better between reassortment and crossing
over, additional recombinants which had inherited the focus
forming marker from a sarcoma and the host range marker from
a leukosis virus were investigated. The RNAs of recombinants
and of parental viruses were compared with respect to electrophoretic mobility, RNase T1 fingerprint pattern, and genetic
complexity. The results favor crossing over and suggest that
the genome of RNA tumor viruses may be polyploid.

RESULTS

THE RNAs OF SEVERAL RECOMBINANT SARCOMA VIRUSES
OBTAINED FROM DIFFERENT HOST RANGE CROSSES

Figure 1A shows an electropherogram of heat–dissociated
60-70S RNA from a recombinant between the focus forming marker
of PR-A and the host range marker of RAV-2. This recombinant
contained only 30-40S RNA of class a, which coincided with the
class a RNA of the PR-C standard (the latter showed a class b
component as well, probably representing a transformation-
defective segregant which had formed during nonclonal passage
of this virus stock) (5,7,8). The RNA of a recombinant between PR-B focus formation and RAV-1 host range was co-
electrophoresed with the PR-A x RAV-2 recombinant of Figure
1A, and the electropherogram is presented in Figure 1B. Both
viruses contained only 30-40S RNA of size class a. Five

other recombinants between the focus forming marker of a sarcoma and the host range marker of a leukosis virus were studied and found to contain only class a RNA. Some of these recombinants showed the presence of class a and class b RNA initially; however, subsequent cloning eliminated class b RNA. We conclude that probably all recombinants carrying the focus forming marker of a sarcoma and the host range marker of a leukosis virus contain only 30-40S RNA of class a.

FURTHER EVIDENCE FOR THE ABSENCE OF CLASS b RNA FROM THE 60-70S COMPLEX OF SARCOMA VIRUS RECOMBINANTS

Heated 60-70S RNA of the recombinants investigated contains, in addition to a major component of 30-40S RNA, minor heterogeneous RNA species of variable concentrations (Figs. 1-4). Therefore, it may be argued that these minor RNAs are distinct subgenomic fragments, including class b RNA of the parental leukosis virus perhaps acquired by reassortment. To test this possibility, heat-dissociated 60-70S ^{32}P RNA of PR-A x RAV-2 (Fig. 1A) was fractionated by sedimentation. Fractions comprising the 30-40S RNA species and fractions comprising the minor heterogenous species sedimenting at <30S and >10S were pooled separately (Fig. 2A) and studied chemically. A sensitive method for partial sequence comparison of RNAs has been developed by Brownlee and Sanger (9) and is based on the electrophoretic and chromatographic properties of RNase T1-resistant oligonucleotides. The technique has been used recently to compare tumor virus RNAs (8). It is shown in Figs. 2B and 2C that the fingerprints of RNA pool 1 (>30S) and of RNA pool 2 (<30S and >10S) were indistinguishable. We conclude that the minor heterogenous RNA species obtained after heat-dissociation of 60-70S RNA consist predominantly of degraded 30-40S RNA of size class a rather than of chemically distinct RNA species. However, the presence of low (<10%) concentrations of small RNA species unrelated to 30-40S RNA cannot be excluded by this experiment.

DIFFERENT RECOMBINANTS DERIVED FROM THE SAME PAIR OF PARENTAL VIRUSES AND SELECTED FOR THE SAME MARKERS HAVE RNAs OF DIFFERENT SIZE

Only two (host range and focus forming markers) of presumably several genes, which may be exchanged between leukosis and sarcoma viruses, have been selected for in the recombinants studied here. If crossing over takes place between RNA tumor virus genomes, it may theoretically occur at any point on the genetic map between the focus forming and the host range markers. In this case, the RNAs of recombinants selected for the same markers, but derived from different crossover events, could differ in their sequences. The first indication of such a difference was the observation that the 30-40S RNA of a **recombinant** between PR-B and RAV-3 (PR-B x RAV-3 #1) had a lower **electrophoretic** mobility and was therefore probably larger than the RNA of parental PR-B (Fig. 3A). The RNA of other preparations of this recombinant was also larger than class a RNA of PR-C and of another recombinant, PR-A x RAV-2 (Figs. 3C,E). By contrast class a RNAs of two different preparations of PR-B (Fig. 3B), class a RNAs of PR-B and PR-C (Fig. 3D), as well as class a RNA of PR-B and of PR-A x RAV-2 (Fig. 3F) were not distinguishable under our conditions. The RNAs of other recombinant clones between the focus forming marker of PR-B and the host range marker of RAV-3 fell into 3 electrophoretic classes: (i) PR-B x RAV-3 #2 had a lower mobility than parental class a RNA of PR-B (Fig. 4A). (ii) PR-B x RAV-3 #3 had a higher mobility than parental RNA (Fig. 4B). This recombinant was produced by transformed cells in 10-20 fold lower titers than other sarcoma viruses, perhaps indicating a defective replicating function. (iii) PR-B x RAV-3 #4 had practically the same mobility as parental PR-B RNA (Fig. 4C). These experiments indicate that the primary structure of recombinant RNAs differs from that of parental RNA.

The apparent molecular weight by which certain recombinant RNAs differ from parental, wild type RNA is estimated to be around 70,000 daltons on the following basis: The electrophoretic differences observed between RNAs were ± one fraction (Figs. 3,4). Class a and class b RNA differ by about 5 fractions under the same condition (*cf* Figs. 1,3) (5,10). The difference between a and b was estimated to be about 350,000 daltons (10). Thus, certain recombinant RNAs differ from wild type RNA by about one-fifth of that or 70,000 daltons. The size differences observed among the RNAs of distinct recombinants were stable after several successive clonings. This suggests that the size variations are not likely to be host modifications similar to those observed earlier in two specific cases which were not stable on passage of the virus in different cells (5).

THE EXACT SIZE OF RECOMBINANT RNA CANNOT BE PREDICTED FROM THE SIZE OF PARENTAL RNAs

Class a RNAs of different nondefective sarcoma viral strains were shown to differ electrophoretically by about one fraction (5); likewise class b RNAs of different leukosis

viruses differ slightly if compared by this method (Fig. 5).
Since the class a RNAs of PR-A, PR-B and PR-C are all electrophoretically indistinguishable (Fig. 3, ref. 5) but the
class b RNAs of RAV-1, RAV-2 and RAV-3 used to form recombinants with these sarcoma viruses are different, it appeared
possible that a direct correlation existed between the size
of class b RNA in the parental leukosis virus and the size of
class a RNA in the recombinant virus. For instance, it was
found that compared to a class b RNA standard (tdPR-C), the
RNAs of RAV-1 and of RAV-2 are slightly larger, while the RNA
of RAV-3 is the same size as the standard. Yet, the RNAs of
two recombinants between PR-B and RAV-3 (#1, Fig. 3 and #2,
Fig. 4 respectively) were actually larger than a recombinant
between PR-A and RAV-2 (cf Figs. 1,3) and a recombinant between PR-B and RAV-1 (cf Fig. 1). Moreover, it was shown
that class a RNAs of different recombinant clones between the
focus forming marker of PR-B and the host range marker of
RAV-3 have different mobilities. It follows that the exact
size of class a RNAs of different sarcoma virus recombinants
cannot be predicted from the known sizes of the parental RNAs.
This observation could be explained if some crossovers occurred at points of the parental genomes which were not strictly
homologous, leading to the acquisition or loss of small
stretches of genetic material in the recombinants (unequal
crossing over).

FINGERPRINT ANALYSES OF SARCOMA VIRUS RECOMBINANTS DERIVED
FROM THE SAME PAIR OF PARENTAL VIRUSES
AND SELECTED FOR THE SAME MARKERS

If crossing over is responsible for the small electrophoretic differences observed among the class a RNAs of four
recombinants between PR-B and RAV-3, it would be expected
that these RNAs also differ in their sequences. This possibility was tested by fingerprinting the RNAs of these four
recombinants of the PR-B x RAV-3 cross (cf Figs. 3,4). It is
apparent that their oligonucleotide patterns are very similar
but differ from each other in at least 2-3 out of about 20
major RNase T1-resistant oligonucleotide spots (Fig. 6A-D).
Some spots which are found in one but not in all other recombinants are indicated by arrows. The pattern of wild type
PR-B is shown in Fig. 6E and that of RAV-3 in Fig. 6F. Their
patterns differ from those of the recombinants more extensively than the recombinant patterns differ from each other.
Although differences observed by fingerprinting are only
qualitative (8), it may be concluded that the recombinants
analyzed differ in RNA sequences. This observation supports
the possibility that crossing over points between focus

forming and host range markers are not at a fixed location.

We have not determined in detail which of the large oligonucleotides of the four PR-B x RAV-3 recombinants are derived unchanged from either parental viral strain and which of these oligonucleotides contain new sequences representing sites at which crossing over may have taken place. However, at least one spot of recombinant #3, circled in Fig. 6C, appeared to be new and not to have a homologous counterpart in either parental virus (Figs. 6E,F). This spot as well as some others in Fig. 6A-D had lower intensities than neighboring spots of presumably similar size (9). This may be due to incomplete transfer of the oligonucleotides from the cellulose acetate strip used for electrophoresis to the DEAE-cellulose thin layer used for homochromatography (9). It may also reflect inhomogeneities in the RNAs. Further work, including complete transfer of oligonucleotides, as used in Figs. 6E,F, will be required to resolve this problem.

THE 60-70S TUMOR VIRUS RNA APPEARS TO BE LARGELY POLYPLOID

If the 30-40S subunits of a given 60-70S tumor virus RNA were identical and the 70S RNA represented a polyploid genome, stable recombinants could arise only by crossing over. The genetic complexity of the 60-70S RNA should then be equal to that of each of the 30-40S pieces. However, if 60-70S RNA were haploid, its complexity would be higher than that of an individual 30-40S subunit. The complexity of an RNA species uniformly labeled with ^{32}P can be estimated if the sizes of several oligonucleotides derived from it are determined, and the radioactivity of these oligonucleotides is compared with the total radioactivity in the intact RNA molecule (11). The average complexity of PR-B RNA as determined from about 20 RNase T1-resistant oligonucleotides, resolved as described in Fig. 6E, amounted to 2.7×10^6 daltons (Table 1). This is in good agreement with the lower of several molecular weight estimates for viral 30-40S subunits obtained by other methods (10). Preliminary experiments suggest that the RNA of a recombinant has a similar complexity. Further work will be required to explain the fluctuations ($\sigma = \pm 0.48 \times 10^6$) observed among complexity estimates based on different oligonucleotides. These may be due to inhomogeneities of the 60-70S ^{32}P RNA prepared from virus harvested at 12 hr intervals (12, 13, 14). Oligonucleotides deriving from preferentially degraded sequences of 60-70S RNA would lead to a higher complexity estimate and oligonucleotides derived from sequences of partially degraded RNA which associate preferentially with 60-70S RNA would lead to a lower complexity estimate. Nevertheless we may conclude that the RNase T1-resistant sequences of the 60-70S tumor virus RNA have an approximate complexity of not more than 3×10^6. Thus, the 60-70S viral RNA appears largely polyploid and consequently recombination is likely to involve crossing over.

DISCUSSION

Recombination involves crossing over. Sarcoma virus recombinants, derived from a sarcoma virus parent with only class a RNA and a leukosis virus parent with only class b RNA, were found to contain only, or almost only, class a RNA. The class a RNA of certain recombinants was either larger or smaller than the parental class a RNA. Further, oligonucleotide patterns of recombinants, presumably derived from different recombination events but selected for the same markers, differed among themselves, and differed even more extensively from those of parental RNA. The 60-70S RNAs of wild type and of recombinant viruses appeared to be largely or completely polyploid. The sum of all these observations favors the conclusion that at least some of the recombination among avian tumor viruses involves crossing over.

If recombinants arose by reassortment of segments in a haploid genome, these recombinants should show only a limited number of fingerprint patterns. In recombinants selected for the same markers the two segments containing these markers must be the same. Sequence diversity could still be caused by genome segments not carrying the selected marker, and of these there are at most two, to give a total of four segments per genome (4). The number of possible variations is then four; however, if there are only three segments per genome the same recombinants could occur in only two fingerprint variations. Since we have already observed four distinct fingerprint patterns in the PR-B x RAV-3 cross, our data would agree with reassortment only if the genome has four (but not three or two) genetically unique segments. Even in the case of four segments there is only a 9% chance of finding all four possible fingerprint patterns in the first four recombinants tested.

Disregarding our suggestive evidence on polyploidy the remaining data on recombinant RNAs could be reconciled with reassortment, if we make the *ad hoc* assumption that class b RNA of leukosis virus is augmented by cellular RNA sequences to yield a class a molecule when it becomes incorporated into a sarcoma virus in the process of recombination. This augmentation by cellular RNA would have to be genetically stable. Such a process could generate the observed size and sequence diversity and cannot be definitely ruled out on the basis of present data.

Is host modification involved in the formation of recombinant RNA? Small differences in the size of class *a* RNA can be observed among recombinants selected for the same markers. These differences could result from host modification of the viral RNA rather than from unequal crossing over. Such modifications may include various degrees of polyadenylation (15) or addition of cellular sequences acquired at the chromosomal sites at which viral DNA is thought to integrate into cellular DNA. Although such changes could account for the electrophoretic differences observed among different recombinant RNAs, it is unlikely that these variations in size amounting to only ±2% of the RNA are also responsible for the changes observed in fingerprint patterns.

Alternatively recombination between exogenous tumor viruses could include interactions with endogenous tumor viruses present in all normal chicken cells (16). This type of "host modification" has not been tested for by our experiments. However, recombination with endogenous virus has been observed only in helper factor positive cells, in which endogenous virus is at least partially expressed (3) but not in the helper factor negative cells used to prepare our recombinants. Also, if genetic interaction with an endogenous virus were responsible for some of the new properties of recombinant RNAs, it would be difficult to explain why such modification of RNA is not regularly observed in single infection.

What is the mechanism of tumor virus recombination? No direct answer can be given to this question from our experiments, except that crossing over appears to occur. Since there is no precedent and no plausible molecular mechanism for high frequency crossing over between viruses containing single-stranded RNA, it appears likely that recombination among avian RNA tumor viruses involves the synthesis of the DNA provirus (17,18). The high frequency recombination among RNA tumor viruses could then be a direct consequence of polyploidy. The progeny of a doubly infected cell would be largely heterozygous, containing different genomes in a 60-70S complex. Transcription of such a heterozygous RNA into DNA would bring homologous DNAs together and could increase the chances of crossing over (3,6,17).

LIST OF VIRUS ABBREVIATIONS

PR-A: Prague Rous sarcoma virus, subgroup A.
PR-B: Prague Rous sarcoma virus, subgroup B.

PR-C: Prague Rous sarcoma virus, subgroup C.
*td*PR-C: Transformation defective variant derived from PR-C.
RAV-1:   Rous associated virus, type 1, subgroup A.
RAV-2:   Rous associated virus, type 2, subgroup B.
RAV-3:   Rous associated virus, type 3, subgroup A.

ACKNOWLEDGMENTS

We thank Sunny Kim, Marie Stanley and Philip Harris for excellent help with these experiments. The work was supported by Public Health Service research grants CA 11426 and CA 13213 from the National Cancer Institute and by the Cancer Program-National Cancer Institute, under Contract No. N01 CP 43212 and Contract No. N01 CP 43242.

REFERENCES

1. Vogt, P. K. (1971). *Virology 46*, 947-952.
2. Kawai, S. and Hanafusa, H. (1972). *Virology 49*, 37-44.
3. Weiss, R. A., Mason, W. and Vogt, P. K. (1973). *Virology 52*, 535-552.
4. Duesberg, P. H. (1970). in "Current Topics in Microbiology and Immunology" *51*, 79-114.
5. Duesberg, P. H. and Vogt, P. K. (1973). *Virology 54*, 207-219.
6. Vogt, P. K. and Duesberg, P. H. (1973). in "Virus Research" eds. Fox, C. F. and Robinson, W. S., Academic Press, New York, pp. 505-511.
7. Martin, G. S. and Duesberg, P. H. (1971). *Virology 47*, 494-497.
8. Lai, M. M-C., Duesberg, P. H., Horst, J. and Vogt, P. K. (1973). *Proc. Nat. Acad. Sci. 70*, 2266-2270.
9. Brownlee, G. G. and Sanger, F. (1969). *Europ. J. Biochem 11*, 393-399.
10. Duesberg, P. H. and Vogt, P. K. (1973). *J. Virology 12*, 594-599.
11. Fiers, W., Lepoutre, L. and Vandendriesche, L. (1965). *J. Mol. Biol. 13*, 432-450.
12. Duesberg, P. H. and Cardiff, B. (1968). *Virology 36*, 696-700.
13. Bader, J. P. and Steck, T. C. (1969). *J. Virol. 4*, 454-459.
14. Erikson, R. L. (1969). *Virology 37*, 124-131.
15. Lai, M. M-C. and Duesberg, P. H. (1972). *Nature 235*, 383-386.
16. Weiss, R. A. (1971). in "RNA Viruses and Host Genome in Oncogenesis" eds. Emmelot, P. and Bentvelzen, P., pp. 117-135, North Holland.

17. Vogt, P. K.(1973). in "Possible Episomes in Eukaryotes," Proceedings of the Fourth Lepetit Colloquium, ed. Silvestri, L., North Holland, pp. 35-41.
18. Weiss, R. A.(1973). in "Possible Episomes in Eukaryotes," Proceedings of the Fourth Lepetit Colloquium, ed. Silvestri, L., North Holland, pp. 130-141.

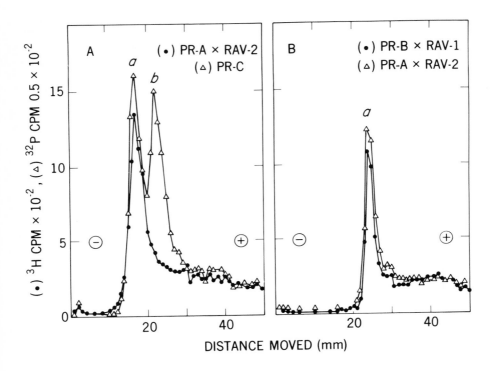

Fig. 1. Electrophoresis of heat-dissociated 60-70S RNA of two cloned recombinant sarcoma viruses, PR-A x RAV-2 and PR-B x RAV-1. (A) Appropriate amounts of radio-labeled PR-A x RAV-2 RNA and PR-C RNA were mixed and heated in electrophoresis sample buffer and subjected to electrophoresis in 2% polyacrylamide as described (5). PR-C had not been cloned recently and contained both class a and class b RNA species. (B) A mixture of the RNAs of two sarcoma virus recombinants PR-B x RAV-1 and PR-A x RAV-2 was analyzed as described for A.

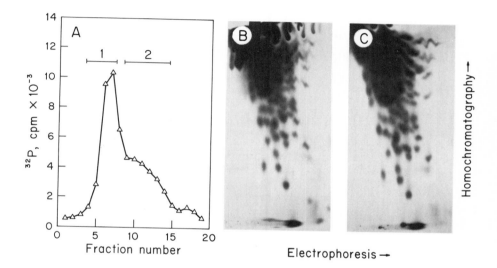

Fig. 2. Sedimentation and fingerprint analyses of heat-dissociated 60-70S ^{32}P-RNA (approx. 2 x 10^6 cpm) of a recombinant sarcoma virus PR-A x RAV-2, harvested at 3-5 hour intervals from infected cells. (A) RNA in 300 μl was heat-dissociated as described for Fig. 1. After addition of NaCl to 0.1 M the solution was layered on a 15-30% glycerol gradient containing 0.1 M NaCl, 0.01 M Tris HCl pH 7.4, 1 mM EDTA and 0.1% sodiumdodecylsulfate. Centrifugation was for 105 minutes at 50,000 rpm in a Spinco SW 50.1 rotor at 20°C. Fractions indicated by the bars in Fig. 2A were combined in two pools and the RNA was ethanol-precipitated. Fingerprinting of RNA pools 1 (B) and 2 (C) was as described previously (8).

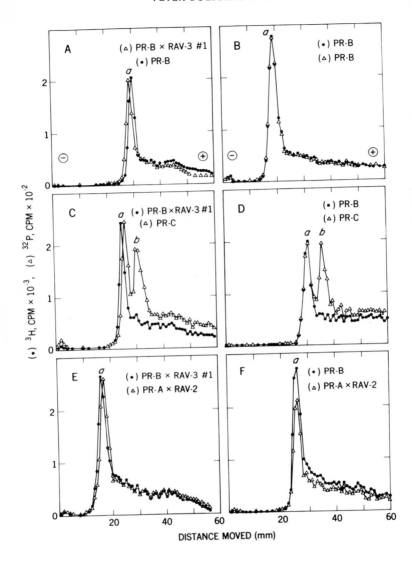

Fig. 3.   Heat-dissociated 60-70S RNAs of different preparations of a cloned recombinant sarcoma virus, PR-B x RAV-3
#1 and of several other wild type and recombinant sarcoma
viruses after electrophoresis as described for Fig. 1.   The
experiments were carried out to demonstrate that class *a* RNA
of PR-B x RAV-3 #1 had a lower electrophoretic mobility than
other class *a* RNAs as described in the text.

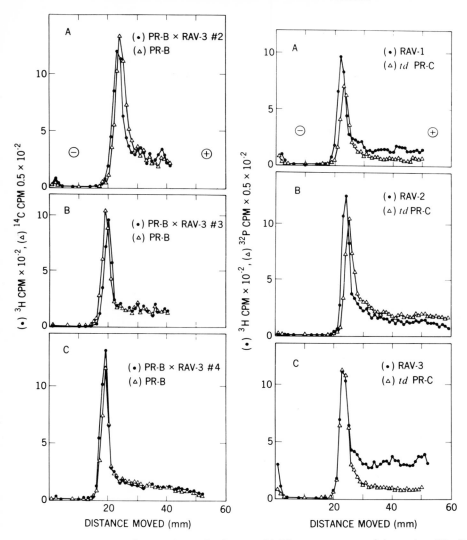

Fig. 4. The RNAs of three different recombinants PR-B x RAV-3 #2 (A), #3 (B) and #4 (C) after heat dissociation and electrophoresis with a standard of PR-B RNA. Conditions were as described for Fig. 1.

Fig. 5. The RNAs of three leukosis viruses RAV-1 (A), RAV-2 (B) and RAV-3 (C), used to form recombinants with PR RSV strains, after heat dissociation and electrophoresis with a standard of *td* PR-C RNA. Conditions were as described for Fig. 1.

Fig. 6. Fingerprint analyses of the RNase T1-digested
60-70S ^{32}P-RNAs of the four recombinants PR-B x RAV-3 #1 (A),
#2 (B), #3 (C) and #4 (D) as well as of PR-B (E) and RAV-3
(F). 60-70S ^{32}P-RNAs of virus harvested at 12 hour intervals
were digested and analyzed as described previously (8) except
that a 3% homo-mixture b (9) was used. The arrows in A-D indicate spots not found in all of the four recombinants
analyzed. The circled spot in C has no homologous counterpart in the patterns of either parental virus (E,F). A
schematic tracing of the large oligonucleotides of PR-B (E)
identifies spots which were analyzed as described in Table 1.

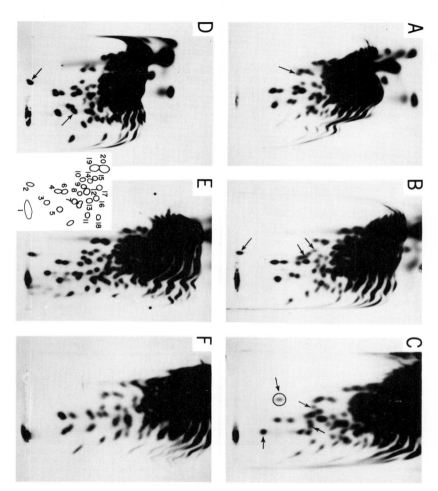

Electrophoresis →

Homochromatography →

TABLE 1

THE COMPLEXITY OF PR-B RNA[*] ESTIMATED FROM THE SIZES
OF RNASE T_1-RESISTANT OLIGONUCLEOTIDES

Oligonucleotide spot no.[†]	CPM		Approximate base composition		Calculated complexity of RNA in daltons $(\times 10^{-6})$	
	Exp.1	Exp.2	Exp.1	Exp.2	Exp.1	Exp.2
1	40,370	39,600	Poly A	Poly A	–	–[‡]
2	8,200	–	$(C_3A_7UG)_2$[§]	$(C_3A_6UG)_2$	3.2	2.9
3	6,500	–	$C_3A_3U_4G$	$C_4A_4U_4G$	1.8	2.1
4	6,060	4,900	$C_6A_4U_3G$	$C_5A_3U_2G$	2.5	2.1
5	7,900	–	$(C_3A_2U_3G)_2$	$(C_3A_2U_4G)_2$	2.4	2.7
6	5,890	4,800	$C_5A_3U_3G$	$C_4A_3U_2G$	2.2	1.9
7	7,050	–	$(C_3A_3U_3G)_2$	$(C_3A_3U_3G)_2$	3.0	3.0
8	5,470	–	$C_4A_4U_3G$	$C_4A_5U_3G$	2.4	2.6
9	4,560	–	$C_4A_3U_3G$	$C_5A_4U_3G$	2.6	3.1
10	4,160	–	$C_5A_3U_2G$	$C_6A_4U_2G$	2.8	3.3
11	4,660	–	C_3AU_5G	C_3AU_5G	2.3	2.3
12	9,000	–	$(C_5A_3U_4G)_2$	$(C_5A_4U_3G)_2$	3.1	3.1
13	5,250	4,500	$C_2A_3U_3G$	$C_3A_4U_3G$	1.8	2.3
14	4,490	–	$C_4A_3U_2G$	$C_5A_4U_2G$	2.4	2.9
15	3,880	–	C_3A_3UG	$C_4A_4U_2G$	2.2	3.0
16	4,150	4,300	C_4AU_3G	–	2.3	–
17	5,940	5,000	$C_3A_4U_3G$	–	1.8	–
18	4,580	–	$C_2A_2U_4G$	$C_3A_2U_6G$	2.1	2.8
19	10,800	8,800	$(C_5A_4UG)_3$	$(C_4A_4UG)_3$	3.3	3.1
20	11,900	9,200	$(C_4A_4UG)_3$	$(C_4A_5UG)_3$	2.7	3.3
				Average[¶]	2.6	2.8

[*] 60-70S ^{32}P-RNA derived from virus harvested at 12-hour intervals was prepared and exhaustively
digested with RNase T_1 as described (8). The digest was resolved by electrophoresis and, after
complete transfer to DEAE-cellulose, chromatographed as shown in Fig. 6. Two identical patterns
were made each using 3.34 x 10^6 cpm (Exp. 1) or 2.86 x 10^6 cpm (Exp. 2) of the digested RNA.
One pattern was used to determine the total radioactivity in a spot and the other to determine
base compositions. An average of 380 cpm/nucleotide was found in Exp. 1. Oligonucleotides were
eluted and base compositions determined by published procedures (9). Further details will be
described elsewhere (Beemon and Duesberg, in preparation). The complexity was calculated using an
average nucleotide MW of 323, calculated from the base composition of PR-B RNA (24.4% C,
23.8% A, 28.8% G, 23.0% U) and the known MW of the nucleotides.

[†] Numbers refer to diagram in Fig. 6E.

[‡] CPM from Exp. 1 and base compositions obtained in Exp. 2 were used in all calculations except
where CPM from Exp. 2 are shown.

[§] Specific activity indicates more than one G per oligonucleotide due to either 2 (or 3) unresolved
spots or to incompletely digested RNA. Heterogeneity of some spots is also suggested by their
autoradiographic appearance; see for example spots #12, 19 and 20.

[¶] Values of presumed multiple spots are considered multiply in the average.

CHARACTERISTICS OF CELLS TRANSFORMED
BY BRYAN ROUS SARCOMA VIRUS

John P. Bader* and Artrice V. Bader+

Chemistry Branch*
Viral Biology Section+
National Cancer Institute
National Institutes of Health
Bethesda, Maryland 20014

ABSTRACT. Cell transformation by the Bryan strain of Rous sarcoma virus (RSV-BH) is characterized by changes in size, density, and water content, in addition to changes in shape and intense cytoplasmic vacuolization. These observations suggest a role for water and cations in transformation, and a possible general sequence of metabolic events leading to malignancy in this system is proposed.

INTRODUCTION

Comparative studies on malignant and non malignant cells have revealed a host of biochemical differences between them, and for each difference an extrapolation to the physiological origin of the malignant process has been attempted. The types of experiments have evolved from the grossest comparisons of tumors and normal tissues, to tumors and tissues of tumor origin, to cells transformed in culture and their nontransformed counterparts, to the current analyses of cells which under some conditions are transformed but under other conditions are nontransformed. Concurrent with the experimental changes evolved changing interests in particular classes of biochemical molecules thought to be primary to the malignant process, until today, it probably can be said without great outcry, attention has focused on the glycosylated molecules of the cell surface membrane. The major difficulty in assigning a malignant role to a suspected molecule is the inability to locate that molecule within the sequence of metabolic changes which accompany the malignant process, i.e., to establish a cause-effect relationship with other biochemical changes.

Infection of chick embryo (CE) cells with the Bryan strain of Rous sarcoma virus (RSV-BH) induces several characteristic morphological changes, including rounding vacuolization and an apparent increase in size (1,2). A mutant of this virus (RSV-BH-Ta) has been isolated which induces similar changes at 37° but not at 41° (3,4). These morphological changes, which accompany changes in cellular growth properties, are not prevented by inhibition of DNA, RNA, or protein synthesis before and after shifting cells from 41° to 37°. Induction of certain metabolic changes, including increased hexose uptake and hyaluronate synthesis, require new RNA and protein synthesis (4), and in this way factors associated with the morphological changes can be distinguished from secondary induced changes.

An investigation into the nature of the morphological changes induced by RSV-BH is described here, and a model for a sequence of metabolic changes culminating in malignancy is outlined.

RESULTS

Morphological Changes. Differences in the morphology of CE cells and cells transformed by RSV-BH are shown in Fig. 1. Transformed cells are rounded or polygonal, appear larger, and are heavily vacuolated, in contrast to the spindle-shaped, smaller, nonvacuolated CE cells. Cells infected with RSV-BH-Ta resemble noninfected CE cells when grown at 41°, but at 37° are indistinguishable from cells transformed by RSV-BH (Fig. 1). The presence of Actino-mycin D, cycloheximide, or puromycin has no effect on the development of the morphological changes occurring after shifting RSV-BH-Ta infected cells from 41° to 37°. Vacuolization is the most obvious change, and is readily observed within 10 to 30 minutes after a temperature shift.

The Vacuoles. The initial observation of the cyto-plasmic vacuolization of Rous cells probably was made by Carrel (5) in 1925, and this vacuolization has been re-discovered about every decade thereafter without any additional information on the nature of the vacuoles or their contents. Electron microscopy of cells sectioned perpendicular to the plane of the cell monolayer (Fig. 2) showed that the vacuoles in fact were intracytoplasmic, and not merely indentations in the cell surface, or accumulations of material under the cell which might result in refractility. The vacuoles by lack of substance were distinguishable from lysosomes or phagocytic vacuoles. A trilaminar structure typical of cell membrane was found bounding the vacuoles. Such material often was more easily resolved in smaller vacuoles, suggesting that the membrane bounding the vacuole was distensible.

The failure of osmium tetroxide or lead acetate to stain the contents of the vacuoles in cell sections suggested that lipids and nucleic acids were absent, or were lost in the processing for electron microscopy. Histochemical staining of cells in monolayer failed to reveal neutral lipids, glycolipids, nucleic acids, proteins glycoproteins, glycosaminoglycans, or polysaccharides. The possibility of that these structures were gas vacuoles, analagous to those found in blue-green algae (6), was dispelled after the addition of neutral red to the cell culture medium. During subsequent incubation, neutral red was rapidly taken into cells and into the vacuoles, demonstrating that, whatever else was in the vacuoles, water was a major component.

The role of specific components of the cell growth medium (Eagle's MEM + 10% tryptose phosphate broth + 5% bovine fetal serum) in the vacuolization process was examined (Table 1). Neither tryptose phosphate broth nor amino acids-vitamins were needed for vacuolization to occur, and the presence of serum was slightly inhibitory. Deletion of glucose resulted in slightly less vacuolization but this decrease was enhanced proportional to the length of preincubation at 41° before shifting to 37°. The development of vacuoles, therefore, could occur in a simple salt solution (Earle's BSS) consisting of Na^+, K^+, Mg^{++}, Ca^{++}, Cl^-, $PO_4^=$, $SO^=$, and HCO_3^-.

Further reduction of components showed that neither HCO_3^- nor $SO_4^=$ were required for vacuolization, and a requirement for $PO_4^{\equiv}$ is questionable. No attempt has been made to eliminate Cl^- from the medium.

305

Among the cations only Ca^{++} was found unnecessary, although effects of deleting K$^+$ or Mg^{++} were variable (Table 2). When deletion of K$^+$ resulted in decreased vacuolization, addition of Rb$^+$ prevented the decrease. Replacement of Na$^+$ with isoosmotic sucrose induced vacuolization at 41°, and enhanced vacuolization at 37°, but replacement of Na$^+$ with Li$^+$ resulted in the complete failure of cells to form vacuoles. These results suggested that vacuolization was a specific response to a change in the cell affecting water and cation uptake.

Another factor found to influence the development of vacuoles was pH. Within the range pH 6.6 to 7.8 there was a progressive increase in vacuolization with increasing pH. The possible relationship of vacuolization and ion composition as a function of pH has not been examined.

Inhibitory effects of cyclic AMP phosphodiesterase inhibitors, dibutyryl cyclic AMP, adenosine, 3'-deoxyadenosine, 2'-deoxyadenosine and various adenine nucleotides on vacuolization have been observed. The reasons for such inhibition are obscure, but an involvement of cyclic AMP in the vacuolization process does not seem remote.

Size Changes. The apparent increase in size of transformed cells, observed by microscopy, was examined more objectively. Diameters of suspended cells were measured, and RSV-BH transformed cells were found to be substantially larger than nontransformed CE cells (Table 3). Likewise cells infected with RSV-BH-Ta were larger when incubated at 37° than when incubated at 41°. On the other hand, cells transformed by another strain of Rous sarcoma virus, the Schmidt-Ruppin strain (RSV-SR), do not usually become vacuolated or appear notably different in size from CE cells. These cells are only slightly larger in average diameter than CE cells.

The noted increase in diameter was confirmed in volume determinations (Table 3), where cells transformed by RSV-BH or RSV-BH-Ta were considerably larger than CE cells, RSV-BH-Ta infected cells incubated at 41°, or RSV-SR infected cells. A general increase in cell mass could account for only a part of the noted increases in sizes of transformed cells, since the density of protein per unit

306

volume of cell was less in the larger transformed cells than nontransformed or RSV-SR transformed cells.

Wet and dry weight determinations were then performed, and RSV-BH and RSV-BH-Ta transformed cells were found to contain a smaller proportion of the total weight as dry weight, i.e. contained more water, than nontransformed or RSV-SR cells (Table 3).

Density Changes. The increased water content of RSV-BH transformed cells was reflected in a decreased density of these cells when banded in density gradients of Dextran T 110 (0-18%). Although all cell groups presented broad banding patterns, the average densities of RSV-BH and RSV-BH-Ta (37°) cells was consistently less than the average densities of the other groups (Table 3).

Differences in densities of RSV-BH-Ta cells were observed within two hours after shifting from 41° to 37° and neither Actinomycin D nor cycloheximide prevented the decrease in density. Therefore, this property of the cells occurred without a requirement for RNA or protein synthesis.

Metabolic Changes. The foregoing observations suggested that an early event in the transformation of cells by RSV-BH was an increased accumulation of water. One might expect such an event to be accompanied by an alteration in cation uptake. A preliminary series of experiments was performed in an attempt to determine whether exogenous ion concentrations could affect the induction of increased hexose which is known to occur in RSV-BH-Ta cells after shifting from 41° to 37° (Table 4).

Substantial effects of deletion of Na^+, K^+, or Mg^{++} were found, all inhibiting the induction of increased ability to take up 2-deoxyglucose (a minimally metabolized glucose analogue). However, effects of these ion deletions were also seen in cells maintained at 41°, and the ionic environment may be important in the maintenance of glucose-transporting molecules as well as their induction. The failure of Li^+ to substitute for Na^+, coupled with the ability of Rb^+ to substitute for K^+, and a requirement for Mg^{++} suggests that Na^+-K^+ ATPase may be involved in the maintenance or enhanced ability of cells to take up hexose.

DISCUSSION

The results presented here suggest a possible physiological mechanism for malignancy in cells transformed by the Bryan high titer strain of Rous sarcoma virus. They are not intended to support a generalized mechanism of carcinogenesis, even to an extension to transformation by a related virus, the Schmidt-Ruppin strain of Rous sarcoma virus. RSV-BH cells in the process of transformation accumulate water. Vacuolization may be a response to increased cellular water, perhaps a mechanism for extrusion of excess water, and in this case probably is an appurtenance to the malignant process. However, uptake of water from physiological solutions is characteristically accompanied by Na^+, and increased cellular Na^+ could affect the transport of other cations, particularly K^+. Changes in intracellular ion concentrations could lead directly to changes in transcription, resulting in qualitative and/or quantitative changes in synthesized proteins, culminating in malignancy. This is not a new idea (7,8).

ACKNOWLEDGMENTS

The authors appreciate the technical assistance of David A. Ray, Nancy R. Brown, and Monica Bigelow in the performance of these experiments.

REFERENCES

1. A. Goldé, *Virology 16*, 9 (1962).
2. J.P. Bader, *Virology 48*, 494 (1972).
3. J.P. Bader and N.R. Brown, *Nature New Biol. 234*, 11 (1971).
4. J.P. Bader, *J. Virol. 10*, 267 (1972).
5. A. Carrel, *C.R. Soc. Biol., Paris 92*, 477 (1925).
6. A.E. Walsby, *Bact. Rev. 36*, 1 (1972).
7. C.D. Cone, *J. Theoret. Biol. 30*, 151 (1971).
8. C.D. Cone and M. Tangier, *Oncology 25*, 168 (1971).

TABLE 1

MEDIUM REQUIREMENTS FOR VACUOLIZATION AFTER A SHIFT OF
RSV–BH–Ta INFECTED CE CELLS FROM 41° TO 37°

Salts	Glucose	AA+vits.	Serum	TPB	41°	41°→37°
+	+	+	+	+	0[a]	+++[a]
+	+	+	+	−	0	+++
+	+	+	−	−	0	++++
+	+	−	−	−	0	++++
+	−	−	−	−	0	+++

Cells infected with RSV–BH–Ta after transfer were grown
for two days at 41°. Growth medium, consisting of Eagle's
MEM (Earle's salts + glucose + amino acids and vitamins),
10% tryptose phosphate broth (TPB), and 5% fetal bovine
serum, was removed. Fresh growth medium, or medium minus
one or more constituents was added. Cultures were
incubated 1 hour at 41°, then half were shifted to a 37°
incubator. Six hours later the degree of vacuolization
was assessed by phase contrast microscopy, and recorded.

[a]0 = no vacuoles; + = detectable vacuoles in less than 10%
of cells; ++ easily detectable in 5–20% of cells; +++ = in
20–50%; ++++ = in greater than 50%.

TABLE 2

CATION REQUIREMENTS FOR VACUOLIZATION AFTER A SHIFT
OF RSV–BH–Ta INFECTED CE CELLS FROM 41° TO 37°

Na^+	K^+	Mg^{++}	Ca^{++}	41°	41°→37°
+	+	+	+	0	+++
+	+	+	−	0	+++
+	+	−	+	0	++
+	−	−	+	0	++
+	−	+	+	0	++
+	−(+Rb^+)	+	+	0	+++
−(+sucrose)	+	+	+	+++	++++
−(+Li^+)	+	+	+	0	0

RSV–BH–Ta infected cells grown at 41° were rinsed, and
medium was replaced with Earle's BSS (containing glucose,
and the above cations + Cl^-, $PO_4^{\equiv}$, $SO_4^=$ and HCO_3^-) or replaced with BSS minus the appropriate cations.

TABLE 3

BIOPHYSICAL AND BIOCHEMICAL PARAMETERS OF NONTRANSFORMED
CELLS AND CELLS TRANSFORMED BY ROUS SARCOMA VIRUSES

	CE	RSV–BH	RSV–BH–Ta 41°	RSV–BH–Ta 37°	RSV–SR
Diameter, average (μm/cell)	19.2	27.4	19.9	25.8	21.2
Volume, average (cc x 10^9/cell)	2.54	5.94	3.44	5.10	3.64
Protein (μg x 10^4/cell)	2.53	4.30	3.00	3.50	2.72
(μg x 10^{-4}/cc cells)	11.4	7.7	10.2	8.6	10.6
% dry weight	16.9	11.6	16.5	12.7	16.1
Density	1.044	1.024	1.042	1.030	1.034

TABLE 4

Effect of deletion of exogenous cations from incubation medium on capacity for uptake of 2-deoxyglucose by RSV-BH-Ta cells.

	cpm x 10^{-2}/culture	
	41°	41°→37°
Salts + glucose	449	813
" minus K^+	360	567
" minus K^+ + Rb^+	410	756
" minus Na^+ + Li^+	300	463
" minus Mg^{++}	375	571
" minus Ca^{++}	460	830

RSV-BH-Ta cells were incubated for 5 hours in Earle's BSS or in BSS deficient in indicated ions. The solutions then were removed, and phosphate-buffered saline containing a full complement of ions plus 2-deoxyglucose-^{3}H (1 µCi/ plate) was added. After a 10 minute incubation at 39°, cultures were rinsed, 0.2% Triton X-100 was added to lyse cells, and radioactivity determined.

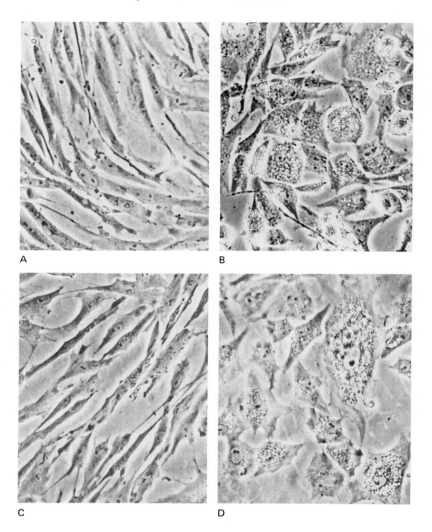

Legend to Fig. 1.

Phase contrast micrographs of cells in culture:
(A) Chick embryo (CE) cells
(B) CE cells transformed by RSV-BH
(C) CE cells infected with a mutant of RSV-BH,
     RSV-BH-Ta and grown at 41°
(D) Same as C, except grown overnight at 37°

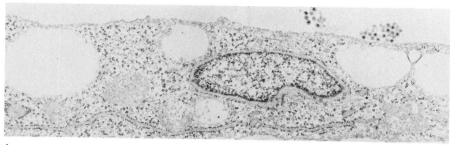

A

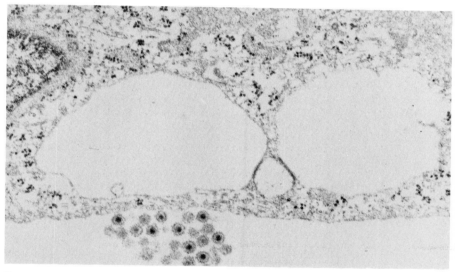

B

Legend to Fig. 2.

    Electron micrographs of cell infected with RSV-BH
displaying vacuoles:
(A) Cytoplasmic vacuolization
(B) Higher magnification of juxtaposed vacuoles
     and bounding membranes

PROTEASES ASSOCIATED WITH MALIGNANT TRANSFORMATION

D.B. Rifkin, N.B. Gilula, J.P. Quigley*, D. Loskutoff,
L. Ossowski, J.C. Unkeless, K. Danø and A. Piperno

Department of Chemical Biology
The Rockefeller University
New York, New York 10021

*Present address: Dept. of Microbiology and Immunology,
Downstate Medical Center, Brooklyn,
New York

ABSTRACT. We have examined the ability of transformed
cells to produce a proteolytic activity in vitro. The
nature of this activity, its association with malignancy,
and its meaning for the transformed phenotype have been
examined.

The ability of tumor cells and the inability of most
normal cells to digest fibrin clots has been well documented during the last fifty years (1, 2). However, the exact
nature of this process and the molecules involved were not
well characterized. Because of the possible significance
of such a biochemical difference between normal and transformed cells, the hydrolysis of fibrin by tumor cells has
been reinvestigated (3, 4).

The assay used is as follows (3): commercial preparations of bovine fibrinogen are purified by precipitation and then iodinated with ^{125}I, the excess ^{125}I is removed by dialysis of the reaction mixture, and known
amounts of ^{125}I-fibrinogen coated onto sterile petri dishes. The fibrinogen film is dried at 45°C overnight and
then converted into fibrin by incubation at 37°C with
Eagle's medium containing 2.5% fetal bovine serum for 2-5
hours. The ^{125}I-fibrinopeptides released during incubation are removed by washing each dish with buffer. The
^{125}I-fibrin which remains coated to the surface of the
petri dish after this treatment is insoluble and can only
be removed by acids, bases, or proteases. The fibrinolytic activity of normal or transformed cells, cellular
extracts or conditioned medium can be then assessed by
monitoring the release of ^{125}I-labelled material from the

surface of the petri dish into the supernatant liquid.

    The initial experiments indicated that cells trans-
formed by RSV, MSV or SV-40 generate a high level of fibrinolysis when grown on ^{125}I-fibrin films, whereas, the normal
parent cells do not (3, 4, 5). The level of proteolysis
is dependent upon the serum used for the growth of the
cells (3, 4, 5). Certain sera promote high levels of proteolysis with a single type of transformed cell while
other sera appear to inhibit the fibrinolytic activity
produced by that cell type. The spectrum of activating
and inhibiting sera is unique for each species of animal
from which the transformed cells were derived. Thus the
serum spectra for mouse cells transformed by a number of
different agents are identical.

    The fibrinolytic activity generated by the transform-
ed cells requires the interaction of two factors; one produced by the cell, and one normally present in the serum
(3, 4, 5). This was initially demonstrated by incubating
serum-free conditioned medium from cultures of transformed cells on ^{125}I-fibrin dishes with aliquots of the appropriate serum (Table 1). Under these conditions neither
serum-free conditioned medium nor serum by itself can hydrolyze the fibrin. Only when serum-free conditioned medium is incubated with the appropriate serum does proteolysis occur. The spectrum of inhibiting and activating sera
is identical when whole cells are assayed the activities
of different sera when tested with serum-free conditioned
medium from the same tumor cells. The inhibitory activity
of certain sera is due to the relative amount of
α_2-macroglobulin in the sera (6).

    The serum molecule necessary for fibrinolysis has been
purified by lysine-sepharose affinity column chromato-
graphy (7). The required factor is the zymogen plasminogen as shown by its chromatographic behaviour, its molecular weight, and its ability to be activated by other
known activators of plasminogen.

    The molecule produced by the transformed cells is
then a plasminogen activator since it converts plasminogen
to its active form plasmin (7, 8). Plasmin is a trypsin-
like protease with a braod substrate specificity. The
spectrum of activating or inhibiting sera for a particular
cell type is identical when either serum-free conditioned

medium from that cell or live cells are tested on ^{125}I-fibrin plates.

The conversion of plasminogen to plasmin is proteoly-tic in nature. The single polypeptide chain of plasmino-gen is hydrolyzed to form two polypeptide chains. There-fore, the plasminogen activator is itself a protease. This enzyme appears to have limited specificity since it does not activate trypsinogen, chymotrypsinogen, or pro-thrombin. The plasminogen activator is sensitive to DFP indicating that it probably has a serine residue at the active center (5, 8). Christman and Acs have shown that the enzyme is stable in 1% SDS (9), and, therefore, can be assayed following purification by SDS-polyacrylamide gel electrophoresis and an approximate molecular weight can be calculated. The plasminogen activator from trans-formed chicken cells has a molecular weight of approxi-mately 40,000 (8), while the molecular weight of the plas-minogen activators from transformed human (5, and hamster (9) cells is approximately 50,000. If ^{3}H-DFP inhibited plasminogen activator and active plasminogen activator are combined, analyzed by SDS-polyacrylamide gel electrophore-sis, and the gel analyzed for the activity of plasminogen activator and ^{3}H-DFP, one major band of radioactivity is found at the same position as plasminogen activator acti-vity (5, 8, 9). From the molecular weight of the enzyme, and the specific activity of the original ^{3}H-DFP, an esti-mate of the amount of plasminogen activator present in the original medium can be made. From these calculations it appears that the level of plasminogen activator is 1-5 γ/l of serum-free conditioned medium (5, 8, 9).

The production of the plasminogen activator is tight-ly correlated with transformation. The induction of this enzyme occurs when chick embryo fibroblasts (CEF) are in-fected with avian sarcoma viruses but not when these cells are infected with avian leukosis viruses (3). These vir-uses, which are able to cause leukemias in vivo, are able to replicate in CEF but are unable to transform CEF. A number of other animal viruses have been used to infect CEF and tested for their ability to induce plasminogen activa-tor after infection of chick embryo fibroblasts. These in-cluded lytic RNA-containing viruses such as NDV, VSV, in-fluenza, sindbis, and sendai, a temperate RNA-containing virus SV_5, and the lytic DNA containing virus, vaccinia

(3). In all cases these viruses fail to induce significant levels of plasminogen activator following infection. Only infection and transformation of CEF by RNA tumor viruses induces the plasminogen activator.

When CEF are infected with a temperature sensitive non-transforming mutant of Rous sarcoma virus, TS-68, cells grown at the restrictive temperature, 41°, are found to contain no plasminogen activator (Table 2). However, at the permissive temperature, 36°, these cells contain high levels of plasminogen activator. An experiment was performed to determine when the plasminogen activator can first be detected after shifting the cells from a non-permissive to a permissive temperature. Petri dishes containing CEF infected with TS-68 and maintained at 41° were transferred to 36° for various periods of time, and the cells assayed for plasminogen activator. The results indicate that plasminogen activator could first be detected between 1-3 hours after the temperature shift. Thus, this enzyme appears quite early in transformation.

A large number of normal and transformed cells have been examined for the production of plasminogen activator (3, 4, 5). In general normal cells have either low or no detectable activity, whereas, the transformed cells contain high levels of the enzyme (Table 3). Thus chicken, mouse, rat, hamster and human cells transformed by RNA or DNA viruses, cells transformed by chemical carcinogens, or spontaneous transformants all promote fibrinolysis. Moreover, benign mammary fibroadenomas do not contain this activity. Cells from ninety-eight out of one hundred and ten primary cultures of rat mammary fibroadenomas produced no soluble plasminogen activator (10). Two normal cell types which have been found to produce a plasminogen activator in culture are embryonic lung cells and embryonic kidney cells (5). Cultures of these cell types from various animal species have been assayed and all have been found to be positive for plasminogen activator production. The production of plasminogen activator by cells from lung and kidney may be related to the highly vascularized nature of these tissues and may serve as a mechanism of preventing clot formation.

The production of a plasminogen activator and the subsequent formation of plasmin might be expected to affect the behavior of transformed cells. Indeed this has been found to be true in a number of experiments. The strategy in these experiments was either to inhibit plasmin activity by including soybean trypsin inhibitor in the growth medium or to prevent the formation of plasmin by removing the plasminogen from the serum. Under these conditions it was shown that the growth of transformed cells in soft agar is reduced by approximately 70% (4, 11), the migration of cells into a wound is reduced by over 50% (11), and significant morphological changes of transformed cells can be observed (4, 11).

It seemed reasonable to propose that the cellular site of action of plasmin resulting in phenotypic alterations is the plasma membrane. Several aspects of membrane structure have been examined and appear to reflect changes related to plasmin activity. One of these is the distribution of the 80 $\overset{o}{A}$ intramembranous particles as visualized by electron microscopy after freeze fracture of cell membranes. If either normal or transformed cells are fixed with glutaraldehyde and their membranes examined, no significant differences can be found in the arrangement of the intramembranous particles. However, if the cells are first treated with glycerol and then fixed, a radical difference between the distribution of the intramembranous particles is now apparent (12). The particles in the normal chick embryo fibroblast membrane are aggregated into groups of particles, while in the membranes of cells transformed by RSV, the particles still maintain their uniform distribution. This reaction does not appear to be dependent upon differences of the growth rate of the two cell types as has been previously reported for Balb/3T3 cells (13). When cultures of cells infected with the temperature sensitive non-transforming mutant of RSV, TS-68, are examined (Figure 1), no aggregation of the intramembranous particles can be seen when the cells are maintained at the permissive temperature 36° (Fig. 1a), while a large amount of aggregation occurred when the cells are maintained at 41°, the non-permissive temperature (Figure 1b). This phenomenon may well be related to partial plasmin hydrolysis of the cell membrane for the following reasons; those sera which allow high levels of plasmin to be formed enhance the distribution of intramembranous particles seen in transformed cell membranes, and, when normal cells are treated with trypsin, the intramembranous particles no

319

longer aggregate but are dispersed in a manner similar
to that seen in the membranes from transformed cells. It
is reasonable to think that trypsin is simply mimicking
the action of plasmin which occurs on transformed cell
membranes. While this data is suggestive it is not con-
clusive. This would require the demonstration that the
intramembranous particle distribution of transformed cells
could be made to resemble the distribution seen with normal cell membranes by the removal of plasminogen. This has
not yet been possible.

In conclusion it appears that transformed cells of
several types produce a plasminogen activator which is capable of converting the plasminogen in the serum used for
cell growth into plasmin. This reaction occurs with great
efficiency and creates a milieu in which transformed cells
in culture are continually exposed to low levels of protease, i.e. plasmin. The generation of plasmin and its
subsequent activity may account for many of the phenotypic
characteristics of malignant cells. Certain preliminary
experiments indicate that alterations of the cellular phenotype may be the result of plasmin hydrolysis of proteins
of the cell plasma membrane.

ACKNOWLEDGEMENTS

This work was supported by grants CA-13138 and CA-
08290 from the National Institute of Health and E-78 from
the American Cancer Society. D.B. Rifkin holds Faculty
Research Award No. PRA-99 from the American Cancer Society.
D. Loskutoff is a Damon Runyon fellow.

REFERENCES

1. A. Fischer, Arch. Entwicklungsmech. Organ. 104, 210
    (1925).
2. T. Astrup, Fed. Proc. 25, 42 (1966).
3. J.C. Unkeless, A. Tobia, L. Ossowski, J.P. Quigley,
    D.B. Rifkin, and E. Reich, J. Exp. Med. 137, 85 (1972).
4. L. Ossowski, J.C. Unkeless, A. Tobia, J.P. Quigley,
    D.B. Rifkin, and E. Reich, J.Exp.Med. 137, 112 (1973).

5. D.B. Rifkin, J.N. Loeb, G. Moore, and E. Reich, J. Exp. Med. <u>139</u>, 1317 (1974).
6. D. Loskutoff and E. Reich, manuscript in preparation.
7. J.P. Quigley, L. Ossowski, and E. Reich, J. Biol. Chem., in press.
8. J.C. Unkeless, K. Danø, G.M. Kellerman, and E. Reich, J. Biol. Chem. In press.
9. J.K. Christman, and G. Acs, Biochim. Biophys. Acta. In press.
10. A. Piperno, A. Tobia, D.B. Rifkin, and E. Reich. Manuscript in preparation.
11. L. Ossowski, J.P. Quigley, G.M. Kellerman, and E. Reich, J. Exp. Med. <u>138</u>, 1056 (1973).
12. N.B. Gilula, and D.B. Rifkin. Manuscript in preparation.
13. R.E. Scott, L.T. Furicht, and J.H. Kersey, Proc. Nat. Acad. Sci. U.S. <u>73</u>, 3631 (1973).

TABLE 1
Fibrinolytic activity of HF from RSV-Infected and Normal
Chick Embryo Fibroblasts: Serum Specificity

Test fluids	Serum supplement in medium	Radioactivity released into solution (% of total) %
Medium	None	1.6
Medium	Chicken	1.1
Normal cell HF	Chicken	1.2
RSV-transformed cell HF	None	2.5
"	Chicken	45
"	Fetal bovine	6.5
"	African green monkey	11
"	Dog	3.7
"	Hamster	2.6
"	Fetal pig	1.7

Petri dishes (35 mm diameter) containing [^{125}I] fibrin
(10 μg/cm^2; total radioactivity 2.5 X 10^4 cpm) were prepared as described in Methods. Serum-free Eagle's medium
or HF (1 ml) was mixed with the indicated serum supplement
to yield a final serum concentration of 2.5% (vol/vol),
added to the [^{125}I]fibrin-coated plates, and incubated at
37°C for 3 h. Aliquots of the incubation medium were removed for radioactivity assays. The control value for
chicken serum medium incubated in the absence of HF is
the only one presented in the table. The controls for all
other sera without HF gave values identical to that found
with the chicken serum control.
(Table 1 taken from: An Enzymatic Function Associated with
Transformation of Fibroblasts by Oncogenic Viruses. I.
Chick Embryo Fibroblast Cultures Transformed by Avian RNA
Tumor Viruses, J.C. Unkeless, A. Tobia, L. Ossowski, J.P.
Quigley, D.B. Rifkin, and E. Reich, J. Exp. Med. 137, 85
(1973).

TABLE 2

Plasminogen Activator in Cells Infected with a Temperature
Sensitive Non-Transforming Virus.

Cell type and temperature of incubation		radioactivity removed (CPM)
Normal cells	41°	535
RSV	41°	10,370
RSV	36°	8,035
TS-68	41°	200
TS-68	36°	14,900
TS-68	41°-36° 1 hr	125
TS-68	41°-36° 2 hr	250
TS-68	41°-36° 4 hr	3,550
TS-68	41°-36° 8 hr	14,900

Secondary chick embryo fibroblasts were infected with
wild type RSV or TS-68 in 60 mm dishes. The cells were
maintained either at $41^{\circ}C$ or $36^{\circ}C$ until confluent. At
that time certain cultures infected with TS-68 were moved
from 41° to 36°. After incubation at 36° for the time indicated, the medium was removed from all plates, the cells
washed twice with isotonic buffer, scraped in isotonic
buffer and spun at 100 xg for 5 min. at 0°. The cell pellet was then dispersed in 0.3 ml of 0.5% Triton X100 in
0.1 M Tris pH 8.0. Aliquots of 100 µl (25% of the total
volume) were then plated at ^{125}I-fibrin coated plates in
2 ml of 0.1 M Tris pH 8.0 containing 2.5% chick serum and
incubated for 3 hr at 37°. At the end of that period the
supernatant was assayed for soluble radioactivity. Total
cpm per plate was 50,000 cpm.

TABLE 3

Fibrinolytic Activity of Various Normal and Transformed
Cells

Cell Type	Radioactivity Released in Growth Medium (% of total)
RSV-transformed chick	75.5
Normal chick	1.5
SV-40 transformed Hamster	33
Normal Hamster	0.3
MSV-transformed Mouse	36
Normal Mouse	0.1
Human Osteosarcoma*	57
Human Melanoma*	70
Human Embryonic fibroblasts	5
Rat mammary Tumor (DMBA induced)	50
Normal Rat lactating tissue	3

Cells were plated on ^{125}I-fibrin coated dishes in Eagle's
medium containing 10% fetal bovine serum, allowed to at-
tach, and the medium removed and replaced with Eagle's
medium containing 2.5% of the best activating serum for
that cell type (3, 5, 5). After incubation at 37° the
medium was counted for radioactivity.

*Serum-free conditioned medium was assayed rather than
 whole cells (5).

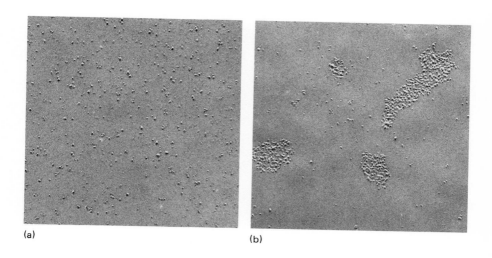

(a)

(b)

Figure 1. Electron micrographs of chick embryo fibroblasts infected with TS-68 virus. Cells were treated with glycerol, fixed with glutaraldehyde, freeze fractured and examined by electron microscopy. (a) Cells maintained at 36°. (b) Cells maintained at 41°. The magnification was 62,500. The direction of shadowing was from the bottom of the figure towards the top.

REVERSAL OF THE TRANSFORMED PHENOTYPE
BY DIBUTYRYL CYCLIC AMP
AND A PROTEASE INHIBITOR

Michael J. Weber

Department of Microbiology
University of Illinois
Urbana, Illinois 61801

ABSTRACT. We have examined the possible roles of cyclic AMP and proteases in the genesis of the transformed phenotype by adding either dibutyryl cyclic AMP or a trypsin inhibitor (TLCK) to cultures of chick cells transformed by Rous sarcoma virus. Hexose transport, adhesiveness and cellular morphology were used as markers for the transformed phenotype. We find that TLCK can convert the transformed cells into nearly perfect phenocopies of normal cells with respect to those three markers, but that dibutyryl cyclic AMP is somewhat less effective.

INTRODUCTION

Malignant cells, in addition to their altered growth behavior, are characterized by alterations in cellular morphology, membrane transport, (1,2,3,4,5) and adhesiveness (6,7,8,9) as well as by a variety of other structural and functional changes, especially in the cell surface (10,11). Although it is known that some viral gene product is required to establish and to maintain this transformed phenotype (12,13) the mechanism by which viral oncogenic activity modifies cellular metabolism is largely unknown.
There has been much recent discussion of the possible roles cyclic AMP and/or proteolytic activity might play in the genesis of the transformed phenotype. Evidence for the involvement of cyclic AMP in viral transformation is based on reports that the levels of cyclic AMP in transformed cells are lower than in their normal counterparts and that addition of dibutyryl cyclic AMP to transformed cells can restore some of their growth or cellular properties to a

327

more "normal" state. (See Reference 14 for review). However, some of this work has been performed with cell lines which have no normal counterpart (such as L cells) and this makes quantitative comparisons of the normal and transformed phenotypes impossible.

Similar evidence for the involvement of proteolytic activity in oncogenesis exists: transformed cells seem to have higher levels of proteolytic activity than do their normal counterparts (15,16,17) and addition of protease inhibitors to transformed cultures causes them to reach a stable population plateau such as is seen with normal cultures (15,18,19). However, growth inhibition with dibutyryl cyclic AMP or with protease inhibitors seems not to occur simply by restoration of normal growth controls (20,21,22), and it is difficult to distinguish between non-specific toxicity and normal growth control when the assay used is the absence of growth (23). Thus, it is important to examine the effects of these agents on cellular manifestations of the transformed phenotype which do not require growth assays for their detection, and to use a system in which a closely-matched normal cell control is available for comparison.

Using chick cells transformed by a temperature conditional mutant of Rous sarcoma virus (RSV-T5) we have examined the effects of dibutyryl cyclic AMP and the trypsin inhibitor, TLCK[1] on three cellular manifestations of the transformed phenotype: increased hexose transport, decreased adhesiveness and rounded morphology. All three of these markers are altered early in transformation, and their appearance is not dependent on growth of the cells (2,3,24). One might suspect, therefore, that all three of these alterations are closely coupled to the first expression of viral oncogenic information. Shifting cells infected with RSV-T5 from the permissive temperature (36.5°C) where they are transformed, to the restrictive temperature (41°C) results in a rapid reversal of the transformed phenotype and provides a control on the kinetics and completeness of "curing" when viral oncogenic information is "switched off." We find that TLCK treatment converts the transformed cells into nearly perfect phenocopies of normal cells but that dibutyryl cyclic AMP is somewhat less effective.

---

[1]TLCK: Tosyl-lysyl-chloromethylketone.

MATERIALS AND METHODS

Cell culture and transport measurements were as described (5). The temperature-conditional mutant of Rous sarcoma virus, RSV-T5, was from Martin (2). Cells were plated at 1.5 x 10^5 cells/35 mm dish and allowed to remain in culture for a minimum of 48 hours before experimental manipulations were begun. DNA was measured by the method of Burton (26).

Adhesiveness was measured by determining the percentage of cells on a dish which could be detached by a stream of culture fluid. Medium was removed from the plate in a pipette and dropped back onto the plate from a height of 20 cm, while the plate was systematically moved back and forth under the stream. The operation was repeated 4 more times so that the entire surface of the plate was hit by the stream. The detachable cells were counted in a Coulter particle counter, and the adherent cells were removed from the dish with trypsin and counted. The technique generally provides data with less than 10% difference between duplicate points. In a typical transformed culture between 50 and 90% of the cells are detachable, whereas in a normal culture fewer than 5% of the cells can be detached by this procedure.

Growth media and sera were from GIBCO, dibutyryl cyclic AMP from Sigma and TLCK from Sigma or Nutritional Biochemicals. Isotope was from New England Nuclear.

Use of TLCK:

There is only a 2 - 4 fold difference between a lethal and an effective dose of TLCK, and thus obtaining reproducible results with the protease inhibitor requires careful control of cell culture conditions. In our experience freshly seeded cells are especially sensitive to the toxic effects of the inhibitor, and thus it is essential to keep cells in culture at least 48 hours prior to treatment, and to use only healthy sub-confluent cultures. In addition, TLCK is unstable, and has a half-life in growth medium of as little as 3 - 5 hours (as measured by inhibition of trypsin hydrolysis of tosyl-arginyl-methylester). Therefore, solutions of TLCK should be made up fresh before each use and the powdered compound should be stored frozen and dessicated.

RESULTS

The effect of varying concentrations of the trypsin
inhibitor TLCK on the transport of 2-deoxyglucose is shown
in Figure 1. Shifting cultures from the permissive to the
restrictive temperature provides a control on the changes
in transport rate when viral oncogenic information is
"switched off." As shown previously (2,3) shifting cultures to the restrictive temperature results in a rapid
restoration of the transport rate, down to the level characteristic of normal, exponentially growing cells. Addition of the protease inhibitor also lowers the transport to
a level and with kinetics similar to those seen with the
temperature shift. However, concentrations of 200 μg/ml
and 400 μg/ml of TLCK caused substantial killing of cells
and detachment from the dish. The effects of 50 and
100 μg/ml were reversible, however, To minimize toxic
side-effects, the lowest effective dose, 50 μg/ml, was
used in subsequent experiments.

Figure 2 shows the effects of varying concentrations
of dibutyryl cyclic AMP on 2-deoxyglucose transport by
the transformed cells. Dibutyryl cyclic AMP at 1 mM or
5mM caused a prompt and complete restoration of the transport rate to the normal level. However at 10 mM, or with
the addition of theophylline, transport was first stimulated and then declined. The reason for the transient
stimulation of hexose transport is not known, but is consistent with other reports that dibutyryl cyclic AMP can
have contrary effects on carbohydrate metabolism (27).
The inhibition of 2-deoxyglucose transport by dibutyryl
cyclic AMP cannot be due to inhibition of cell growth since
the cyclic nucleotide does not inhibit cell growth in this
system in the absence of theophylline, and generally, it
stimulates cell growth (24,28).

Analysis of the effects of the cyclic nucleotide
analogue and the trypsin inhibitor on cellular adhesiveness is shown in Figure 3. In order to facilitate comparison with the effects on hexose transport, the data
are plotted as the fraction of the cells which can be detached, so that as adhesiveness increases, the curve
decreases. It can be seen that cultures shifted to the
restrictive temperature (41°C) rapidly increased their
adherence to the dish. Addition of dibutyryl cyclic AMP
had only a small effect on the ability of cells to adhere

to the culture dish. The most dibutyryl cyclic AMP has increased adhesiveness, in our experience, is by a factor of two. TLCK, on the other hand, increased adhesiveness to levels which approached those seen in the culture shifted to the restrictive temperature. In other experiments, in which TLCK was re-added at 25 μg/ml every 12 - 24 hours, the difference between the TLCK-treated cultures and the cultures shifted to 41°C was reduced even more.

Cellular Morphology

Figure 4 shows phase micrographs of a transformed culture, (A); a normal, uninfected culture, (B); a culture treated with dibutyryl cyclic AMP, (C); and a culture treated with TLCK, (D). It can be seen that the dibutyryl cyclic AMP-treated culture, though more elongated and flattened than the transformed culture, does not display the cellular morphology of a normal culture. Rather, the cells seem bloated and perhaps slightly epithelioid. This result is obtained regardless of whether theophylline or papaverine or no phosphodiesterase inhibitor is used, and with either 1 mM or 5 mM dibutyryl cyclic AMP. Treatment of cells with TLCK, however, converts them into morphological phenocopies of normal cells. The TLCK-treated cultures frequently cannot be distinguished from normal cultures in a single-blind test. These results indicate that TLCK can restore cellular morphology to normal but that dibutyryl cyclic AMP cannot.

Virus Replication

Do dibutyryl cyclic AMP and TLCK alter the transformed phenotype by acting on some step specific to oncogenesis, or do they directly interfere with virus replication? To answer this question, we examined virus production in cells treated with either TLCK or dibutyryl cyclic AMP plus theophylline. It can be seen (Table 1) that both agents seem to cause a transient inhibition of virus production (although this result is not always obtained) but by 40 hours there is little inhibition of virus replication over and above the effect on total cellular protein synthesis. At this time, the transport, adhesion and morphology changes have already occurred. Thus, the effects of TLCK and dibutyryl cyclic AMP on transport, adhesiveness and morphology are not directly mediated by inhibition of virus replication

DNA Content

Cells treated with TLCK or with dibutyryl cyclic AMP plus theophylline have been reported to be arrested in their growth, presumably in a state analogous to density-dependent inhibition of growth. Density-inhibited cells are arrested in the G1 stage of the cell cycle, and have a diploid amount of DNA. Cells treated with dibutyryl cyclic AMP plus theophylline, or treated with TLCK have at least a 4N amount of DNA (Table 2), and thus are not in a typical G1 state. This agrees with the findings of Paul (20), Smets (21) and Schnebli (22).

Effects on Normal Cells

TLCK and dibutyryl cyclic AMP lowered the rate of hexose transport of transformed cells to the level characteristic of normal exponentially growing cells. However, the inhibitors had little effect when added to normal cells. Hexose transport was never reduced to the very low level seen with density-inhibited cells (Table 3). These data suggest that, although the transformation-specific change in hexose transport is regulated by cyclic AMP levels, the change in hexose transport associated with density-dependent inhibition of growth may occur by another mechanism.

Effects of Sodium Butyrate

Figure 5A is a phase micrograph of a culture treated for 42 hours with 1 mM sodium butyrate. The cells have flattened and taken on an appearance which is similar, although not identical, to that induced by dibutyryl cyclic AMP. Sodium butyrate had little effect on hexose transport but could cause an increase in cellular adhesiveness (Table 4). Thus, the effects of dibutyryl cyclic AMP on adhesion and morphology, but not on transport, can be partially attributed to the release of sodium butyrate from the cyclic nucleotide analogue.

Effects of Cycloheximide

Since TLCK is inhibitory to growth, we investigated the possibility that the effects of the protease inhibitor could be attributed to its toxicity. Figure 5B is a phase micrograph of a culture treated for 30 hours with cycloheximide at 2 µg/ml. The cells have flattened out, but rather than taking on the elongated appearance of normal cells, they have become stellate. Thus, cycloheximide causes a morphological change but does not cause the cells to return to normal in this respect. Cells treated with cycloheximide showed no increase in adhesiveness at concentrations from 0.02 to 5 µg/ml (Table 4). They did, however, show a drop in hexose transport capacity, presumably due to turnover of the transport system. However, 0.05 µg/ml cycloheximide, which inhibited protein synthesis as well as did 50 µg/ml TLCK was much less effective at inhibiting hexose transport (Table 4). Thus it seems unlikely that the effects of TLCK can be attributed entirely to its inhibition of protein synthesis.

DISCUSSION

The data presented here demonstrate that addition of the trypsin inhibitor TLCK to cultures of chick cells transformed by Rous sarcoma virus restores their rate of hexose transport, their adhesiveness and their morphology to near normal. Although TLCK is toxic to the cells and inhibits their growth, it does not appear that simple growth inhibition can account for these findings, since cycloheximide did not have the same effects. We therefore interpret these data as providing evidence for the involvement of a proteolytic activity at an early stage in the genesis of the transformed phenotype. However, this interpretation must be tempered with caution, since we do not know with certainty whether the effects of TLCK are due entirely to its action as a protease inhibitor.

We also have found that treatment of transformed cells with dibutyryl cyclic AMP lowers their hexose transport rate to the level characteristic of normal, growing cells. However, the cyclic nucleotide does not cause a return to a completely normal morphology or adhesiveness under our conditions. Three explanations seem possible to us:

1. Dibutyryl cyclic AMP might not be a good cyclic AMP analogue to use in this system since it does not completely mimic the effects of cyclic AMP. For example, the effects of sodium butyrate might mask the action of cyclic AMP on the transformed phenotype.

2. Reversal of the morphological and adhesive manifestations of the transformed phenotype may require higher concentrations of cyclic AMP than does reversal of the high rate of hexose transport. Using dibutyryl cyclic AMP we were perhaps unable to achieve internal concentrations of cyclic AMP high enough to cause complete reversal of these transformed characteristics.

3. It is possible that the transformation-specific decline in cyclic AMP levels occurs after the activity of a protease, and after a branchpoint in the pathway of oncogenic activity, as shown in Figure 6. In this model, a viral gene product activates a protease (or is a protease) which acts on the cell surface to cause a decrease in adhesion, a change in cellular morphology and a drop in cyclic AMP pools. The drop in cyclic AMP pools is directly responsible for the activation of hexose transport, and only partially responsible for changes in morphology and adhesion. Inhibition of protease activity by TLCK completely restores the transformed phenotype because it acts on a primary event. Dibutyryl cyclic AMP restores hexose transport to normal but does not completely restore adhesion and morphology. A partial effect of cyclic AMP could occur for example, if cyclic AMP sensitive elements, such as microtubules, and cyclic AMP insensitive elements, perhaps microfilaments, were both involved in the control of cellular shape and adhesiveness.

Experiments designed to distinguish between these hypotheses are currently in progress.

ACKNOWLEDGMENTS

I would like to thank Ms. Shirley Yau for skilled and dedicated technical assistance and Arthur Hale for valuable discussions. Supported by USPH Grant CA-12467

REFERENCES

1. Hatanaka, M. and Hanafusa, H. Virology 41,647.(1970).
2. Martin, G. S., Venuta , S., Weber, M.J. and Rubin, H. Proc. Nat. Acad. Sci. 68,2739 (1971).
3. Kawai, S. and Hanafusa, H. Virology 46,470 (1971).
4. Isselbacher, K. PNAS 69,585 (1972).
5. Weber, M. J. J. Biol. Chem. 248,2978 (1973).
6. Coman, D. R. Cancer Res. 4,625 (1944).
7. Coman, D. R. Cancer Res. 21,1436 (1961).
8. Edwards, J. G., Campbell, J. A. and Williams, J. F. NNB 231,147 (1971).
9. Johnson, G. S. and Pastan, I. NNB 236,247 (1972).
10. Burger, M. M. Fed. Proc. 32,91 (1973).
11. Herschman, H. In Membrane Molecular Biology. Fox, C. F. and Keith, A. (Eds.) Sinauer Assoc. Stanford, Conn.
12. Dulbecco, R. and Eckhart, W. PNAS 67,1775 (1970).
13. Martin,,G. S. Nature 227,1021 (1970).
14. Schultz, J. and Gratzner, H. G.,(Eds.) The Role of Cyclic Nucleotides in Carcinogenesis. Academic Press, New York (1973).
15. Schnebli, H. P. Schweizerische Medizinische Wochenschrift 102,1194 (1972).
16. Bosmann, H. B. Biochim. Biophys. Acta 264,339 (1972).
17. Unkeless, J. C., Tobia, A., Ossowski, L., Quigley, J. P., Rifkin, D. B. and Reich, E. J. Exptl. Med. 137,85 (1973).
18. Schnebli, H. P. and Burger, M. M. Proc. Nat. Acad. Sci. USA 69,3825 (1972).
19. Goetz, I. Weinstein, C. and Roberts, E. Cancer Res. 32,2469 (1972).
20. Paul, D. NNB 240,179 (1972).
21. Smets, L. A. NNB 239,123 (1972).
22. Schnebli, H. P. Cold Spring Harbor Symposium on Growth Control in Animal Cells. In Press.
23. Chou, I., Black, P. H. and Roblin, R. Cold Spring Harbor Symposium on Growth Control in Animal Cells. In Press.
24. Weber, M. J. In Preparation.
25. Shaw, W., Mares-Guia, M. and Cohen, W. Biochemistry 4,2219 (1965).
26. Burton, K. Biochem. J. 62,315 (1956).

27. Hilz, H. and Tarnowski, W. BBRC 40,973 (1970).
28. Hovi, T. and Vaheri, A. Nature New Biol. 245,175 (1973).

TABLE 1

EFFECT OF TLCK AND DIBUTYRYL CYCLIC AMP ON VIRUS PRODUCTION BY CELLS TRANSFORMED BY RSV-T5

hours	no treatment		TLCK, 50 µg/ml		1 mM dib-cAMP, 1mM theophylline, 25 µg/ml PGE$_1$	
	FFU[a]/ml	FFU/ml/ /mg	FFU/ml	FFU/ml/ /mg	FFU/ml	FFU/ml/ /mg
6	0.09	0.6	0.01	0.14	0.0	0.0
17	0.15	0.6	0.2	1.4	0.02	0.3
32	1.0	2.1	0.1	0.4	0.4	1.2
41	1.2	2.2	0.2	0.9	0.6	1.1
51	0.7	1.1	0.5	2.2	0.5	0.9

[a]FFU = focus forming units x 10^{-5}

TABLE 2

Cell type	DNA content (µg/10^6 cells)
RSV-T5 at 36°C	2.9 $\pm$ 0.5
RSV-T5 at 41°C	2.8 $\pm$ 0.2
RSV-T5 at 36°C + 50 µg/ml TLCK, 40 hrs.	5.5 $\pm$ 0.5
RSV-T5 at 36°C + 1 mM dib-cAMP, 1 mM theophylline, 25 µg/ml PGE$_1$, 40 hrs.	6.7 $\pm$ 1.4

TABLE 3

EFFECT OF TLCK AND DIBUTYRYL CYCLIC AMP[a] ON HEXOSE TRANSPORT IN NORMAL AND TRANSFORMED CELLS

Cell type	2-deoxyglucose transport (nMoles/min/mg protein)	Percent untreated control
transformed	1.60	100
transformed + 50 μg/ml TLCK	0.55	34
transformed + 1 mM dib-cAMP, 1 mM theophylline, 2.5 μg/ml PGE$_1$	0.64	40
transformed + 1 mM dib-cAMP	0.38	24
transformed + 5 mM dib-cAMP	0.37	23
normal, growing	0.38	24
normal + 50 μg/ml TLCK	0.43	27
normal + 100 μg/ml TLCK	0.52	32
normal + 1 mM dib-cAMP, 1 mM theophylline, 2.5 μg/ml PGE$_1$	0.45	28
normal + 1 mM dib-cAMP	0.37	23
normal + 5 mM dib-cAMP	0.28	18
density-inhibited	0.10	6

[a]Cells were treated with the inhibitors for 45 hours.

337

TABLE 4

HEXOSE TRANSPORT AND ADHESION IN CULTURES TREATED WITH SODIUM BUTYRATE, TLCK OR CYCLOHEXIMIDE[a]

	Percent inhibition of protein synthesis[b]	Percent inhibition of 2-deoxyglucose uptake	Percentage of detachable cells[c]
1 mM sodium butyrate	23	15	46
50 µg/ml TLCK	60	67	22
0.05 µg/ml cycloheximide	60	21	71
0.5 µg/ml cycloheximide	94	75	69

[a]Cells were treated with the inhibitors for 45 hrs.
[b]Protein synthesis was measured by Lowry assay of protein increase over 45 hrs.
[c]Control cultures had 76% detachable cells.

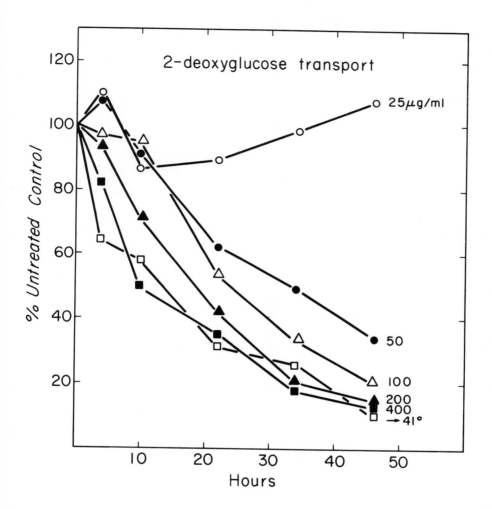

Fig. 1. Inhibition of 2-deoxyglucose uptake by various concentrations of TLCK. Cells transformed by RSV-T5 at 36.5°C were changed to medium containing TLCK and at various times duplicate plates were taken for transport measurements. One set of cultures was shifted to 41°C (open squares).

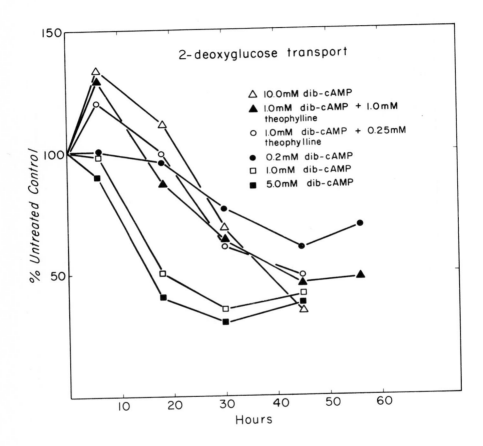

Fig. 2. Inhibition of 2-deoxyglucose uptake by dibutyryl cyclic AMP and theophylline.

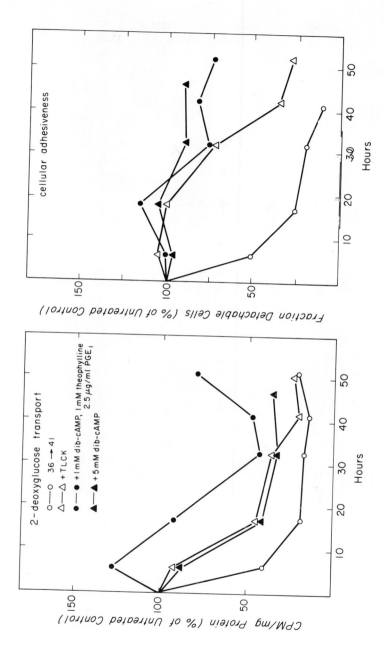

Fig. 3. Effect of dibutyryl cyclic AMP or TLCK on 2-deoxyglucose transport and on cellular adhesiveness.

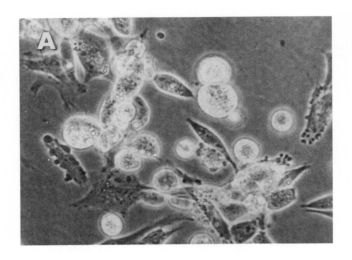

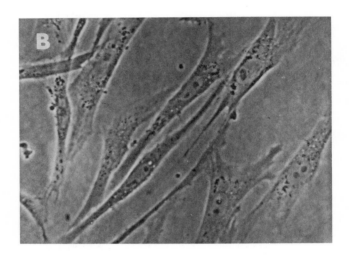

Fig. 4. Effects of dibutyryl cyclic AMP and TLCK on cellular morphology. Phase micrographs at 430 x of a transformed culture (A); a normal culture (B); a culture treated for 40 hours with 1 mM dibutyryl cyclic AMP (C); a culture treated for 40 hours with 50 μg/ml TLCK (D).

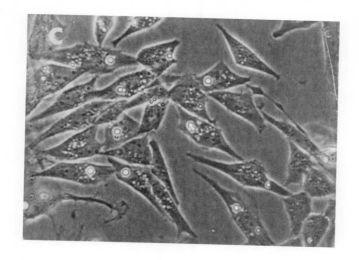

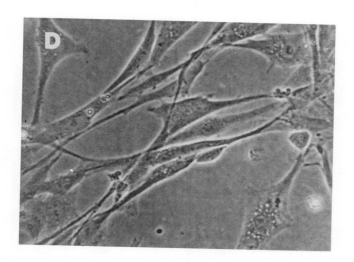

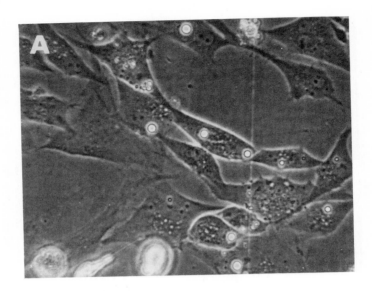

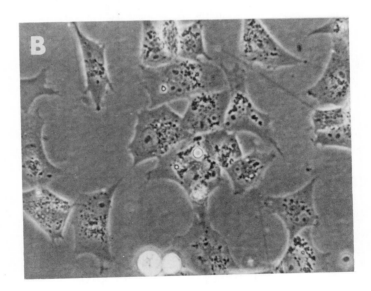

Fig. 5. Effects of sodium butyrate (A) or cycloheximide (B) on cellular morphology. Phase micrographs
(430 x) of cultures treated 40 hours with 1 mM sodium
butyrate or 2 μg/ml cycloheximide.

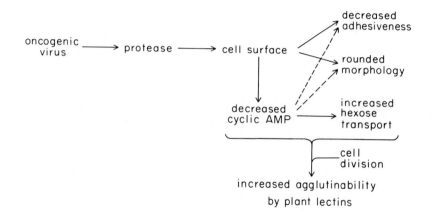

Fig. 6. Model for the pathway by which viral oncogenic activity generates the transformed phenotype.

PLASMINOGEN ACTIVATORS OF NORMAL AND ROUS SARCOMA VIRUS-TRANSFORMED CELLS

Allan R. Goldberg and Sondra G. Lazarowitz

The Rockefeller University
New York, New York 10021

ABSTRACT. Evidence of increased protease levels in cells transformed by Rous sarcoma virus has been obtained by two independent techniques which measure plasminogen activator levels. Limited proteolytic cleavage of the HA (hemagglutinin) polypeptide, the largest glycoprotein of influenza virus, to polypeptides HA1 and HA2 occurs when influenza virus is grown in the presence of serum-free media in transformed cells but not in normal cells. This cleavage, which takes place at the cell surface, is brought to completion by the addition of pure chicken plasminogen to the serum-free medium. Differences in plasminogen-activator levels also have been observed by means of an agarose-overlay assay using casein as a substrate. Both normal and transformed chick cells hydrolyze casein in the presence of chick serum, however transformed cells show a markedly faster rate of hydrolysis than untransformed cells in the presence of serum at low concentrations. Pure chicken plasminogen can substitute for chicken serum in this assay. The activated plasmin can be inhibited by bovine pancreatic trypsin inhibitor (Kunitz), soybean trypsin inhibitor, TLCK, and pure fetuin from fetal calf serum.

INTRODUCTION

Extensive studies of neoplastic and normal cell surfaces during recent years have revealed significant differences. One such area of investigation that has received considerable attention is the increased sensitivity of transformed cells to agglutination by certain plant lectins. It is generally true that in the presence

347

of low levels of wheat germ agglutinin (1) or Concanavalin A (2) transformed cells agglutinate, whereas normal cells agglutinate very poorly if at all. Changes in agglutinability found during transformation or reversion of transformed cell lines to a morphologically normal state, usually are paralleled by changes in growth properties (3-6). Several laboratories have demonstrated that proteolysis of the surface membrane of resting, normal cells leads to overgrowth and enhanced agglutinability (7,8). Schnebli and Burger (9) have reported that incubation of transformed cells with inhibitors of proteases causes those cells to grow to saturation densities similar to those observed for normal cells. The corollary of this observation is that transformed cells incubated with a protease inhibitor should become markedly less agglutinable. Recent experiments in this laboratory have substantiated this prediction (10,11). In addition it was shown that Rous sarcoma virus (RSV) transformed chick embryo fibroblasts (CEF) do elaborate substances which can cause normal CEF to both undergo multiplication and to become agglutinable (10). These results imply that transformed CEF release proteases. It is likely that the overgrowth-stimulating activity reported by Rubin (12) is equivalent to the enzyme activity observed in this laboratory.

CASEIN OVERLAY ASSAY FOR THE DETECTION OF PLASMINOGEN ACTIVATOR PRODUCTION

A rapid screening assay for proteases was sought to determine if normal and transformed cells produce such enzymes, and also to determine if a qualitative or quantitative difference exists between normal and transformed cells with regard to the production of proteases (13). Casein, in the form of non-fat milk, was chosen as a convenient, inexpensive general substrate and visible indicator which could be incorporated into a liquid in vitro assay or an agarose-overlay assay for the direct testing of cells growing in monolayer. When monolayers of RSV-transformed CEF were overlayed with serum-free medium containing casein and agarose only occasional small clear plaques were evident over zones of piled-up cells indicating production, at a low level, of an enzyme capable of digesting casein (Table 1). Sera normally used for the growth of CEF were tested in the overlay. Caseinolysis was greatly amplified in the presence of chicken serum but not in the presence of calf or fetal calf serum. Since serum alone had no effect on casein it was surmised that a zymogen of a serum protease might be activated by the cellular protease which had only limited specificity for casein. Plasminogen seemed a likely candidate for this role since the production by cells of proteases which can activate plasminogen to plasmin is well-known (13). When RSV-transformed CEF were overlayed with agarose containing chicken plasminogen at a concentration of 1-2 μg/ml in place of serum, total digestion of the substrate occurred within 12 hr (Fig. 1). In contrast, normal CEF required > 55 μg/ml of plasminogen in the overlay assay for equivalent activity.

It has been shown previosuly that plasminogen is the only component of serum responsible for the observed caseinolysis in the overlay assay (13). Though calf and fetal calf serum were ineffective in promoting caseinolysis, calf and fetal calf plasminogen can be converted to plasmin by the activator secreted by RSV-transformed CEF.

The activation reaction appears to be specific for plasminogen. Other zymogens such as pepsinogen, trypsinogen, and chymotrypsinogen can not be activated by the cell-produced activator.

Avian sarcoma viruses of subgroups A, B, and C can elevate plasminogen activator levels to the same extent upon infection of CEF. In contrast, non-transforming avian leukosis viruses of the same subgroups do not affect plasminogen activator levels. These findings are in agreement with the experiments reported by Unkeless et al. (14) and Ossowski et al. (15,16).

When RSV infection of CEF was carried out at a MOI of 10, activator levels reached a plateau at 20-24 hours, just prior to the appearance of morphological transformation. Studies are in progress to correlate the appearance of elevated plasminogen activator levels with the maturation of virus and with various criteria associated with transformation such as increased agglutinability and altered glucose transport.

Several known macromolecular inhibitors of plasmin action such as soybean trypsin inhibitor and bovine pancreatic trypsin inhibitor (Kunitz) can inhibit the

plasmin-mediated caseinolysis (13). Pure fetuin from
fetal calf serum also was found to be inhibitory.
In addition a wide variety of synthetic trypsin and
chymotrypsin inhibitors, such as TLCK, TPCK, NPGB,
and APB inhibited caseinolysis at concentrations ranging
from 1×10^{-3} M to 1×10^{-5} M.

PROTEOLYTIC CLEAVAGE BY PLASMIN OF THE HA POLYPEPTIDE OF INFLUENZA VIRUS: HOST CELL ACTIVATION OF SERUM PLASMINOGEN

The cleavage of the hemagglutinin (HA) polypeptide,
the largest glycoprotein of the WSN strain of influenza
virus, to polypeptides HA1 plus HA2, has been used as
another sensitive indicator of the production of
plasminogen activators by cells (17,18). Studies of the
synthesis of influenza virus specific proteins demonstrated that the HA polypeptide (75,000-80,000 dalton
glycoprotein) is a primary viral gene product, whereas
HA1 (50,000-60,000 daltons) and HA2 (23,000-30,000
daltons) are derived from the proteolytic cleavage of
HA (19-21). In cells infected with the WSN strain of
influenza A_0 virus, the cleavage appears to occur while
the HA polypeptide is associated with the cell plasma
membrane (19,22). The proteolytic nature of this
cleavage is suggested by the observations that: (a) in
vitro incubation of virions with trypsin results in the
cleavage of the HA polypeptide to HA1 plus HA2 (25);
and, (b) diisopropylphosphofluoridate (DFP), an inhibitor
of cellular proteases, inhibits the appearance of HA1
and HA2 in fowl plague virus-infected CEF (23). The
hemagglutinin of WSN virions grown in Madin-Darby bovine
kidney (MDBK) cells in the absence of serum has been
shown to consist of $\geq 85\%$ uncleaved HA polypeptide
(24,25). In contrast, the HA polypeptide of WSN
virions grown in the presence of 2% calf serum was
demonstrated to be $\geq 90\%$ HA1 plus HA2. However, in
vitro incubation of virions containing uncleaved HA
polypeptide in the presence of 2% calf serum did not
result in cleavage to HA1 plus HA2 (25). It thus
appeared that serum alone was not responsible for the
cleavage of the HA polypeptide, but rather an interaction
between a serum component and a cellular factor caused
proteolysis of the HA polypeptide.

It was surmised that plasminogen might be a likely candidate for this role. To determine whether plasminogen might be a factor in the cleavage of the HA polypeptide when WSN is grown in MDBK cells in the presence of calf serum, the structural proteins of WSN virions grown with either reinforced Eagle's medium (REM) or REM containing 2.0 µg/ml purified calf plasminogen as growth medium were compared. As shown in Fig. 2A, the hemagglutinin of virions grown in unsupplemented REM is exclusively uncleaved HA polypeptide. Neither HA1 nor HA2 are detectable by either amino acid or glucosamine label. However, growth in the presence of low levels of plasminogen results in complete cleavage as shown in Fig. 2B. Chicken plasminogen can effectively substitute for calf plasminogen. Furthermore, plasminogen appears to be the only serum component involved in this conversion since the presence in the growth medium of 2% plasminogen-free calf serum does not result in the cleavage of the HA polypeptide. Cleavage is inhibited by the presence of plasmin inhibitors in the growth medium.

Comparison of the HA polypeptide of influenza virions grown in normal vs. RSV-transformed CEF also has shown that plasminogen activator activity is elevated in transformed cells (26). Figs. 3-5 illustrate a $\geq$ 10-fold difference in the amount of plasminogen in the growth medium necessary to produce proteolytic cleavage of the HA polypeptide in RSV-transformed CEF vs. normal CEF. The observation that less plasminogen is needed for the cleavage of the HA polypeptide in the growth medium of RSV-transformed CEF than in the medium of normal CEF is indicative of a higher level of plasminogen activator in transformed cells. Ten-fold or greater differences in activator levels are apparent upon examination of early influenza harvest (4-10 hours post-infection) as well as late harvests (10-20 hours post-infection) from CEF transformed by two different mutants of Schmidt-Ruppin RSV at permissive temperature (37°). Little or no cytopathic effects of influenza virus infection are evident by 10 hours post-infection. Therefore, influenza virus infection is not simply causing the preferential release of sequestered plasminogen activator from RSV-transformed CEF. It is of interest that infection by influenza virus serves to turn off the production of RSV.

CONCLUSION

The casein-agarose overlay assay allows the screening of cellular mutants which possess a temperature-sensitive lesion in plasminogen activator, thereby allowing thorough analysis of the role of plasminogen activators in the metabolism of both normal and transformed cells. It will also be of interest to select RSV mutants which are unable to elevate the level of plasminogen activators upon infection of susceptible cells. Complementation analysis using the casein-agarose assay and alterations in the polypeptide composition of influenza virions to compare these mutants with known transformation-mutants should help to elucidate which RSV functions and how many are involved in the maintenance of transformation.

ACKNOWLEDGMENTS

This work was supported by research grants CA-13362 from the National Cancer Institute and AI-05600 from the National Institute of Allergy and Infectious Diseases, and a Brown-Hazen grant from The Research Corporation. A.R.G. is a Richard King Mellon Foundation Fellow in The Rockefeller University. This research was done in part while A.R.G. was a Special Fellow of the Leukemia Society of America. S.G.L. is a National Institutes of Health Predoctoral Fellow 5 F01 GM-48628.

REFERENCES

1. M. M. Burger and A. R. Goldberg, Proc. Nat. Acad. Sci. U.S.A. 57, 359 (1967).
2. M. Inbar and L. Sachs, Proc. Nat. Acad. Sci. U.S.A. 63, 1418 (1969).
3. R. E. Pollack and M. M. Burger, Proc. Nat. Acad. Sci. U.S.A. 62, 1074 (1969).
4. B. Ozanne and J. Sambrook, Lepetit Colloq. Biol. Med. 2, 248 (1971).
5. L. A. Culp and P. H. Black, J. Virol. 9, 611 (1972).
6. H. C. Renger and C. Basilico, Proc. Nat. Acad. Sci. U.S.A. 69, 109 (1972).

7. M. M. Burger, Nature, 227, 170 (1970).
8. B. Sefton and H. Rubin, Nature 227, 843 (1970).
9. H. P. Schnebli and M. M. Burger, Proc. Nat. Acad. Sci. U.S.A. 69, 3825 (1972).
10. A. R. Goldberg in "Conference on Biomedical Perspectives of Agglutinins of Invertebrate and Plant Origins," Annals of the New York Academy of Sciences meeting, New York, May 21-23, 1973; in press (1974).
11. A. R. Goldberg, Abstracts of the Annual Meeting of the Amer. Soc. Micro., p. 218 (1973).
12. H. Rubin, Proc. Nat. Acad. Sci. U.S.A. 67, 1256 (1970).
13. A. R. Goldberg, Cell 2, (1974).
14. J. C. Unkeless, A. Tobia, L. Ossowski, J. P. Quigley, D. B. Rifkin, and E. Reich, J. Exp. Med. 137, 85 (1973).
15. L. Ossowski, J. C. Unkeless, A. Tobia, J. P. Quigley, D. B. Rifkin, and E. Reich, J. Exp. Med. 137, 112 (1973).
16. L. Ossowski, J. P. Quigley, G. M. Kellerman, and E. Reich, J. Exp. Med. 138, 1056 (1973).
17. A. R. Goldberg and S. G. Lazarowitz, J. Cell Biol. 59, 112a (1973).
18. S. G. Lazarowitz, A. R. Goldberg and P. W. Choppin, Virology 55, 172 (1973).
19. S. G. Lazarowitz, R. W. Compans and P. W. Choppin, Virology 46, 830 (1971).
20. H.-D. Klenk, C. Scholtissek, and R. Rott, Virology 49, 723 (1972).
21. J. J. Skehel, Virology 49, 23 (1972).
22. R. W. Compans, Virology 51, 56 (1973).
23. H.-D. Klenk and R. Rott, J. Virol. 11, 823 (1973).
24. D. B. Rifkin, R. W. Compans and E. Reich, J. Biol. Chem. 247, 6432 (1972).
25. S. G. Lazarowitz, R. W. Compans and P. W. Choppin, Virology 52, 199 (1973).
26. A. R. Goldberg and S. G. Lazarowitz, in preparation (1974).

TABLE 1

Serum-dependent Caseinolytic Activity of[†] PR-RSV
Transformed Chick Embryo Fibroblasts

Serum	Caseinolytic Activity
None	±*
Chicken	++++
Monkey	++
Human	++
Horse	+
Calf	0
Fetal Calf	0
Rabbit	0
Swine	0

The overlay assay is described in detail (13). Transformed or normal cells were overlayed with Eagle's or
Scherer's medium containing 0.4% agarose, 1.5-2.0%
commercial non-fat dried milk, and serum at 2.5%
(v/v) in a total volume of 3.0 ml. Caseinolytic
activity was scored at 15 hours. Parallel control
plates lacking cells showed no caseinolytic activity.

*Occasional small clear plaques were evident over zones
of piled-up cells in the absence of serum.

[†] Prague strain of RSV - subgroup C.

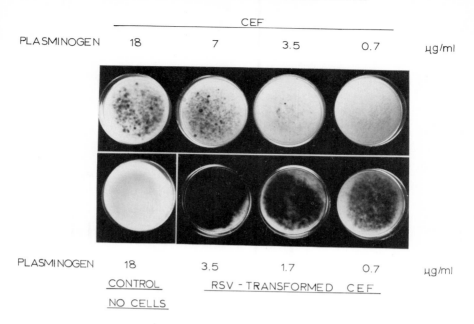

Fig. 1. Titration of Plasminogen Activator Levels of Chick Embryo Fibroblasts and RSV-Transformed Chick Embryo Fibroblasts. The overlay assay was performed as described (13). Subconfluent cultures containing either CEF or PR-RSV-C transformed CEF in equal numbers were used. Incubation was at $39°$ for 12 hours. The plates were illuminated with an indirect fluorescent light and were photographed through a blue filter against a black background. On the scale of 0 to ++++ used to indicate the extent of caseinolysis 0 represents no clearing, + represents faint mottling (e.g. 3.5 μg plasminogen/ml incubated with CEF), ++ represents approximately 25% clearing (e.g. 7 μg plasminogen/ml incubated with CEF), +++ represents approximately 50% clearing (e.g. 18 μg plasminogen/ml incubated with CEF), and ++++ represents complete clearing (e.g. RSV transformed CEF shown above). Plasminogen at 50 μg/ml, in the absence of cells, was never found to result in any caseinolysis during a three day incubation. Thus, the level of plasmin contaminating the plasminogen preparations is too low to detect by means of the casein-agarose overlay assay.

355

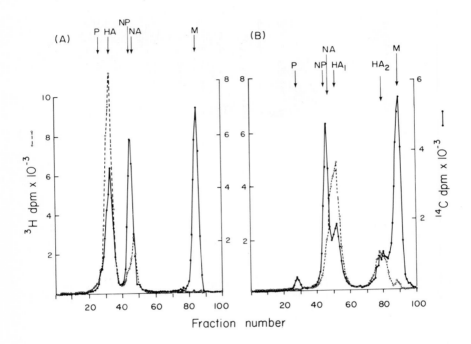

Fig. 2. Effect of plasminogen in the growth medium on the cleavage of the HA polypeptide. Polyacrylamide gel electropherograms of (^{3}H) glucosamine- and (^{14}C) amino acid-labeled WSN virions grown in MDBK cells in the presence and in the absence of plasminogen. Details of virus growth and purification procedures are in Ref. 18. (A) Virions grown in unsupplemented REM; (B) virions grown in REM containing 2.0 µg/ml plasminogen. Migration is from left to right. The ^{3}H:^{14}C ratio is the same in both panels. ^{3}H, o——o ; ^{14}C, ●——● .

Influenza Virus

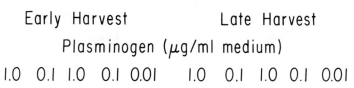

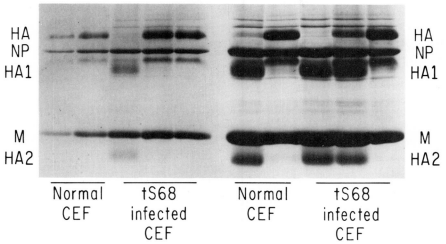

Fig. 3. Coomassie blue stained SDS/Tris/glycine gel slab. Confluent monolayers of CEF and CEF fully transformed by tsNY68SR-A were washed twice with phosphate-buffered saline (PBS) to assure removal of growth medium and were inoculated at a MOI of ~10 PFU/cell. After adsorption for 2 hr, the inoculum was removed, and the cells washed once with PBS. The monolayers were incubated for 2 hr in REM, and were then washed once more with PBS. Fresh REM containing various levels of plasminogen was added to the monolayers and incubation proceeded for 6 more hours. Early harvests were collected at 10 hours. Fresh REM containing plasminogen was added to the same cells for an additional 10 hours at which time late harvests were collected. Virus was purified as described (18) and then was subjected to electrophoresis on polyacrylamide gel slabs.

Influenza Virus
Early Harvest (4-10 hrs postinfection)
Calf Plasminogen (μg/ml medium)
1.0 0.1 0.01 1.0 0.1 0.01

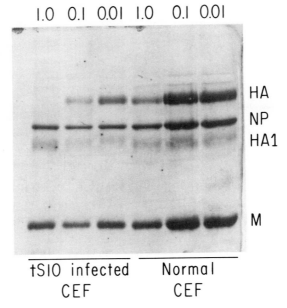

HA

NP

HA1

M

tS10 infected
CEF   Normal
CEF

Fig. 4. Coomassie blue stained SDS/Tris/glycine gel slab. Influenza virus early harvest from infection of CEF and CEF transformed by tsNY10SR-A.

Influenza Virus
Late Harvest (10-20 hrs postinfection)
Calf Plasminogen (μg/ml medium)
1.0   0.1   0.01   1.0   0.1   0.01

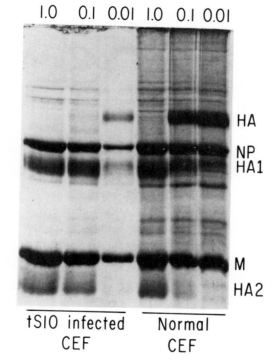

HA

NP
HA1

M

HA2

tS10 infected   Normal
CEF   CEF

Fig. 5. Coomassie blue stained SDS/Tris/glycine gel slab. Influenza virus late harvest from infection of CEF and CEF transformed by tsNY10SR-A.

VIII

CONTROL MECHANISMS FOR PHAGE

REGULATION OF LYSOGENY AND THE EVOLUTION OF TEMPERATE
BACTERIAL VIRUSES

David Botstein and Miriam M. Susskind

Department of Biology
Massachusetts Institute of Technology
Cambridge, Massachusetts 02139

ABSTRACT

(1)   There are several barriers to successful superinfection of P22 lysogens of <u>Salmonella</u> <u>typhimurium</u>.
These include exclusion at the level of adsorption,
injection, gene expression, and late phage development.

(2)   The repression-immunity system of phage P22 is bipartite.   The central, novel element of this system is a non-
specific antirepressor active against many phage
repressors.

(3)   Functional hybrids between the <u>Salmonella</u> phage P22
and the coliphage λ can readily be formed.   Analysis of
these hybrids indicates that P22 and λ have common
evolutionary ancestry.

An hypothesis concerning the evolution of temperate
viruses is presented.

INTRODUCTION

Temperate bacteriophages have evolved several
different mechanisms for preventing growth of superinfecting phages in the lysogenic host.   These mechanisms,
which can broadly be defined as superinfection exclusion
systems, are often not essential for maintenance of
the lysogenic state by the prophage; they are, however,
presumed to have a broader evolutionary significance for
lysogeny.   In the following sections, a brief review of
various exclusion mechanisms will be presented, with
special reference to those of phage P22, a temperate
phage of <u>Salmonella</u> <u>typhimurium</u>.   P22 is a particularly
suitable model for this discussion, since it specifies

363

many of the types of exclusion systems to be discussed.
The superinfection exclusion mechanisms specified by
P22 prophage are summarized in Table 1.

Clearly, all the superinfection exclusion mechanisms
have similar results. Therefore, it is usually necessary
to eliminate all but the system one wishes to study.
This is done by either using mutant prophages missing one
or more of the exclusion systems, or by using superinfection phages insensitive to one or more of the
systems.

Exclusion at the level of phage adsorption. Adsorption of phage to bacteria involves interaction with
specific receptors on the cell surface. In Salmonellae,
the O-antigen moeity (polysaccharide side-chains) of
the lipopolysaccharide layer of the cell envelope serves
as the receptor site for many temperate phages. Lysogenization of certain Salmonella strains by certain
temperate phages results in specific alterations in
the chemical structure of the O-antigen synthesized
by the cell (see Wright and Kanegasaki (1) for
review). This may reduce or abolish the ability of
some phages to adsorb; frequently, O-antigen alteration
by prophage specifically causes loss of the receptor
site for homologous phage. If adsorption is prevented, the infectious process cannot be initiated
and the cells continue to multiply as if the phage
were not present.

Studies of various Salmonella phages show that
phage-encoded functions are responsible for O-antigen
alteration. For example, O-antigen alteration by P22,
which results in a reduction in the rate of adsorption
of P22 to the lysogenic cell, is specified (at least
in part) by the prophage a_1 gene. The closely related
Salmonella phage ε^{34}, which causes a similar O-antigen
alteration (addition of glucose residues to galactosyl
moieties in the polysaccharide chain), has been shown
to have two genes that direct discrete steps in the
glucosylation process. In the case of ε^{34}, O-antigen
alteration by the prophage completely abolishes adsorption of ε^{34} to the lysogenic cell.

364

Table 1

SUPERINFECTION EXCLUSION MECHANISMS SPECIFIED

Level of exclusion	System	Result of Superinfection
adsorption	O-antigen alteration	lysogen survives
injection	sieA	lysogen survives
gene expression	immunity	lysogen survives
late phage development	sieB	lysogen dies, but no phage are produced

Exclusion at the level of injection. P22 prophage specifies an exclusion mechanism which apparently blocks entry of DNA from any of several temperate Salmonella phages that adsorb to the lysogenic cell, including P22 itself (2). This exclusion system, specified (at least in part) by the P22 sieA gene (for superinfection exclusion) (3), has been shown to block expression of all superinfecting phage functions that have been tested, including functions that are expressed by the resident prophage (4, 5, 1). The superinfecting phage DNA apparently does not enter the cell cytoplasm, since it is unavailable for marker rescue (5, 6) and for degradation by a host DNA restriction system (2). At least some of the superinfecting DNA leaves the phage head, since it is attacked to some extent by endonuclease. The hypothesis that the sieA exclusion system prevents complete injection of superinfecting phage DNA is consistent with the observation that the sieA system has no effect on either induction of resident prophage or zygotic induction of prophage transferred to the cell via bacterial conjugation.

Immunity-repression: Exclusion at the level of gene expression. All temperate phages have immunity systems which repress vegetative development of the prophage and, by the same token, prevent growth of superinfecting homologous phage. Superinfection of an immune lysogen with homologous phage has no effect on the cell, since the superinfecting phage can express only those genes already expressed by the prophage. Phage immunity-repression systems will be discussed in greater detail below. At this point, it should be noted that two criteria allow immunity systems and other superinfection exclusion systems to be distinguished unambiguously. First, exclusion mechanisms other than the immunity system are in all cases non-essential to maintenance of the prophage state. Secondly, immunity systems are necessaruly specific for superinfecting phage whose genomes are homologous to that of the prophage (at least in the immunity region itself); the other exclusion mechanisms mentioned here are either non-specific for the genetic nature of the DNA or (see below) specific for phages differing from the prophage.

Modification-restriction of DNA. DNA modification-restriction systems often account for the inability of phage propagated in one host strain to grow in a related host strain. Operationally, bacterial strain A is considered to have a modification-restriction system if it restricts the growth of phage previously grown for one cycle in host B, but fails to restrict phage upon one cycle of growth in host A. Temperate coliphage P1 specifies such a modification-restriction system in the prophage state (7).

In molecular terms, host-controlled modification involves chemical alteration of DNA molecules, and restriction involves specific degradation (endonucleo-lytic attack followed by solubilization) of improperly modified (unmodified) DNA. Though recognition of short nucleotide sequences is involved, restriction systems are active against a wide variety of (unmodified) DNA's differing in genetic content. The mode of entry of the DNA into the cell (whether by injection from phage particles, bacterial conjugation, or transformation) is usually not a factor (see (8)).

Exclusion at the level of late phage development. P22 prophage directs another exclusion mechanism, specified (at least in part) by the prophage sieB gene, that blocks superinfection by certain temperate Salmonella phages, including the closely related phage L, but does not interfere with superinfection by P22 itself (3). In P22sieB$^+$ lysogens, vegetative development of L appears to be normal until approximately 20 minutes after infection (mid-way through the normal latent period), when there is a rapid and complete cessation of DNA, RNA, and protein synthesis (9). The culture then undergoes slow, partial lysis, but studies with lysis-deficient phage mutants indicate that this is a secondary effect of the damage sustained by the cell, rather than its cause. The superinfected cells are killed, and no progeny phage are produced. If, on the other hand, the superinfecting phage elects the lysogenic rather than the lytic (vegetative) response, the sieB exclusion system in no way interferes with the establishment of lysogeny. This fact most clearly demonstrates that some aspect of the late vegetative development of the superinfecting phage is involved in triggering early arrest of macromolecular synthesis during sieB exclusion.

As mentioned above, P22 itself is not sensitive to exclusion by the sieB mechanism. This insensitivity to exclusion is due to a determinant, esc^+_{P22}, on the P22 genome. Phages carrying the esc^+_{P22} determinant can rescue sieB-sensitive phages (such as phage L) in mixed superinfection of $sieB^+$ lysogens; insensitivity is thus dominant to sensitivity in this case. The P22 escape function is under negative control by the P22 repression-immunity system, so that an excluding $P22sieB^+esc^+_{P22}$ prophage does not itself rescue super-infecting sieB-sensitive phages. However, the efficiency of the exclusion mechanism is limited by the ability of superinfecting L phage to recombine with the excluding prophage to produce recombinants with the immunity type of L and the esc^+_{P22} determinant of P22 (3, 9).

The sieB exclusion mechanism is probably not unique, since the rex exclusion system of coliphage λ (10) and the old exclusion system of coliphage P2 (11) appear to be quite similar.

6. The immunity-repression system. Unlike barriers to adsorption and injection, which affect the survival of lysogens in the event of superinfection but are of no intrinsic importance in maintainance of the lyso-genic state, the immunity-repression system of a tem-perate phage is present as an intrinsic and essential feature of the way in which lysogeny is maintained. The critical event in lysogenization is the repression of the lytic phage functions. As a matter of first principle, any direct genetic regulation by repressors which recognize DNA sites should apply not only to the prophage but also to homologous superinfecting phage. The hallmark of true immunity (as opposed to other superinfection exclusion mechanisms) is that immunity-repression is specific; i. e., only phages with homolo-gous repressors are prevented from growing in an immune lysogen.

The first lysogenic immunity system to be understood in this way was that of bacteriophage λ. The
situation in λ is quite simple: a single gene (cI)
specifies a single repressor. Expression of the cI
gene suffices to repress the lytic functions of any
and all λ DNA molecules in the cytoplasm. The cI repressor is the only barrier to superinfection by λ maintained
by λ lysogens (12).

However, it is not true that all temperate phages
regulate lysogeny in the same simple way. What follows
is a summary of our understanding of the immunity-
repression system of phage P22. The immunity system
of P22 is bipartite, consisting of two elements whose
activity is continuously required for the maintenance
of lysogeny.

The first indication that P22 immunity is bipartite was found by Bezdek and Amati (13), who observed
(using mutant phages lacking both the sieA and sieB
functions) that some recombinants between P22 and the
closely related phage L exhibit immunity patterns
different from either parent. The recombinant phages
with new immunity specificities are themselves temperate and lysogenize normally; such lysogens are
immune to superinfection by homologous phage. Two
kinds of recombinants with new immunity are found in
such crosses, as if two determinants of immunity (now
called immI and immC) segregate in the cross. The
actual immunity patterns of P22, L, and the recombinants is shown in Table 2.

More recently, Chan and Botstein (14) found that
P22 lysogens whose prophages had deletions of either
immI or immC (which are on opposite ends of the prophage map) are sensitive to superinfection by wild-
type P22. The pattern of immunity of prophage deletions
is also found in Table 2.

The patterns of immunity in Table 2 clearly show
that both immI and immC are determinants of immunity
in phage P22. P22 can grow in any lysogen whose prophage differs from P22 at either immI or immC. However,

phage L cannot grow in lysogens unless they differ at immC.

Use of hetero-immune related phages is only one way of analyzing the properties of the immunity-repression system of a phage. Another way is to examine the properties of phage mutants which either have defects in the repression system (resulting in failure to establish or to maintain lysogeny) or have defects in recognition f the repressing elements (resulting in ability to express lytic functions and to grow in immune lysogens -- defined as virulence).

Analysis of temperature-sensitive mutants with defects in the maintenance of lysogeny provides a third line of evidence that P22 immunity-repression is bipartite: there are two genes whose function is continuously required for the maintenance of lysogeny. Phage carrying temperature-sensitive mutations in the c_2 gene (15) form stable lysogens at permissive temperature, but these lysogens are induced if exposed to non-permissive temperature. Since these c_2 mutations are recessive, we can operationally define the product of the c_2 gene as the c_2-repressor. Similarly, phage carrying temperature-sensitive mutations in the mnt gene (16) form stable lysogens at permissive temperature but are induced at non-permissive temperature; mnt mutants are also recessive, and thus we can operationally define an mnt-repressor. The c_2 gene lies in the immC region, and the mnt gene lies in the immI region. Thus, the two determinants of immunity specificity are associated with two repressors, each of which is continuously required for the main-tenance of the lysogenic state. Inactivation of either mnt or c_2 repressor results ultimately in the derepression of the phage lytic functions.

Current understanding of the way in which this complicated system of repression works is summarized in Table 3 and Figure 1. The immC region of phage P22 contains what is essentially a lambda-like repressor-operator-promoter region: the c_2-repressor is flanked by its operator/promoters, Vx and K5 (17, 18). Vx mutants are constitutive for genes to the left of the

TABLE 3

PHENOTYPES OF REGULATORY MUTANTS OF P22

Mutation	Mutant Phenotype	map location	function
c_2-ts (recessive)	failure to establish or to maintain lysogeny 40°; 30° lysogens are induced at 40°	immC	c_2-repressor
Vx (cis-dominant)	partial virulent constitutive to left of c_2	immC	operator/promoter site of repression by c_2-repressor to the left
K5 (cis-dominant)	partial virulent constitutive to right of c_2	immC	operator/promoter site of repression by c_2-repressor to the right
VxK5=virB (cis-dominant)	virulent, non-inducing	immC	--
mnt-ts	failure to maintain lysogeny (40°) 30° lysogens induced at 40°	immI	mnt-repressor
Vy (cis-dominant)	weak virulent, inducing. constitutive for ant	immI	operator/promoter site of repression by mnt-repressor
ant (recessive)	suppresses mnt and Vy mutations; fails to make antirepressor	immI	antirepressor antagonizes c_2-repressors
Vyc_2=virA (dominant)	virulent, inducing	immI	--

c_2 gene; K5 mutants are constitutive for genes to the right of the c_2 gene. VxK5 double mutants are virulent (called virB) because they fail to recognize the c_2-repressor. This system exerts simple negative control of the prophage -- lytic functions fail to be expressed because of the action of c_2-repressor on flanking operators. Superinfecting P22 phages fail to grow because they have Vx and K5 operators identical to those of the prophage; hetero-immune phages with different operator sites are able to grow in the presence of c_2-repressor.

The immI region of P22 is, however, also required for immunity and maintenance of lysogeny. Recent results from the laboratories of Levine and Botstein (19) suggest that the mnt-repressor acts on an operator/promoter (Vy), which is located adjacent to the mnt gene itself. Vy mutants are constitutive for a new gene called ant, which specifies an antirepressor that antagonizes the c_2 repressor. Thus, if one induces an mnt-ts lysogen, antirepressor is made, which removes the c_2 repressor, which in turn allows lytic functions to be expressed. Similarly, Vy mutants are virulent since, on infection of a lysogen, they fail to be repressed by the mnt-repressor, make antirepressor, and grow.

Several predictions of this model have been tested. First, ant mutations should suppress all the phenotypes of Vy and mnt mutations. Vy-ant double mutants should not be virulent, and they are not; mnt-ts-ant double mutant lysogens should not be induced upon temperature shift, and they are not. Second, the model makes specific predictions about what should happen when various kinds of virulent mutant P22 phages grow in immune P22 lysogens. The virB type (which are double mutants VxK5 in the immC region) should be insensitive to c_2-repressor; when they grow, the prophage should remain repressed and not contribute to the yield of progeny. On the other hand, the virA mutants (Vy mutants in the immI region) should only be able to grow by making antirepressor constitutively, resulting in removal of c_2-repressor activity. This should allow all P22 phages to grow and be

represented in the yield. This prediction has been
confirmed: when virB virulents grow in lysogens, 10%
of the yield or less is prophage-type; when virA virulents grow, more than 35% of the yield is prophage-
type.

The third prediction of the model is that growth
of P22 phage in heteroimmune lysogens where immI is
the only difference between superinfecting phage and
prophage should be abolished if the superinfecting
phage is ant⁻. This prediction has also been confirmed -- in particular, P22 ant⁻ mutants cannot grow
in immI$_L$immC$_{P22}$ lysogens nor in immI$_{deletion}$immC$_{P22}$
lysogens, whereas P22 wild-type grows in both kinds
of lysogens. It should be pointed out that all of
the immunity phenomena in Table 2 are readily
explained if one assumes that phage L, unlike P22,
has no ant, Vy, or mnt genes, and that immI$_L$ is simply
the absence of these elements. In fact, the inability
of phage L to grow on immI$_{deletion}$immC$_L$ lysogens is
strong evidence that L has no antirepressor.

Properties of P22 antirepressor. The outstanding
new feature of the P22 bipartite immunity is the P22
antirepressor, the product of the ant gene. Since
we have mutations in the ant gene which are nonsense
(amber) and temperature-sensitive, and since ant⁻
mutations are recessive, the antirepressor most
probably is a protein. The P22 antirepressor seems
to be rather non-specific with respect to the phage
repressors which it will antagonize; it works in
vivo on at least three Salmonella phage repressors
and on the coliphage λ repressor. Antirepressor does
not work at the same level as does the "inducer"
produced after irradiation of lysogens with ultraviolet light; mutants of both λ and P22 in which the
repressor is insensitive to induction by ultraviolet
irradiation are fully sensitive to P22 antirepressor.

The activity of the antirepressor can be seen in
crude extracts; the capacity of λ phage repressor to
bind specifically to λ phage DNA is reduced or absent
in the presence of extracts containing P22 antirepressor.

Table 2

PATTERNS OF IMMUNITY SPECIFICITY

superinfecting phage		P22 P22	L L	P22 L	L P22	P22 deletion	deletion P22	deletion L
immI	immC							
P22	P22	−	+	+	+	+	+	+
L	L	+	−	−	+	+	+	−
P22	L	+	+	−	+	+	+	+
L	P22	−	+	+	−	+	−	+

374

It should be noted that mutations in the anti-repressor gene do not cause any phenotype in growth or lysogeny of the P22 phage. This is in marked contrast to the situation with the cro gene of λ, which, on first glance, might be thought to be a gene coding for an antirepressor. However, cro⁻ mutants are unable to enter the lytic cycle in the presence of a functional repressor (20); this is definitely not the case with P22 ant⁻ strains. Apparently the only function of P22 antirepressor is to allow the induction of many heteroimmune prophages when P22 superinfects. Possibly this enhances the ability of P22 to assimilate by recombination segments of other temperate phage genomes which might confer advantage to the new hybrid phage thus formed.

Construction and properties of P22-λ hybrid phages. Our explanation of the bipartite immunity properties of phage P22 clearly indicate that the c_2-repressor has the primary role of controlling expression of the lytic phage functions. The immC region of P22 resembles in detail the immunity region of coliphage λ; Figure 2 shows that this resemblance is only part of an extensive resemblance between P22 and λ in the way in which clusters of genes specifying phage functions are arranged on the genetic maps of these two temperate bacteriophages (21).

Although P22 and λ normally grow on bacterial hosts of different species (Salmonella typhimurium and Escherichia coli, respectively), it has been possible to construct viable hybrids between the two phages. Two different methods have been used: Gemski et al. (22) constructed a Salmonella-coli hybrid host which supports the growth of both phages; Botstein and Herskowitz (23) used episomes to transfer (as prophage) one of the phages into the natural host of the other.

A particular class of P22-λ has become useful in the analysis of the regulatory systems which the two phages must have at least grossly in common. These hybrids, called λimmP22, are fundamentally lambdoid phages in which the control region between the attachment site (see Figure 2) and the lysis genes

is substituted to varying degrees by analogous material
from P22. The λ genes which can be substituted
include: the recombination genes; the genes regulating
immunity (cI, cII, and cIII; note that this includes
the repressor gene cI of λ which, due to an unfortunate
historical accident, is called c_2 in P22); the DNA
replication genes O and P (genes 18 and 12 of P22),
the late control gene Q (gene 23 in P22) and the lysis-
control gene S (gene 13 in P22). Important sites of
genetic activity on the DNA are also substituted;
these include the operators v2 and v1v3 (replaced by
Vx and K5 of P22), the origin of replication, and the
late promoter for late transcription, which lies
between genes Q and S of λ (see (24) for review of
λ regulation).

Using the λimmP22 hybrids, one can determine the
specificities of the various regulatory elements.
Results of such studies have yielded the following
information:

a.   The immunity specificity of P22 is different
from that of λ, and a variety of lambdoid phages including 80, 81, 434, 424, and 82. Surprisingly, however,
λimmP22 hybrids are all homo-immune to the lambdoid
phage 21. The identity of repressors is confirmed in
DNA heteroduplexes between λimmP22 and λimm21: there
is homology at the position at which the repressor
gene (and its operators) lie. Thus, we believe that
the repressor and operators of P22 and those of
phage 21 are descended from the same ancestor.

b.   The specificity of the regulatory gene N of
P22 is different from that of all the lambdoid phages
tested. The N gene of P22 (called gene 24) will work
on the sites of action of both phages λ and 21 as well
as those of P22, whereas the N genes of λ and 21 are
each specific for their own sites.

c.   The DNA replication genes of P22 will only
replicate phages with the DNA replication region derived
from P22. Since the origin of replication of λ is
thought to lie between genes P and O, we interpret
this as meaning that the P and O gene products will

not recognize the P22 origin, and that genes 18 and 12 of P22 specify products which will not recognize the λ origin. There are also important mechanistic differences. For example, P22 replication genes cause host DNA replication to stop; λ DNA genes do not.

   d.   The late regulators (gene Q of λ; gene 23 of P22) seem to share a common specificity despite the fact that they are probably not entirely homologous. This means that the λ Q gene can cause activation of transcription from the late promoter derived from P22 and gene 23 of P22 can cause activation from the late promoter of λ. Furthermore, crosses between mutants in the Q gene and mutants in the 23 gene yield functional (i. e., non-mutant) recombinants.

   All of this information leads to two important conclusions. First, somehow P22 and the lambdoid group of bacteriophages share some common ancestry, despite their different host species. Some of these specificities have remained intact since the divergence of the two species, others have not. Second, most of the clusters of genes (recombination, immunity, early control, DNA replication, late control) have retained, over evolutionary time, both the capacity to function in the hybrids and the capacity to recombine with other clusters to form these hybrids in the first place. These capacities have been retained despite quite striking divergence in the mechanism of the functions themselves. (The DNA replication genes are a good example of this.)

Evolutionary Considerations

   Superinfection exclusion. The most striking features of the exclusion and immunity barriers to superinfection present in wild-type P22 lysogens are their large number and the diversity in their mechanisms. There clearly has been substantial selection pressure for ways to prevent superinfection. For those exclusion systems which act against homo-immune phage types (O-antigen alteration, sieA), the source of this selection pressure is easily understood. Vy (virA) virulent phages can arise as single-step mutations;

377

if the mutation arises in a $sieA^+$ prophage, the virulent mutant cannot continue to grow, but if the prophage is $sieA^-$, the newly arisen virulent mutant can propagate itself. In practice, ordinary $sieA^-$ lysogens are unstable as cultures because spontaneous Vy mutants of the prophage arise, can grow, and eventually destroy the culture. Thus, long-range stability of lysogeny maintained by the bipartite immunity system (which allows single-step virulents to arise) ultimately depends in part on superinfection exclusion systems. It is relevant that phage L, which has no sieA system, also has no functional antirepressor gene and does not spontaneously mutate to virulents in a single step.

The selective value of the sieB exclusion system, which is active only against certain heteroimmune Salmonella phages, is less clear.

Bipartite immunity. Most wild strains of bacteria, especially Salmonellae, are lysogens of one or more temperate phages (25). Sometimes these prophages specify alterations of the cell surface, producing sites for the adsorption of particular other phages. Lysogeny of one phage thus may be essential to produce a sensitive host for a second; this is explicitly the case for the Salmonella phage ε^{34}, which adsorbs only to cells lysogenic for phage ε^{15} (26). Therefore, ε^{34} has an obvious evolutionary interest in the survival of ε^{15}.

Any phage (A) which is dependent upon another phage (B) for its adsorption profits from inducing that phage when it grows. Induction of prophage allows two modes of further growth of phage A: encounter with a sensitive strain or encounter with an insensitive strain that can be lysogenized with phage B to become sensitive. Of course, this argument can be applied to any phage that is dependent in any way on a helper prophage.

Although it is not known in the case of P22 that a particular prophage is required for sensitivity to P22, P22 is known to be closely related to ε^{34} (C. Van Beveren and A. Wright, unpublished results). The antirepressor of P22 could have evolved in some other background (such

as that of ε^{34}) and been acquired recently by P22.
Its retention, however, implies continued selective
advantage and requires another explanation nevertheless.

Segmental evolution of temperate bacteriophages: an hypothesis. We would like to
suggest that the evolution of at
least the temperate bacterial viruses proceeds by the
local diversification of functional gene clusters with
concommitant maintenance of functional compatibility
and genetic homology such that the ability to reassort
segments is indefinitely retained. This view, first
clearly stated by Hershey (27), is supported by a
great deal of evidence. First, within the lambdoid
temperate bacteriophages of E. coli, one can readily
discern a pattern of alternating homologies and non-
homologies in the DNA (28, 29). It should be pointed
out that almost all combinations of these phages form
viable hybrids. More striking is the fact that viable
hybrids can be formed between P22 and λ (23, 22; Hilliker
and Botstein, unpublished results); functional compatibility and adequate stretches of genetic homology
have been retained even though these phages grow on
different host species. Furthermore, over evolutionary time the specificities of some of the genes
(repressor and Q) have not changed, whereas others
(DNA replication genes and lysis genes) have.

If the evolution of phages proceeds in this segmental way, then it is incorrect to view a single
phage type as the product of evolution; the individual
functional segment is the unit and the entire set of
segments in the product of evolution. The role of an
antirepressor, according to this scheme, is to facilitate the reassortment of the functional segments to
fit changing environmental conditions. Antirepressor,
by inducing the prophage and allowing it to replicate,
increases recombination; its relative nonspecificity
for particular phage repressors is nicely consistent
with this role.

There is no reason to believe that this form of
evolution is limited to bacterial viruses. In fact,

the segmented nature of many animal virus genomes (alluded to elsewhere in this volume) might reflect a form of group/segmental evolution. One might expect, therefore, that functional hybrids between viruses of quite divergent host species might frequently be encountered.

ACKNOWLEDGEMENTS

This paper summarizes the unpublished work of many others, principally Sandra Hilliker, Ira Herskowitz, Andrew Wright, and Kenneth Lew. We thank Van Jarvik for technical assistance, and Ann Skalka for bringing to our attention Hershey's ideas on phage evolution.

DB holds a Career Development Award from the National Institutes of Health (#5 K04 GM70325-02) and MMS is a fellow of the Damon Runyon Memorial Fund (Fellowship #798). Research was supported by the American Cancer Society under grant #VC18B and by the National Institutes of Health under grant #GM18973.

REFERENCES

1. Wright, A. and Kanegasaki, S. (1971). Physiol. Rev. 51, 748-784.

2. Susskind, M. M., Botstein, D., and Wright, A. (1974a). Virology, in press.

3. Susskind, M. M., Wright, A., and Botstein, D. (1971). Virology 45, 638-652.

4. Walsh, J. and Meynell, G. G. (1967). J. Gen. Virol. 1, 581-582.

5. Rao, R. N. (1968). J. Mol. Biol. 35, 607-622.

6. Ebel-Tsipis, J. and Botstein, D. (1971). Virology 45, 629-637.

7. Luria, S. E. (1953). Cold Spr. Harbor Symp. Quant. Biol. 18, 237-244.

8. Boyer, H. W. (1971). Ann. Rev. Microbiol. 25, 153.

9. Susskind, M. M., Botstein, D., and Wright, A. (1974b). Virology, in press.

10. Garen, A. (1961). Virology 14, 151-163.

11. Lindahl, G., Sironi, G., Bialy, H., and Calendar, R. (1970). Proc. Nat. Acad. Sci. USA 66, 587-594.

12. Ptashne, M. (1971). In The Bacteriophage Lambda (A. D. Hershey, ed.), Cold Spring Harbor Laboratory, Cold Spring Harbor, New York, pp. 221-237.

13. Bezdek, M., and Amati, P. (1968). Virology 36, 701-703.

14. Chan, R. K. and Botstein, D. (1972). Virology 49, 257-268.

15. Levine, M. and Smith, H. O. (1964). Science 146, 1581-1582.

16. Gough, M. (1968). J. Virol. 2, 992-998.

17. Bronson, M. J. and Levine, M. (1971). J. Virology 7, 559-568.

18. Bronson, M. J. and Levine, M. (1972). Virology 47, 644-655.

19. Levine, M. (1972). Current Topics in Microbiol. and Immunol. 58, 135-156.

20. Echols, H. (1971). In The Bacteriophage Lambda (A. D. Hershey, ed.), Cold Spring Harbor Laboratory, Cold Spring Harbor, New York, pp. 247-270.

21. Botstein, D., Chan, R. K., and Waddell, C. H. (1972). Virology 49, 268-282.

22. Gemski, P., Jr., Baron, L. S., and Yamamoto, N. (1972). Proc. Nat. Acad. Sci. USA 69, 3110-3114.

23. Botstein, D. and Herskowitz, D. (1974). Nature, in press.

24. Herskowitz, I. (1973). Ann. Rev. Genet. 7, 289-324.

25. Adams, M. H. (1959). Bacteriophages (New York: Wiley Interscience).

26. Uetake, H. and Hagiwara, S. (1961). Virology 13, 500-506.

27. Hershey, A. D. (1971). In Carnegie Institution Year Book 70, Cold Spring Harbor Laboratory, Cold Spring Harbor, New York.

28. Simon, M. N., Davis, R. W., Davidson, N. (1971). In The Bacteriophage Lambda (A. D. Hershey, ed.), Cold Spring Harbor Laboratory, Cold Spring Harbor, New York, pp. 313-328.

29. Fiandt, M., Hradecna, Z., Lozeron, H. A., and Szybalski, W. (1971). In The Bacteriophage Lambda (A. D. Hershey, ed.), Cold Spring Harbor Laboratory, Cold Spring Harbor, New York, pp. 329-354.

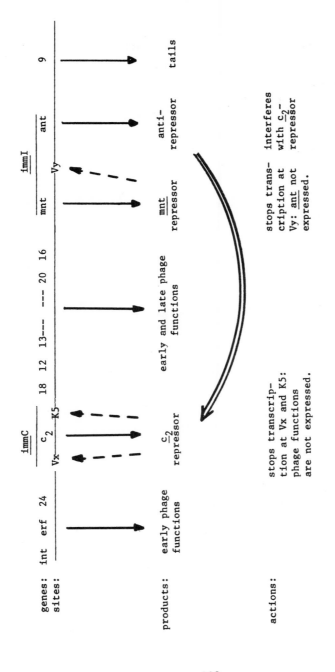

FIGURE 1

MODEL FOR BIPARTITE IMMUNITY OF PHAGE P22

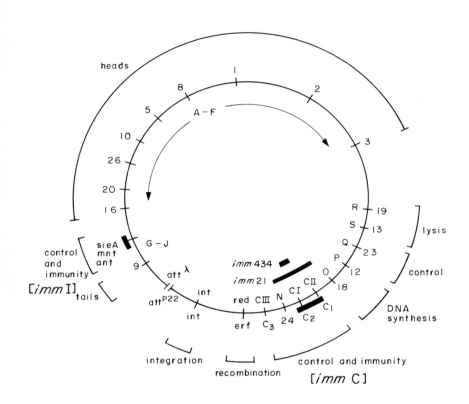

RECIPROCAL TRANSACTIVATION IN A TWO CHROMOSOME PHAGE SYSTEM

Kathleen Barrett[1], Stephen Barclay[2], Richard Calendar[1]*,
Björn Lindqvist[3] and Erich Six[4]

ABSTRACT. Satellite phage P4 carries genes for DNA replication and control of gene expression, but relies on a
helper phage for most of the genes which cause morphogenesis of the phage particle. P4 transactivates these needed
genes from a repressed prophage helper. The helper genome
appears to also provide a transactivating gene product,
which causes two late genes of satellite phage P4 to be
expressed earlier and more actively. These P4 late gene
products may determine phage head size. Transactivation
similar to the phenomena we report here may also be observed in the adenovirus-adeno associated virus system, and
perhaps also in the interaction between the Y chromosome
and other chromosomes.

INTRODUCTION

Helper-dependence of satellite phage P4. Satellite phage
P4 and its helper, temperate coliphage P2, have occupied
our attention for several years, because they provide an
unusual opportunity to observe chromosome-chromosome interactions in a system amenable to extensive genetic analysis.
Figure 1 outlines the unusual life cycle of satellite phage
P4. This virus can infect E. coli strains carrying P2 or a
related helper prophage and produce a burst of progeny P4
containing no helper phage (<0.1 per cell) (1,2). Satellite phage P4 can also infect nonlysogenic strains, but

---

Present addresses: [1]Molecular Biology Dept., University of
California, Berkeley, Ca.94720; [2]McArdle Laboratories for
Cancer Research, University of Wisconsin; [3]Institute of
Medical Biology, University of Tromsø, Norway; [4]Micro-
biology Dept., University of Iowa Medical Center.

*Reprint requests should be addressed to Richard Calendar.

such an infection produces no progeny. Instead, P4 DNA
replicates and can insert into the host genome to yield a
repressed prophage (2,3). These data indicate that P4
carries genes for integration and immunity to superinfection, but lacks the genes needed for phage particle synthesis and cell lysis. These conclusions can be confirmed
by using conditional-lethal mutants in the P2 prophage helper (Figure 1 c and d) (Six, in preparation). No P4 progeny are produced when P4 infects E. coli carrying a P2
"late" mutant, which affects phage particle synthesis or
cell lysis. The required late genes include 11 tail synthesis genes, six head synthesis genes, and one lysis gene,
all of which fall into four transcription units (Figure 2).
When P4 infects a strain carrying a P2 "early" mutant prophage, the burst of P4 is of normal size and occurs after
a slightly extended latent period. P4 can make plaques on
strains which carry P2 early mutant prophages. Thus the
two known P2 early genes are not needed for replication of
P4 DNA. Furthermore, these results suggest that P4 carries
its own function for transactivation of helper late genes,
since P2 early mutants cannot replicate their DNA or express P2 late genes.

Transactivation of genes from the helper prophage. Satellite phage P4 causes genes of the helper prophage to be
expressed by a mode which is different than that used during normal P2 infection, by two criteria: first, the prophage helper DNA is not replicated extensively (11; Lindqvist, unpublished experiments). This contrasts with
normal P2 infection, where a mutation in either of the two
P2 early genes blocks both DNA replication and late gene
expression (5,12). Second, P4 transactivation of helper
late genes appears not to lift the immunity to superinfection which normally blocks late gene expression (2). This
is illustrated in Figure 3. P2 multiplication is blocked
during P4 infection of a P2-lysogenic strain (Figure 3a),
although a P2 "dismune" prophage--one which carries a different immunity specificity--cannot block P2 multiplication
during P4 infection (Figure 3b). Thus, during a P4 infection the immunity system of P2 appears not to be altered
(Figure 3 c and d). Therefore, gene expression in the
P2-P4 system appears unusual, in that the same set of genes
(P2 late genes) can probably be activated by two different
mechanisms, one caused by P2 early genes and one caused by

satellite phage P4 genes.

In order to understand the mechanism of P4 transactivation we have begun to characterize P4 DNA and the genes which it carries. Double-stranded P4 DNA (m.w. 7×10^6 daltons) can be extracted from purified particles (seen in Figure 4), and compared to the double-stranded DNA of helper phage P2 (m.w. 22×10^6 daltons) (13,14). By DNA-DNA hybridization analysis, these two DNA species are less than 1% homologous (15). This fact shows that P4 is not a deletion of P2, and is consistent with the notion that P4 gene products might activate P2 genes by a different mechanism. The P4 genome is large enough to code for ten average proteins (m.w. 35,000 daltons), and from the preceeding discussion, one could guess that these proteins aid in P4 DNA replication, control of P2 gene expression, and P4 prophage integration. In addition, we suppose that P4 carries a gene for determination of small head size, since P4 size heads (diameter=45 nm) are not found in P2 infected cells, which contain only P2 size heads with d=62 nm (16; D.H. Walker, Jr., personal communication). To date we have characterized P4 mutants of three types: recessive amber suppressible mutants which block P4 DNA replication, a dominant temperature-sensitive mutation which shuts off all macromolecular synthesis, and clear plaque type mutants which block lysogenization (3,16).

The 15 P4 amber mutants isolated to date fall into a single complementation group, called the A gene (16). These mutants synthesize DNA at less than 1% the rate observed after infection with P4 wild type. However, helper phage genes are transcribed (transactivated) at 40% the level found during P4 wild type infection, and phage heads are formed in normal quantity (15,16). The A gene product may be identical with an enzyme which transcribes a polydeoxycytidylic acid template, yielding polyriboguanylic acid as product (17). This enzyme may make an RNA primer which is required to initiate rounds of P4 DNA synthesis. Recessive conditional-lethal mutants affecting transactivation have not yet been isolated. Such mutants would probably affect a factor which interacts with the host transcription apparatus. The host RNA polymerase must participate in P4 transactivation because the drug rifamycin, which prevents initiation of RNA chains by binding to the beta subunit of RNA polymerase (18), eliminates P4 transactivation of the P2 genome (15).

387

RESULTS

Kinetics of transactivation. Further information on the transactivation process has been obtained from a kinetic analysis of P2 and P4 protein synthesis (Barrett and Calendar, manuscript in preparation). When satellite phage P4 infects E. coli in the absence of helper, four phage induced proteins can be detected by gel electrophoresis (Figure 5). Two of these are synthesized early after infection (Figure 6). The larger P4 early protein is the gene A product, while the smaller one may be the transactivating factor. The two smallest P4 proteins are synthesized late after infection (Figure 6). These late P4 proteins may be needed for morphogenesis, since one of them is found in the P4 head (Barrett and Calendar, in preparation) The expression of these P4 late proteins is greatly reduced by amber mutations in P4 gene A, implying that P4 DNA replication is needed for expression of P4 late genes.

A surprising property of the transactivation phenomenon can be observed when P4 protein synthesis in the presence of a helper genome is compared with P4 protein synthesis in the absence of the helper (Figure 6). In the presence of P2 helper the P4 late proteins appear about thirty minutes earlier and in 5-10 fold larger quantities (Barrett and Calendar, manuscript in preparation). This transactivation occurs at the transcriptional level, and not at the translational level, because the amount of P4 specific RNA is higher when P4 infects a P2-lysogenic strain than when P4 infects a nonlysogenic strain (15). Thus, the P2 helper genome transactivates satellite phage P4 late genes. This reciprocal or echoing transactivation between P2 and P4 genomes is depicted in Figure 7. We believe that transactivation of P4 late genes is caused by a product of a P2 early gene which has not yet been defined by conditional-lethal mutation. The first evidence for this proposal is the properties of P2 prophage deletions which cover the early region, but retain the late region (Figure 8). These deletions abolish the ability of P4 to form plaques. Table 1 summarizes the effects of several such mutations on the growth of P4. In each case, the latent period of P4 is greatly lengthened. This slowdown is probably caused by the absence of a diffusible product. The existence of this diffusible product was surmised from the result of a complementation experiment described in

Figure 9. In this experiment the defective prophage is the only source of the T (tail) gene product. However, the defective prophage cannot supply the T gene product at the normal time after infection by P4 alone (Figure 9, left panel). Furthermore, superinfecting P2 amT$_5$ cannot transactivate the repressed, defective prophage (Figure 9, right panel). However, superinfecting P4 and P2 amT$_5$ together can transactivate T gene product from the P2 early deletion prophage (Figure 9, center). We cannot say what molecular events cause this early transactivation, but a P2 early gene product seems to be needed. In the absence of this P2 gene product, P4 must exploit the helper late genes and activate its own late genes "on its own". This solo transactivation requires extra time. Figure 7b summarizes our current view of reciprocal transactivation, with each arrow indicating a trans or cis activation for which we have evidence. Any single arrow can be removed from this scheme while still maintaining a workable system. In the slow growth of P4 on strains carrying P2 early deletion prophage, only the arrows originating on the P4 genome are operative. If P4 wild type were to function in this fashion, it could probably have survived in nature without being discovered through its plaque forming ability. Such nonplaque forming "shadow viruses" may be common.

Transactivations in animal viruses and eukaryotic cells. The reciprocal transactivation between phage P2 and P4 may be analogous to certain phenomena observed in animal cells. For example, adeno-associated satellite virus (AASV) antigens are expressed only in the presence of a helper virus (20-23). This potentiation of AASV by its helper may represent the same sort of transactivation which we are observing (Figure 10), especially since the AASV mRNA and antigens are expressed simultaneously with adenovirus late proteins (19,20). Cell lines which carry the Epstein-Barr virus can also help AASV (21), and these cells may be partially analogous to lysogenic E. coli.

It seems likely that transactivation occurs between genes on mammalian chromosomes, although this proposition is only easy to test in the sex chromosome system. Hamerton (24) has in fact suggested that the role of the Y chromosome is to transactivate certain genes on the X chromosome and on the autosomes (Figure 10). Although there is minimal evidence to support this hypothesis (25), the idea is an attractive one in light of the fact that Y-linked genetic markers are so rare. The fact that a single autosomal mutation in goats can largely replace the action of the Y chromosome indicates that the Y chromosome might function simply in <u>trans</u>activation (24).

ACKNOWLEDGEMENTS

This work was supported by Public Health Service Research Grants AI 04043 and AI 08722 from the National Institute of Allergy and Infectious Diseases; CA 14097 and Training Grant CA 05028 from the National Cancer Institute and CA 07175 and T01-CA 05002 from the National Cancer Institute to the McArdle Laboratory. Grants from the Norwegian Government to the University of Tromsø supported the transcription studies. The guidance of William F. Dove was instrumental in the genetic work, while the preparation of the manuscript was aided by the advice of M. David Hoggan and Morgan Harris.

REFERENCES

1. E.W. Six, *Bacteriol. Proc.* p.138 (1963).
2. E.W. Six and C. Klug, *Virology 51*, 327 (1973).
3. B.H. Lindqvist and E.W. Six, *Virology 43*, 1 (1971).
4. G. Lindahl, *Virology 39*, 839 (1969).
5. G. Lindahl, *Virology 42*, 522 (1970).
6. G. Lindahl, *Virology 46*, 620 (1971).
7. G. Lindahl, *Molec. Gen. Genet. 128*, 249 (1974).
8. G. Lindahl and M.G. Sunshine, *Virology 49*, 180 (1972).
9. M.G. Sunshine, M. Thorn, W. Gibbs, R. Calendar and B. Kelly, *Virology 46*, 691 (1971).
10. M. Schnös and R.B. Inman, *J. Mol. Biol. 55*, 31 (1971).
11. E.W. Six and B.H. Lindqvist, *Virology 43*, 8 (1971).
12. B.H. Lindqvist, *Molec. Gen. Genet. 110*, 178 (1971).
13. R.B. Inman and G. Bertani, *J. Mol. Biol. 44*, 533 (1969).
14. R.B. Inman, M. Schnös, L.D. Simon, E.W. Six and D.H. Walker, *Virology 44*, 67 (1971).
15. B. Lindqvist, in preparation.
16. W. Gibbs, R.N. Goldstein, R. Wiener, B. Lindqvist and R. Calendar, *Virology 53*, 24 (1973).
17. K. Barrett, W. Gibbs and R. Calendar, *Proc. Nat. Acad. Sci. U.S. 69*, 2986 (1972).

18. A. Heil and W. Zillig, *FEBS Letters*, *11*, 165 (1970).
19. B.J. Carter and J.A. Rose, *J. Virol. 10*, 9 (1972).
20. N.R. Blacklow, M.D. Hoggan and W.P. Rowe, *J. Exp. Med. 125*, 755 (1967).
21. N.R. Blacklow, M.D. Hoggan and M.S. McClanahan, *Proc. Soc. Exp. Biol. Med. 134*, 952 (1970).
22. N.R. Blacklow, R. Dolin and M.D. Hoggan, *J. Gen. Virol. 10*, 29 (1971).
23. R.W. Atchison, *Virology 42*, 155 (1970).
24. J.L. Hamerton, *Nature 219*, 910 (1968).
25. U. Mittwoch, In: *Genetics of Sex Differentiation*, Academic Press, London, (1973).
26. J.A. Lengyel, R.N. Goldstein, M.G. Sunshine, M. Marsh and R. Calendar, *Virology 53*, 1 (1973).
27. J. Lengyel, R. Goldstein, M. Marsh and R. Calendar, *Virology*, in press (1974).
28. D.K. Chattoraj and R.B. Inman, *Proc. Nat. Acad. Sci. U.S. 71*, 311 (1974).
29. L.E. Bertani and G. Bertani, *Proc. Nat. Acad. Sci. U.S. 71*, 315 (1974).
30. L.E. Bertani, *Virology 36*, 87 (1968).
31. U. Laemmli, *Nature 227*, 680 (1970).

TABLE 1

P4 production on E. coli carrying absolute
defective P2 prophage mutants

Prophage type	Time for synthesis of normal P4 burst, minutes	Burst size, phage/cell
P2 parent	55	225
del 5a-4	150	250
del TR410	200	200
"point" mutation 1-4	120*	100*

The E. coli strain carrying the "P2 parent" prophage
is E. coli C(P2 c5 int₁) constructed by L.E. Bertani (30).
The "point" mutation 1-4 is a heat induction survivor isolated by L.E. Bertani. This strain cannot provide B gene
function after heat induction (L.E. Bertani, personal communication). Cells were grown in LB   broth at 30° and
infected at m.o.i.=0.1 at 37° (deletions) or at m.o.i.=10
at 42° (point mutation).

*This experiment at 42° gives a shorter latent period and
smaller burst than the other experiments performed at 37°.

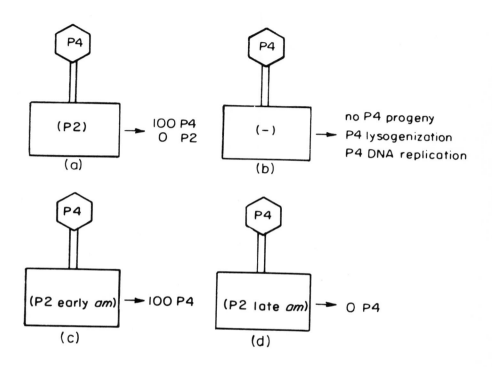

Figure 1. Satellite phage P4 infections in E. coli
(a) lysogenic for P2, (b) nonlysogenic, and (c,d) lysogenic
for P2 amber mutations in early and late genes, where late
genes involve morphogenesis and lysis, while early genes
affect DNA replication and positive control of late gene
expression. These infections (c) and (d) are made under
conditions which are nonpermissive for the P2 mutants employed. Results (a,b) are described in detail by Six and
Klug (1), while (c,d) come from Six, manuscript in preparation.

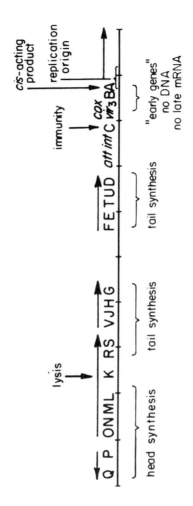

Figure 2. Genetic map of phage P2 constructed from crosses between vegetatively multiplying phage (4-9). The arrows indicate the polar effects of certain amber mutations. These polar effects are thought to indicate units of transcription. The early gene B lies to the left of the replication origin (10,28,29), but gene A could lie to the left or right of it. Replication is unidirectional, from left to right, beginning at 11% from the right end of the mature DNA, plus or minus 500 base pairs (10).

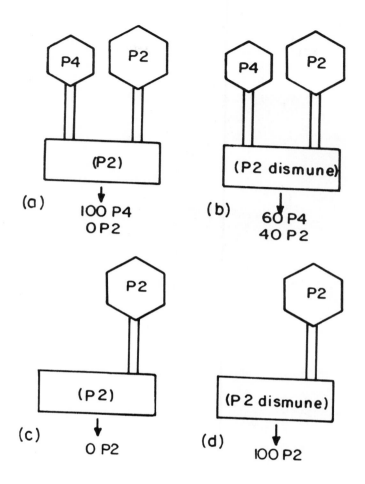

Figure 3. Immunity to P2 superinfection caused by P2 and P2 dismune prophage in the presence and absence of satellite phage P4. P2 "dismune" is a phage which carries all the essential genes of P2 except for the immunity gene, which is replaced by an immunity gene of different specificity. Infections were made at a multiplicity of 5-10 phage per cell for each type in Luria broth, and are described in detail by Six and Klug (2).

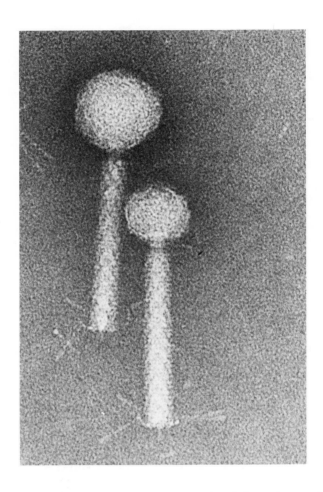

Figure 4. Temperate phage P2 (left) and satellite phage P4 (right), negatively stained with phosphotungstate. The tail structures are 135 nm long, while the P2 head is 62 nm in diameter, and the P4 head is 45 nm in diameter. Electron micrograph by Robley C. Williams, University of California, Berkeley.

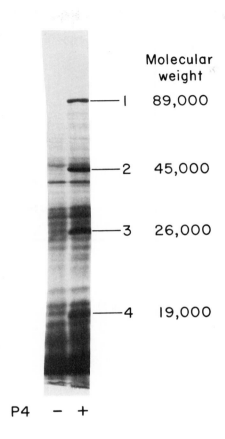

	Molecular weight
1	89,000
2	45,000
3	26,000
4	19,000

P4   −   +

Figure 5. Proteins induced after infection with satellite phage P4. E. coli uvrA was treated with ultraviolet light to reduce host protein synthesis. P4 was allowed to infect these cells, and a two minute pulse of ^{14}C-amino acids was administered after 70 minutes of infection at 37°. The cells were then boiled in 2% sodium dodecyl sulphate, 3% mercaptoethanol, and proteins were seperated by electrophoresis by the Laemmli procedure (31).

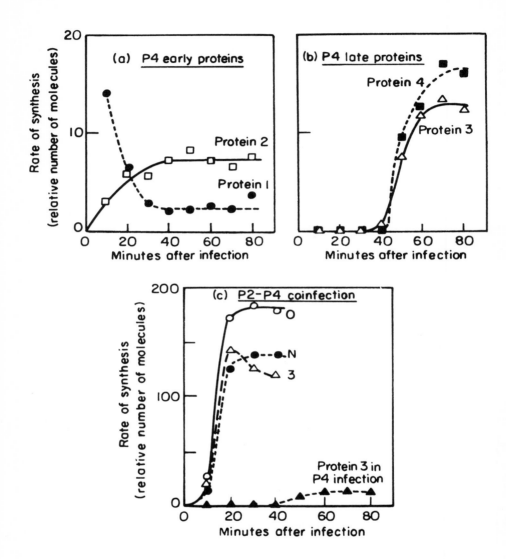

Figure 6. Kinetics of synthesis of P4 proteins in a nonlysogenic host (a,b) and in cells coinfected with both P4 and P2 (c). Proteins N and O are head synthesis proteins encoded in the helper phage genome (26), while proteins 1-4 are the P4 gene products depicted in Figure 5.

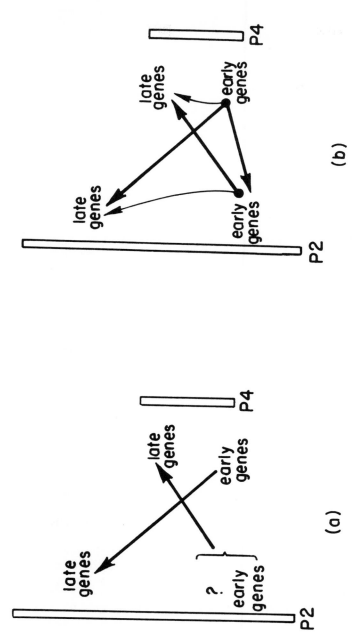

Figure 7. Schemes for reciprocal transactivation between the P2 and P4 genomes. Each arrow represents a transactivation which is caused by a gene product encoded in the genome where the arrow originates and acting on the genome where the arrow points.

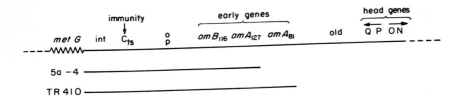

Figure 8. Map of deletions in the early region of P2 prophage. The deletions were selected by heat induction of an integration–deficient prophage (S. Barclay, in preparation).

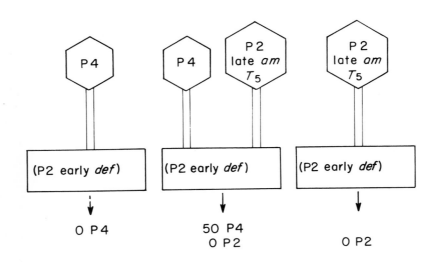

Figure 9. Complementation test designed to show whether the defective prophage is mutant in a site or in a gene which is needed for rapid transactivation of the P2 T gene by P4. E. coli C carrying the early defective mutant 1-4, described in Table 1, was grown in Luria broth at 32° and infected with the appropriate phage at m.o.i.=10 for each phage. The P2 late amber mutation is amT_5, which affects tail synthesis (6,27). Phage were assayed 160 minutes after infection, which is at the end of the P4 latent period on E. coli C (P2). On the strain carrying defective prophage 1-4, P4 are not produced until about 300 minutes.

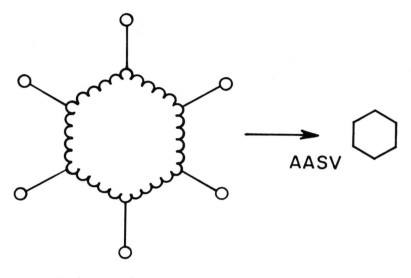

AASV

Adenovirus

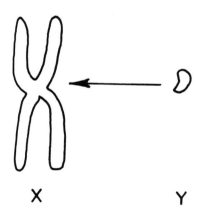

X   Y

Figure 10. Probable <u>transactivations</u> found in eukaryotic cells. The <u>transactivating</u> factor is synthesized by
the genome at the base of the arrow, and the <u>transacti-
vation</u> occurs at the tip of the arrow.

IN VITRO CONSTRUCTION OF BACTERIAL PLASMID REPLICONS CONTAINING PROKARYOTIC AND EUKARYOTIC GENES

Stanley N. Cohen[*], Annie C.Y. Chang[*], John F. Morrow[+]
Herbert W. Boyer[#], Howard M. Goodman[Δ], Robert B. Helling[#×],
Louise Chow[Δ], and Leslie Hsu[*]

Departments of [*]Medicine and [+]Biochemistry
Stanford University School of Medicine
Stanford, California 94305

Departments of [#]Microbiology, and [Δ]Biochemistry
and Biophysics
University of California
San Francisco, California 94143

ABSTRACT. A procedure for the in vitro construction of plasmid chimeras containing genes originating from diverse sources is described. EcoRI restriction endonuclease-generated fragments of bacterial plasmids isolated from Staphylococcus or E. coli, or of amplified DNA coding for the 18S and 28S ribosomal RNA of Xenopus laevis, have been linked to the pSC101 plasmid replicon and introduced into E. coli by transformation. The constructed plasmid chimeras can be cloned as stable replicons in E. coli, where they synthesize RNA and/or protein products specified by their component genes.

INTRODUCTION

Biochemical and genetic investigations carried out during the past decade have established that genes specifying antibiotic resistance in the Enterobacteriaceae can be carried by autonomously replicating units of extrachromosomal DNA (i.e., plasmids) (Recent reviews: refs. 1,2,3). Certain of these plasmids are capable of self-transfer among related bacteria, while others require either a

---

[+]Present Address: Carnegie Institution of Washington, Department of Embryology, Baltimore, Maryland 21210

[×]Present Address: Department of Botany, University of Michigan, Ann Arbor, Michigan

transducing bacteriophage or a conjugally proficient plasmid to accomplish transfer. Recently, it has been shown
that plasmid replicons can also be introduced into Escherichia coli by transformation, using purified plasmid DNA
(4); moreover, clones of bacteria that have been transformed with plasmids contain circular DNA molecules which
have the genetic and structural properties of the parent
plasmid. Consequently, transformation has proved to be a
useful tool for the cloning of bacterial plasmids and for
investigating the characteristics of different species of
plasmid DNA (4,6,7,8).

CHARACTERISTICS OF TRANSFORMATION PROCEDURE

The requirements for transformation of E. coli by
plasmid DNA (4) are shown in Table 1. Transformation is
accomplished by plasmids of various incompatability groups,
and by closed circular, open (nicked) circular, and caten-
ated forms of plasmid DNA; however, denaturation or sonication of the DNA destroys its ability to transform.
Transforming efficiency is unaffected by treatment of plasmid DNA with ribonuclease, pronase, or phenol, but is
abolished by treatment with pancreatic deoxyribonuclease
if carried out prior to the 42° heat pulse step responsible
for DNA uptake (4). Unlike transformation of E. coli with
chromosomal DNA (5), plasmid transformation does not require that recipient cells be deficient in the recBC
nuclease, and genetic determinants carried by the plasmid
can be selected in recipient cells that have been transformed by as little as 10^{-5} to 10^{-6} µg of DNA. Plasmid
DNA isolated from transformants (Figure 1) can itself be
used to transform other bacteria.

Recent experiments have shown that certain DNA fragments generated from larger plasmids by shearing (6) or by
treatment by the EcoRI restriction endonuclease (9) can be
introduced by transformation into E. coli, where they can
recircularize and become functional plasmid replicons.
One such plasmid (i.e., pSC101) (6,7) that was formed
after transformation of E. coli by a sheared fragment of
the larger antibiotic resistance plasmid, R6-5 (10,11)
carries the genetic information necessary for its own replication and for expression of resistance to tetracycline.
This plasmid has proved to be valuable in the construction
of plasmid chimeras in vitro because of the fortuitous lo-

cation of its single cleavage site for the EcoRI endonuclease.

EcoRI RESTRICTION ENDONUCLEASE

The EcoRI restriction endonuclease (12,13) cleaves double stranded DNA so as to produce short overlapping single stranded ends. On a random basis, the nucleotide sequence cleaved is expected to occur once in every 4,000 to 16,000 nucleotide pairs (12); thus, most EcoRI generated fragments contain one or more intact genes. The nucleotide sequences cleaved by the enzyme are unique and self-complementary (12,14,15) so that DNA fragments produced can be associated by hydrogen bonding with either end of any other EcoRI-generated fragment. After hydrogen bonding, the 3' hydroxyl and 5' phosphate ends can be joined by DNA ligase (14,15). Thus, the enzyme appeared to be useful for construction of DNA molecules having segments originating from diverse sources. Molecular chimeras produced by the joining of different EcoRI generated DNA fragments could potentially be introduced into bacterial strains by transformation, provided that at least one of the fragments carries a capability for replication and selection in transformed bacteria. As noted above, the pSC101 plasmid was useful for this purpose, since insertion of a DNA segment at its single EcoRI cleavage site does not interfere with either its replication functions or expression of its tetracycline resistance genes. Our initial plasmid construction experiments involved the linkage of this replicon to a EcoRI-generated fragment of another "synthetic" antibiotic resistance plasmid, pSC102.

CONSTRUCTION OF PLASMID CHIMERAS IN VITRO

The pSC102 plasmid, which carries resistance to kanamycin, neomycin, and sulfonamide was formed by reassociation and in vivo ligation of several EcoRI-generated fragments of the larger plasmid, R6-5 (8). Agarose gel electrophoresis (Figure 2C) indicates that the pSC102 plasmid is cleaved into its three component fragments by the EcoRI restriction endonuclease. The molecular weight of 17.4×10^6 daltons for the sum of three fragments is consistent with the size of the pSC102 plasmid determined by electron microscopy and sucrose gradient sedimentation.

The pSC101 plasmid is cleaved by the EcoRI restriction endonuclease into a single linear DNA fragment (Figure 2D) as noted above.

A mixture of EcoRI cleaved pSC101 and pSC102 plasmid DNA was treated with DNA ligase, and the ligated molecules were used to transform E. coli. Transformants that were resistant to both tetracycline and kanamycin contained a new plasmid (pSC105) which on cleavage with the EcoRI endonuclease (Figure 2A) is seen to contain fragment II of pSC102 (i.e., the fragment that carries kanamycin resistance) plus the DNA fragment that comprises the entire pSC101 tetracycline resistance plasmid.

This procedure for the in vitro construction of recombinant plasmid molecules has also proved useful for the formation of plasmids that include DNA derived from different bacterial species. Such experiments have been carried out with a penicillinase-producing plasmid of Staphylococcus aureus (pI258, molecular weight ~ 20×10^6 daltons (16, 17,18). This staphylococcal plasmid appeared to be especially appropriate for interspecies genome construction, since its genetic and molecular properties have been widely studied, and it carries several different genetic determinants that were potentially detectable in E. coli. Moreover, agarose gel electrophoresis indicated that this plasmid is cleaved by the EcoRI restriction endonuclease into four easily identifiable fragments (19).

Molecular chimeras containing both staphylococcal and E. coli DNA were constructed by ligation of a mixture of EcoRI cleaved pSC101 and pI258 DNA, and were then used to transform a restrictionless strain of E. coli ($C600r_k^-m_k^-$) (19). Transformants that expressed the penicillin resistance determinant carried by the staphylococcal plasmid were selected, and the plasmid DNA isolated from such clones was characterized. Cesium chloride gradient analysis of an E. coli-Staphylococcus plasmid chimera isolated from one such transformant (pSC112) is shown in Figure 3. The buoyant density of the intact plasmid chimera ($\rho = 1.700$ g/cm^3) is intermediate between that of the pSC101 plasmid ($\rho = 1.710$ g/cm^3) and the density of the parent staphylococcal plasmid ($\rho = 1.691$ g/cm^3). Upon treatment with the EcoRI endonuclease, the pSC112 plasmid is cleaved into separate fragments having buoyant density characteristics of the component DNA species. Further study of this plasmid by agarose gel electrophoresis and electron microscope heteroduplex analysis (19) confirmed that it contains DNA sequences derived from both E. coli and Staphylococcus.

CONSTRUCTION OF MOLECULAR CHIMERAS CONTAINING BOTH PROKARYOTIC AND EUKARYOTIC GENES

In the experiments described thus far, genetic determinants carried by DNA fragments linked to the pSC101 plasmid replicon were utilized to select for transformants that contain plasmid chimeras. More recent experiments by Morrow, Cohen, Chang, Boyer, Goodman and Helling (20) involve the in vitro construction of plasmid chimeras composed of both prokaryotic and eukaryotic DNA, and recovery of the recombinant DNA molecules from transformed E. coli in the absence of selection for genetic properties expressed by the eukaryotic DNA. The amplified ribosomal DNA (rDNA) coding for 18S and 28S ribosomal RNA of Xenopus laevis was used as a source of eukaryotic DNA for these experiments, since this DNA has been well characterized and can be isolated in quantity (21,22). Moreover, the repeat unit of X. laevis rDNA is susceptible to cleavage by the EcoRI endonuclease, resulting in the production of DNA fragments of characteristic size (Figure 4) that can be linked to the pSC101 plasmid (20).

A mixture of EcoRI cleaved pSC101 DNA and X. laevis rDNA was ligated, and used to transform E. coli strain C600 $r_k^-m_k^-$. Tetracycline resistant transformants were selected, and the plasmid DNA isolated from 55 separate clones was analyzed by agarose gel electrophoresis, cesium chloride gradient centrifugation, and/or electron microscopy to determine the presence of X. laevis rDNA linked to the pSC101 plasmid replicon. The results of these experiments are summarized in Table 2. Thirteen of the 55 tetracycline-resistant clones selected contained one or more EcoRI-generated fragment having the same size as the fragments produced by cleavage of X. laevis rDNA. The observed variation in size of the EcoRI generated X. laevis rDNA fragments contained in plasmid chimeras was consistent with the observed size heterogeneity of the fragments generated by EcoRI cleavage of the amplified X. laevis rDNA repeat unit (20).

Agarose gel electrophoresis (Figure 4) of EcoRI cleaved DNA comprising several representative E. coli-

407

X. laevis plasmid chimeras listed in Table 2 demonstrates
the presence of DNA fragments characteristic of X. laevis
rDNA. Comparison of the buoyant densities of rDNA isolated from X. laevis and of EcoRI digests of these four
plasmid chimeras isolated from E. coli (Figure 5) indicates
that each plasmid contains at least one EcoRI generated
DNA fragment about equal in buoyant density to amplified
X. laevis rDNA (ρ = 1.729 g/cm^3). In addition, cleavage
by the restriction endonuclease enables identification of
a fragment having the buoyant density of pSC101 DNA
(ρ = 1.710 g/cm^3) as a component of each plasmid chimera.

Electron microscope analysis (Figure 6) of a heteroduplex formed between X. laevis DNA, and the one of the
constructed plasmid chimeras (CD42) isolated from E. coli
confirms that this bacterial plasmid contains DNA nucleotide sequences originating in X. laevis rDNA. Moreover,
in this and other heteroduplexes, two separate plasmid DNA
molecules were seen to form duplex regions with the single
strand of X. laevis rDNA, consistent with the observation
(23,24) that the rDNA sequences of X. laevis are tandemly
repeated.

Additional heteroduplex analysis (Figure 7) of
EcoRI-generated fragments of X. laevis rDNA cloned in E.
coli indicates that the 3.9 and 4.2 megadalton fragments
are identical, except for a 300,000 to 500,000 M.W. segment absent in the smaller fragment. This segment of DNA
appears as an internal deletion loop located about 40% of
the distance between the two EcoRI sites. These data confirm the relationship between the 3.9 and 4.2 megadalton
fragments of amplified X. laevis rDNA inferred earlier on
the basis of DNA-RNA hybridization experiments (20), and
further demonstrate the heterogeneity of the X. laevis
rDNA repeat unit. While our heteroduplex data do not permit determination of whether the deleted DNA segment is
located in the 18S ribosomal RNA cistron carried by these
fragments (20) or in the spacer region (22,23) of the
repeat unit, the similar extent of annealing observed for
the 3.9 and 4.2 megadalton rDNA fragments with 18S X.
laevis ribosomal RNA (20) may provide some support for the
latter interpretation.

Plasmid chimeras containing both E. coli and X. laevis
DNA replicate stably in the bacterial host as part of the
pSC101 plasmid replicon, and can be recovered from transformed E. coli by procedures commonly used for the isola-

tion of bacterial plasmids. Moreover, ^{3}H-labelled RNA isolated from bacteria harboring these plasmids hybridizes in vitro to amplified X. laevis rDNA isolated directly from the eukaryotic organism (20), indicating that transcription of this eukaryotic DNA occurs in its prokaryotic host.

SUMMARY

The experiments presented here demonstrate that plasmids which have been constructed in vitro and which contain both prokaryotic and eukaryotic genes can be introduced into E. coli, where they exist as stable replicons. The procedure described offers a general approach that utilizes bacterial plasmids for the cloning of DNA molecules from various sources, provided that both molecular species have cohesive termini made by a restriction endonuclease and that insertion of a DNA segment at the cleavage site of the plasmid does not interfere with expression of genes essential for its replication and selection. The ability to clone specific fragments of DNA from a complex genome provides a potentially valuable tool for the study of organization and function of eukaryotic genes.

ACKNOWLEDGEMENTS

This paper reviews a series of investigations that have been carried out collaboratively by the various authors. These studies were supported by grants AI 08619, GM 14378 and CA14026 from the National Institutes of Health, by Grant GB 30581 from the National Science Foundation, and by Grant NP-112H from the American Cancer Society. RBH was a USPHS Special Fellow.

REFERENCES

1. R.C. Clowes, Bacterial. Rev. 36, 361 (1971).
2. D.R. Helinski, Ann. Rev. Micro. 27, 437 (1972).
3. N. Willets, Ann. Rev. of Genetics 6, 257 (1972).
4. S.N. Cohen, A.C.Y. Chang and L. Hsu. Proc. Nat. Acad. Sci. U.S.A. 69, 2110 (1972).
5. S.D. Cosloy and M. Oishi, Proc. Nat. Acad. Sci. U.S.A. 70, 84 (1973).
6. S.N. Cohen and A.C.Y. Chang, Proc. Nat. Acad. Sci. U.S.A. 70, 1293 (1973).

7. J. van Embden and S.N. Cohen, J. Bacteriol. 116, 699 (1973).

8. P. Guerry, J. van Embden and S. Falkow, J. Bacteriol. 117, 619 (1974).

9. S.N. Cohen, A.C.Y. Chang, H.W. Boyer, and R.B. Helling, Proc. Nat. Acad. Sci. U.S.A. 70, 3240 (1973).

10. R.P. Silver and S.N. Cohen, J. Bacteriol. 110, 1082 (1972).

11. P.A. Sharp, S.N. Cohen, and N. Davidson, J. Mol. Biol. 75, 235 (1973).

12. J. Hedgepeth, H.M. Goodman, and H.W. Boyer, Proc. Nat. Acad. Sci. U.S.A. 69, 3448 (1972).

13. P.J. Greene, M.C. Betlach, H.M. Goodman, and H.W. Boyer in Methods in Molec. Biol., ed. R.B. Wickner, (Marcel Dekker, Inc. N.Y.) (1974) in press.

14. J.E. Mertz and R.W. Davis, Proc. Nat. Acad. Sci. 69, 3370 (1973).

15. V. Sgaramella, Proc. Nat. Acad. Sci. U.S.A. 69, 3389 (1972).

16. M.G. Rush, C.N. Gordon, R.N. Novick, and R.C. Warner, Proc. Nat. Acad. Sci. U.S.A. 63, 1304 (1969).

17. R.P. Novick and D. Bouanchaud, Ann. N.Y. Acad. Sci. 182, 279 (1971).

18. M. Lindberg and R.P. Novick, J. Bacteriol. 115, 139 (1973).

19. A.C.Y. Chang and S.N. Cohen, Proc. Nat. Acad. Sci. U.S.A. 71, in press (1974).

20. J.F. Morrow, S.N. Cohen, A.C.Y. Chang, H.W. Boyer, H.M. Goodman, and R.B. Helling, Proc. Nat. Acad. Sci. U.S.A. 71, in press (1974).

21. I.B. Dawid, D.D. Brown, and R.H. Reeder, J. Mol. Biol. 51, 341 (1970).

22. M.L. Birnstiel, M. Chipchase, and J. Speirs, Prog. Nucl. Res. Mol. Biol. 11, 351 (1971).

23. P.C. Wensink and D.D. Brown, J. Mol. Biol. 60, 235 (1971).

24. D. Hourcade, D. Dressler, and J. Wolfson, Proc. Nat. Acad. Sci. U.S.A. 70, 2926 (1973).

Table 1

Requirements for transformation by R-factor DNA

DNA species	Transformants/μgDNA
R6-5 (F-like)	
Closed circular	9.2×10^4
+DNase (before)	<0.3
+DNase (after)	7.7×10^4
+RNase (before)	9.6×10^4
+Pronase (before)	8.1×10^4
Phenol extraction	9.9×10^4
Isolated from transformed bacteria	7.0×10^4
Catenated	3.2×10^4
Open-circular	5.6×10^4
Denatured	<0.3
Sonicated	<0.3
No DNA	*
No bacteria	<0.3
R64-11	
Closed circular	9.4×10^3
No DNA	*
No bacteria	<0.3

*No colonies were observed when 10^9 bacteria were assayed in the absence of DNA.

Conditions for isolation of plasmid DNA, and for transformation under the various conditions listed in the table have been described elsewhere (4). Transformation efficiency was determined after a 2 hr. incubation in antibiotic free medium, to allow full expression of drug resistance. The terms "before" and "after" refer to the period of incubation of plasmid DNA and $CaCl_2$-treated cells at 42°.

411

Table 2

X. laevis – E. coli Recombinant Plasmids

Plasmid DNA	Molecular Weight of EcoRI Plasmid Fragments Estimated by Gel Electrophoresis (x 10^{-6})	Molecular Weight From Contour Length (x 10^{-6})	Buoyant Density of Intact Plasmid in CsCl (g/cm^3)
CD 4	5.8, 4.2, 3.0	13.6	1.721
CD 7	5.8, 4.2	–	–
CD 12, CD 20, CD 45, CD 47, CD51	5.8, 3.0	–	–
CD 14	5.8, 4.2, 3.0	–	–
CD 18	5.8, 3.0	9.2	1.720
CD 30	5.8, 3.9	10.0	1.719
CD 35	5.8, 3.9, 3.0	–	–
CD 42	5.8, 4.2	10.6	1.720
pSC101	5.8	6.0	1.710

The procedures employed for plasmid DNA isolation, agarose gel electrophoresis, cesium chloride gradient centrifugation, and calculation of molecular weight and buoyant density of DNA have been described elsewhere (20).

412

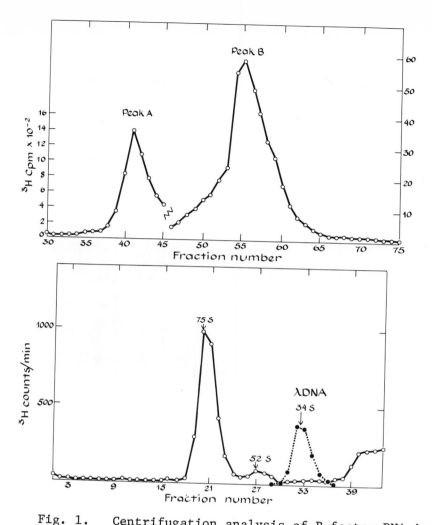

Fig. 1.   Centrifugation analysis of R factor DNA isolated from transformed cells.
(Top)   Tritium-labelled DNA isolated from transformed cells
by a detergent-lysis procedure was centrifuged to equilibrium in ethidium bromide.   Fractions were collected and
assayed for radioactivity.   After removal of ethidium bromide from the covalently closed circular DNA contained in
peak A (fractions 40-43), this DNA was analyzed in a 5-20%
linear sucrose gradient in the presence of ^{14}C-labelled
DNA marker.   The DNA species observed have the molecular
properties of the transforming plasmid.   Experimental details have been described elsewhere (4).   Note the change
in scale in the top figure.

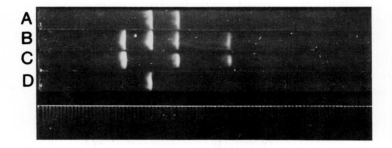

Fig. 2.   Agarose gel electrophoresis of EcoRI digests of plasmids. DNA fragments subjected to electrophoresis in agarose gels as described elsewhere (9) were
stained with ethidium bromide, and the fluorescing DNA
bands were photographed under long wave-length ultraviolet
light.   A. pSC105 DNA.   B. Mixture of pSC101 and
pSC102 DNA.   C. pSC102 DNA.   D. pSC101 DNA.

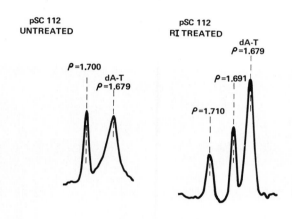

Fig. 3.   Analytical ultracentrifugation of the
E. coli-Staphylococcus aureus plasmid chimera, pSC112.
Densitometer tracings are shown.
(Left) Untreated plasmid chimera showing a buoyant density
intermediate between E. coli and Staphylococcus.
(Right) Cleaved plasmid showing the component EcoRI gener-
ated fragments. The experimental conditions have been de-
scribed elsewhere (19).

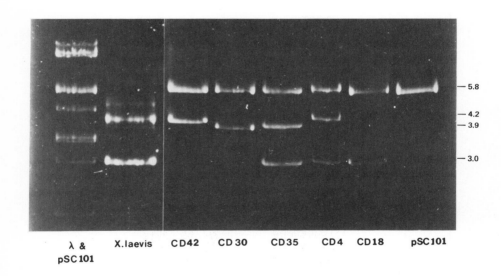

λ &   X.laevis   CD42   CD30   CD35   CD4   CD18   pSC101
pSC101

Fig. 4.   Agarose gel electrophoresis of EcoRI endonuclease-generated fragments. A source of the DNA and the
calculated molecular weights of the major fragments present in EcoRI-treated X. laevis rDNA and the plasmid chimeras shown are indicated in the Figure. All values are
10^{-6}. Experimental details are described by Morrow et al.
(20).

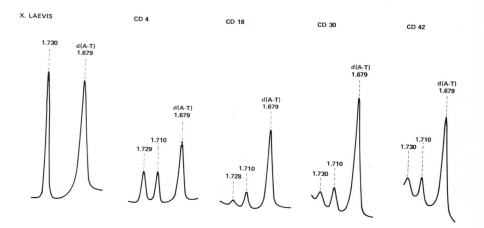

Fig. 5. Analytical ultracentrifugation of EcoRI cleaved DNA isolated from E. coli transformants carrying plasmid chimeras, and X. laevis rDNA. Densitometer tracings of photographs taken during centrifugation are shown. Details are provided elsewhere (20).

417

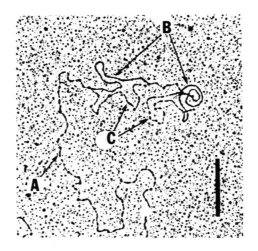

Fig. 6.   Electron photomicrograph of heteroduplex of X. laevis rDNA and two separate molecules of a tetracy-cline-resistance plasmid chimera (CD42) isolated from E. coli.
A. Single strand of X. laevis rDNA.   B. Double-strand-ed regions of homology between plasmid CD42 and X. laevis rDNA.   C. Single stranded regions corresponding in length to the DNA segment of the CD42 plasmid that was de-rived from pSC101. Experimental conditions were as indi-cated by Morrow et al. (20).

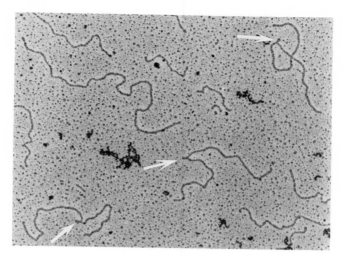

Fig. 7.   CD30 and CD42 plasmid DNA were digested
separately with restriction endonuclease EcoRI, extracted
with phenol and dialysed against TE buffer at 4°C.
(0.01 M Tris, pH 8.5 0.001 M EDTA). Equal amounts of the
two DNA samples were mixed, denatured with 0.1 N NaOH at
room temperature for 10 minutes, and then neutralized with
2M Tris pH 7.2 (1.8 M Tris – HCl + 0.2 M Tris – base).
Annealing was carried out by dialysing the solution against
70% formamide in 10 x TE at a DNA concentration of 3 μg/ml
for 2 hours at room temperature; hybridization was terminated by dialysing against TE buffer at 4°C. The solution
was spread by the formamide technique (spreading solution:
45% formamide, 50 μg/ml cytochrome C, 10 x TE, 0.5 μg/ml
DNA; hypophase: 15% formamide, 1 x TE). DNA was picked
up on parlodion coated copper grids, stained with uranyl
acetate and shadowed with Pt-Pd alloy. Pictures were
taken with a Philips 300.1 electron microscope. Arrows
point to the deletion loops observed in heteroduplexes of
the two X. laevis rDNA fragments (4.2 and 3.9 x 10^6 daltons) present in CD42 and CD30. The deletion loop always
appears as a fold-back "blip" (presumably due to its high
GC content); it measures around 6-9% of CD42 X. laevis
rDNA (4.2 x 10^6 daltons) and maps at 40% of the distance
between the two EcoRI sites. Such heteroduplexes occur in
about 50% of molecules. No deletion loops were observed
when CD42, CD30, or pSC101 DNA samples were separately re-
natured, and the homoduplexes were examined by electron
microscopy.

CHROMOSOMAL MUTATIONS AFFECTING THE ABILITY OF *SACCHAROMYCES CEREVISIAE* TO HARBOR OR EXPRESS THE "KILLER" EXTRACHROMOSOMAL GENOME

Reed B. Wickner

Laboratory of Biochemical Pharmacology
National Institute of Arthritis, Metabolism,
and Digestive Diseases
National Institutes of Health, Bethesda, Maryland 20014

Some strains of the eukaryote *Saccharomyces cerevisiae* (baker's yeast) carry a plasmid, called the "killer plasmid," whose presence is associated with virus-like particles and two species of double-stranded RNA (1-8). This plasmid is dependent on host genes for both its replication or maintenance and its expression.

Makower and Bevan in 1963 (1), first reported that some strains of yeast, called "killers," secrete a substance which is lethal to certain other strains, called "sensitives" (Fig. 1). Killers are resistant to the effects of the toxic substance.

The following phenotype notation is used: K^+ or K^- refers to the killing ability of a strain; R^+ or R^- denotes its resistance to killing. A single phenotype, *e.g.*, the K^-R^+ phenotype, may result from any of several different genotypes.

Somers and Bevan (3) showed that killing ability and resistance require the presence of an extrachromosomal genetic element, the "killer plasmid," which is distinct from mitochondrial DNA and, I have found (15), is probably distinct from two other genetically defined plasmids of *S. cerevisiae* (9, 10). This killer plasmid is passed to all progeny during mitosis and meiosis, but cells may be "cured" of the plasmid by growth of the cells at elevated temperatures (11) or by growth in low concentrations of cycloheximide (12).

Bevan and coworkers (5, 7) and Vodkin and Fink (6, 8) have shown that all killer strains carry two species of ds RNA, called "L" and "M," with the molecular weights 2.5×10^6 and 1.5×10^6, respectively (Table I). All nonkiller strains lack "M" (7, 8) while certain cytoplasmically-inherited killer mutants lack "M" but have a third species called "S" (8). It is not yet certain, however, whether these ds RNA's are the killer plasmid. Bevan *et al.* (7) have also reported finding virus-like particles in all killer strains. Their relation to the killer plasmid or the ds RNA is not yet clear, however, and transmission of killing ability without mating has not yet been observed.

I have begun studying the role of "host" genes in the killer system (13). Several distinct recessive chromosomal genes are essential to the replication or maintenance of the killer plasmid (Table II). They are pets (12), M (3), mak-1 (13), mak-2 (13), and mak-3 (15). If any of these five genes are defective, the killer plasmid is lost and cannot be recovered by mating with a wild type sensitive strain. Strains carrying mutations in any of these genes have the K⁻R⁻ phenotype. In the case of pets, the chromosomal gene defect leads to loss of both the killer plasmid and the mitochondrial genome; in all other cases, only the killer genome is lost. Vodkin *et al.* (8) and Bevan *et al.* (7) have found that M⁻ or pets⁻ cells lose the "M" ds RNA component, but retain the "L" component. This is consistent with the findings that killer strains always carry "M" and "L" (7, 8), while nonkillers always lack "M" but may still have "L".

Three other recessive chromosomal genes are required for the expression of the plasmid functions but are not needed for maintenance or replication of the plasmid (Table II) (13). Two of these, which I call kex-1 and kex-2 for killer expression, have the phenotype K-R+. These strains maintain and replicate the complete killer plasmid, but are unable because of the chromosomal mutation, to produce the killer toxin. The third gene is called rex-1 for resistance expression. Rex⁻ strains maintain and replicate the plasmid normally and produce the killer substance, but are no longer resistant to it. They survive only by being grown and stored at a pH at which the killer toxin is inactive.

Rex⁺ killers have an obvious selective advantage compared to strains which do not carry the killer plasmid. The former kill the latter. Rex⁻ killers, having the K⁺R⁻ phenotype, are suicide-prone. Thus, mutation of a single host gene, by changing the expression of a visiting genome, converts a selective advantage into a selective disadvantage.

Three of these chromosomal genes, pets, mak-1, and kex-2, have been mapped. Pets is near the mating-type locus on chromosome III (12); mak-1 is tightly centromere-linked on chromosome XV; and kex-2 is on chromosome XIV but not meiotically-linked to any known markers on this chromosome (15). None is very close to previously mapped genes, so we do not know what else they may do for the host cell.

A number of different types of plasmid mutants have also been isolated. One type of altered plasmid is called "suppressive." These strains have lost both the ability to kill and to resist being killed but have acquired the ability to exclude the normal plasmid (14), a sort of immunity to infection conveyed by a defective virus. These are the plasmid mutants which have lost ds RNA "M" but have a smaller species "S" (8). Interestingly, some host strains can give rise to this type of mutant plasmid, while others cannot (15). The genetic basis for this strain difference is now under investigation.

Another class of mutants of the killer plasmid is called "latent" (13, 15). These strains may have any defective phenotype, lacking either killing ability or resistance or both, but all have normal chromosomal maintenance and expression genes.

Their interesting property is that they all give rise to K^+R^+ diploids when mated with any strain whatever, even with ones apparently lacking the plasmid (Fig. 2). In fact, even crossing these mutants with themselves gives rise to K^+R^+ diploids. One possible explanation is that these strains carry the complete killer plasmid, but that this plasmid is in some "latent" or "inexpressible" state. Study of the ds RNA species present in these strains is now underway.

In summary, the "killer" of the eukaryote *S. cerevisiae* is a genetically easily manipulated system which may shed much light on the nature of virus-host relationships of the double-stranded RNA viruses.

REFERENCES

1. Bevan, E. A., and Makower, M.: The inheritance of a killer character in yeast (*Saccharomyces cerevisiae*). *Proc. Int. Congr. Genet. XI*, 1, 202 (1963).

2. Woods, D. R., and Bevan, E. A.: Studies on the nature of the killer factor produced by *Saccharomyces cerevisiae*. *J. Gen. Microbiol.*, 51, 115-126 (1968).

3. Somers, J. M., and Bevan, E. A.: The inheritance of the killer character in yeast. *Genet. Res.*, 13, 71-83 (1969).

4. Bevan, E. A., and Somers, J. M.: Somatic segregation of the killer (k) and neutral (n) cytoplasmic genetic determinants in yeast. *Genet. Res.*, 14, 71-77 (1969).

5. Berry, E. A., and Bevan, E. A.: A new species of double-stranded RNA from yeast. *Nature*, 239, 279-280 (1972).

6. Vodkin, M. H., and Fink, G. R.: A nucleic acid associated with a killer strain of yeast. *Proc. Nat. Acad. Sci. U. S. A.*, 70, 1069-1072 (1973).

7. Bevan, E. A., Herring, A. J., and Mitchell, D. J.: Preliminary characterization of two species of dsRNA in yeast and their relationship to the "killer" character. *Nature*, 245, 81-86 (1973).

8. Vodkin, M., Katterman, F., and Fink, G. R.: Yeast killer mutants with altered double-stranded ribonucleic acid. *J. Bacteriol.*, 117, 681-686 (1974).

9. Cox, B. S.: ψ, A cytoplasmic suppressor of super-suppressor in yeast. *Heredity*, 20, 505-521 (1965).

10. Lacroute, F.: Non-Mendelian mutation allowing ureido-succinic acid uptake in yeast. *J. Bacteriol.*, 106, 519-522 (1971).

11. Wickner, R. B.: "Killer character" of *Saccharomyces cerevisiae*: curing by growth at elevated temperature. *J. Bacteriol.*, 117, 1356-1357 (1974).

12. Fink, G. R., and Styles, C. A.: Curing of a killer factor in *Saccharomyces cerevisiae*. *Proc. Nat. Acad. Sci. U. S. A.*, 69, 2846-2849 (1972).

13. Wickner, R. B.: Chromosomal and nonchromosomal mutations affecting the "killer character" of *Saccharomyces cerevisiae*. *Genetics*, in press.

14. Somers, J. M.: Isolation of suppressive sensitive mutants from killer and neutral strains of *Saccharomyces cerevisiae*. *Genetics*, 74, 571-579 (1973).

15. Wickner, R. B., unpublished results.

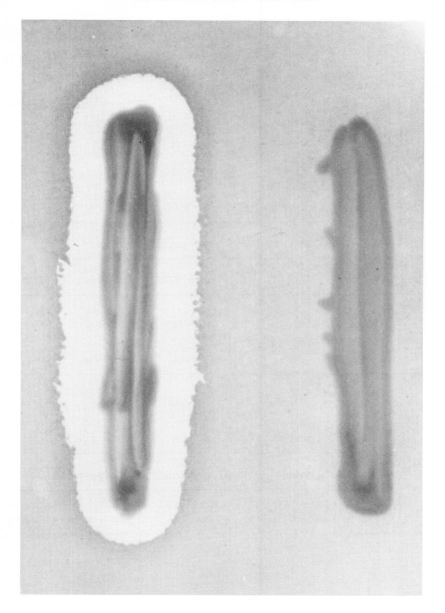

FIG. 1. The effect of a killer strain (left) and a non-killer strain (right) of *Saccharomyces cerevisiae* on the growth of a lawn of a sensitive strain.

FIG. 2. "Latent" mutants give rise to killer diploids on mating with any strain.

```
                              Other strain
"Latent" mutant               lacking plasmid
                       X                             ⟶   K⁺R⁺ diploids
(K⁻R⁺ or K⁺R⁻ or K⁻R-)        (wild type K⁻R⁻
                               or cured K⁻R⁻
                               or mak⁻ K⁻R⁻)
```

TABLE I

Double-stranded RNA in "killer" yeast

ds RNA Species	Molecular Weight	Type of Strain		
		K⁺R⁺	Wild Type K⁻R⁻	Suppressive K⁻R⁻
L	2.5×10^6	+	+ or −	+
M	1.5×10^6	+	−	−
S	0.5×10^6	−	−	+

TABLE II

Chromosomal genes involved in the "killer" system

Mutant Gene	Maintenance or Replication of		Expression of	
	Killer Plasmid	Mitochondrial DNA	Killing	Resistance to Killing
pets	−	−		
M, mak-1, mak-2, mak-3	−	+		
kex-1, kex-2	+	+	−	+
rex-1	+	+	+	−

IX

ONCOGENIC HERPES VIRUS

ASPECTS OF THE PATHOGENESIS OF LYMPHOMA IN COTTON-TOP MARMOSETS FOLLOWING INOCULATION OF EB VIRUS

George Miller, Thomas Shope[*] and Donald Coope
Departments of Pediatrics and
Epidemiology and Public Health
Yale University School of Medicine
New Haven, Connecticut 06510

ABSTRACT. The oncogenicity of EB virus has been tested directly in an experimental animal, the cotton-top marmoset. Of 17 animals given 10^4 to 10^5 transforming units of virus, 5 developed malignant lymphoma, 3 lymphoid hyperplasia, 7 inapparent infection, and 2 failed to develop antibodies. Neither lymphoproliferative disease nor EBV antibody was detected in 7 uninoculated or mock-inoculated animals. Four of five animals with lymphoma had received immunosuppressive drugs. Cell lines which expressed EB viral capsid antigen were derived from 4 pathologic lymph nodes, two with lymphoma and two with hyperplasia. Biologically active EBV and particles with typical morphology have been recovered from the one cell line studied. An imprint prepared from one malignant lymphoma demonstrated that nearly all the tumor cells contained EB nuclear antigen.

The experimental disease shares many features with Burkitt lymphoma. Nonetheless the results do not prove the oncogenicity of EB virus in man. This proof will probably rely on an epidemiologic demonstration that removal of the virus leads to disappearance of the disease.

---

[*] Present address: Department of Pediatrics, Wayne State University School of Medicine, Detroit, Michigan 48201

INTRODUCTION

Epstein-Barr virus (EBV) is intimately associated with three human diseases, namely, infectious mononucleosis, Burkitt lymphoma (BL), and nasopharyngeal carcinoma (NPC). In mononucleosis the association appears causal: mononucleosis represents a primary infection with EBV (1), antibodies to EBV confer protection against mononucleosis (2), and virus can be readily recovered from blood and oropharyngeal secretions of acute cases (3, 4). The nature of the association of EBV with Burkitt lymphoma and nasopharyngeal carcinoma is still under close study. The available evidence demonstrates that the virus is regularly, although not invariably, present in Burkitt tumors. Lymphoblastoid lines established from the tumors contain EB viral particles in a small proportion of cells (5); cloning studies indicate that all cells contain viral specific information (6). Some lines obtained from Burkitt tumors do not produce viral particles or antigens representing viral capsids but they express a nuclear antigen and an antigen complex detectable by complement fixation (7, 8). Furthermore the prototype non-producer line, Raji, contains a complete, or nearly complete, copy of the viral genome intimately associated with cell chromosomes, perhaps integrated in cell DNA (9, 10, 11).

Direct evidence has been obtained for the presence of the viral genome in tumor biopsies. If all reported series are summarized, 93 African BL biopsies contained the EBV genome and 2 biopsies, indistinguishable by histology, have been EBV genome free (12). Biopsies of lymphoma with histologic characteristics of BL obtained from 4 American patients have not contained EBV genomes (13). Recently 14 BL biopsies have been shown to contain EB nuclear antigen in a majority of the cells (14).

Similar results have been obtained for nasopharyngeal cancer. Cell lines containing viral particles and antigens have been established from lymphoid elements of the tumors (15). The genome has also been detected in most tumors by nucleic acid hybridization (16). Both EB nuclear antigen and viral genomes have been found in the epithelial cells of one nasopharyngeal carcinoma biopsy (17). This important finding would indicate that the EBV genome can be detected in non-lymphoid cells.

Seroepidemiologic studies also point to an association of EBV with Burkitt lymphoma and NPC. Specific EBV antibody titers are up to 10-fold higher in sera from patients in the endemic areas than in control populations matched for age (18). A serologic reaction unique to tumored patients has not been identified; however 90% of sera from patients with advanced Burkitt lymphoma contain antibody against the EBV "early antigen"; this reactivity is detected in the sera of less than 10% of normal persons (19).

The association of the virus and antiviral antibodies with the tumors does not prove causality, for it could be argued that the tumor provides a good substrate for replication of a latent or endogenous virus. Two observations seem to argue against the passenger virus hypothesis. First, EBV genomes have not been found in a variety of lymphoproliferative diseases, including EBV genome free BL, within and outside the endemic area. The absence of EBV in these tumors suggests that the ubiquitous virus does not invariably superinfect lymphoma. Second, Burkitt lymphomas from Africa are uniclonal on the basis of 3 markers found in the biopsies, namely, surface immunoglobulin, glucose 6 phosphate dehydrogenase, and EB nuclear antigen (20). Therefore, if EBV is a passenger the primary carcinogen must preferentially transform an EBV genome carrying clone.

One needs to resolve the paradox of the geographic limitations of BL and NPC and the world-wide presence of the virus. Several hypotheses have been proposed to accommodate this finding (21). EBV strains from different parts of the world might differ in subtle aspects. Fine structural details of various EBV's have not yet been worked out. Genetic differences among the host populations might be very important. A variety of environmental factors, such as other diseases or chemical carcinogens might influence the outcome. For example, Burkitt has proposed that the coexistence of malaria might account for the geographic distribution of the tumor (22). One hypothesis which has received experimental support is that EBV coexists in BL and NPC with RNA tumor virus (23). This finding does not shed light on which of the two agents, if either, might be the primary carcinogen.

Studies of the biologic properties of EBV also provide evidence for its possible role as a human oncogenic virus. EB virus causes leukocytes of man and several species of non-human primates to grow continuously in vitro (24-26). This process is referred to as immortalization in an effort to stay clear of the term transformation which is applied to many biologic phenomena, and to indicate that there are few measurements which allow a comparison with transformation of cell monolayers by papovaviruses. EBV is responsible since immortalization is inhibited by EBV specific antibody, since certain EBV antigens and the EBV genome appear in the immortalized cells and since mature EBV can be recovered from the immortalized cells, if they originate from the blood of marmosets or squirrel monkeys (27).

It was of interest to determine whether immortalization, observed in vitro, had a counterpart in the intact animal. Three general approaches to this question have been made. First, cell lines and biopsies from a variety of sources have been heterotransplanted in immunodeficient rodents (28). In such animals the grafted cells grow widely and produce a fatal disease but there is no infection of the host with the virus, and the tumor cells are of donor origin. In the second approach primate cells have been transformed in vitro and autochthonous EBV converted cells then replaced. This method has resulted in a lymphoma in one of 4 marmosets; similar experiments in 5 gibbons and 4 squirrel monkeys have not resulted in tumors (29-31). Finally, cell-free

EBV has been tested for oncogenicity in vivo. This technique has produced negative results in rhesus monkeys, gibbons, and squirrel monkeys. However, we found that cotton-top marmosets developed lymphoma when given cell-free virus and M. A. Epstein and his collaborators induced a lymphoproliferative disease in one owl monkey given a lysate of an EBV carrier Burkitt lymphoma cell line (29, 32). The studies of the direct oncogenicity of EBV involved few animals of a limited number of species. The variable results obtained so far could be explained by differences in the susceptibility of different hosts, differences in the viral strains or differences in the amount of virus inoculated.

In this report we describe in more detail experimental infection and disease in cotton-top marmosets following inoculation of EBV based on recent results.

METHODS

Marmosets: Wild animals, a mixture of juveniles and adults, males and females, from Colombia, South America, were purchased from a commercial dealer. The blood of most animals contained a species of microfilaria; an acanthocephalid, Prosthenorchis elegans, was located in the terminal ileum of many marmosets.

Virus: Four animals received autologous cells transformed in vitro by an infectious mononucleosis strain of EBV, designated 883L (27). Eleven received cell-free virus prepared in marmoset cells (line B95-8) transformed by the 883Lvirus. Two of the latter group received virus obtained from a clone of B95-8 cells (Clone 29) (33). Three animals received EBV which originated from a throat washing. In one instance the virus was derived from a line of marmoset cells transformed by EBV from the throat of a mononucleosis patient. In two instances virus was in the form of a filtered gargle from an immunosuppressed renal transplant recipient. The infectivity of virus in the inocula was measured by

immortalization of leukocytes from human cord blood
with an endpoint dilution assay. Inoculations were made
intravenously, intraperitoneally, and subcutaneously.

Antibody: Antibody levels against EB viral capsid antigen
were determined with the indirect immunofluorescence
technique. The P_3J-HR-1 subline of EBV carrier cells
from a Burkitt lymphoma was the test antigen.

Examination of Lymph Nodes for EBV Antigens and
Particles: Imprints from lymph nodes obtained at biopsy
or necropsy were examined for viral capsid antigen and
nuclear antigen. Reference antibody positive and antibody negative human sera were used to detect the antigens.
Fragments of lymphoid tissues were fixed in gluteralde-
hyde and thin sections examined for viral particles.

EB Virus Recovery: To establish lymphoblastoid cell
lines from marmoset tissues fragments of organs were
placed in stoppered tubes with or without feeder cells of
human placental fibroblasts. Tissue fragments were also
placed on stainless steel grids. Cells shed from the grid
platforms into the fluid phase of the culture were sub-
cultured on placental feeder layers. Cell lines which
formed were studied for viral capsid antigen, nuclear
antigen, and extracellular virus by the immortalization
assay.

RESULTS

Summary of Results of the Inoculation: Seventeen animals
have been given EBV; four received transformed cells
and 13 were inoculated with cell-free virus (Table 1).
Five animals developed malignant lymphoma, reticulum
cell sarcoma type. In 3 instances the disease was fatal,
and 2 other moribund animals were sacrificed. Palpable
abdominal tumors were detected in three additional animals from 7 to 42 days after inoculation. In these animals a surgical biopsy was performed 7-10 weeks after

inoculation. Marked lymphoid hyperplasia was identified grossly and by histopathology. The animals subsequently recovered. Seven animals did not develop palpable abdominal nodes but antibodies to EBV appeared. These are classified as inapparent infection. Two animals developed neither palpable nodes nor antibodies. We have observed seven control animals held in adjacent cages. Two received supernatant fluid from Raji cells, one received culture medium, four received no inoculations. None developed EBV antibodies. No lymphoid pathology was noted in the four control animals which have been necropsied after observation periods of 1 year or longer.

Nine of 17 EBV inoculated animals received an immunosuppressive regimen consisting of azathioprine and prednisilone for 3 to 21 days. (Table 2). Lymphoma occurred four times in immunosuppressed monkeys and once in an untreated animal; hyperplasia has been observed twice in animals receiving no drugs and once in a treated animal.

Pathology: The most consistent gross pathologic finding was marked enlargement of the mesenteric chain of lymph nodes. These were frequently matted and adherent to the adjacent bowel. Characteristically, lymph nodes near the terminal ileum were most extensively involved. In two animals with lymphoma enlarged mediastinal lymph nodes were also identified.

When the lesion was classified as a malignant lymphoma the architecture of the involved lymph node was totally obscured by diffuse infiltration of reticulum cells. There was also compression and occasionally obliteration of the capsule of the lymph node. Reticulum cells filled the perinodal sinusoids and infiltrated the adjacent fat. Nodes involved with lymphoma invariably showed large zones of necrosis. In hyperplastic nodes there was still preservation of follicular structures and the capsule was intact. However these nodes showed an increase in size and follicles were filled with pale reticulum cells. Hyperplastic nodes contained areas of hemorrhage but were not necrotic. (Fig. 1-3).

In two animals which received immunosuppressive drugs and EBV the spleen was markedly enlarged and the splenic architecture obscured by hemorrhage and necrosis. In the remaining animals the spleen was normal. In animals with malignant lymphoma microscopic infiltrates of reticulum cells and other mononuclear cells were identified in the lung, kidney, and liver as well as invading the mucosa of the small intestine.

Pathology unrelated to EBV inoculation was noted in both inoculated and control animals. The small bowel of nearly all autopsied animals contained parasitic granulomas due to the burrowing acanothocephalid. In some instances there was local perforation of the bowel and abscess formation.

Antibody Responses: Thirteen of 17 inoculated animals and none of 7 control animals developed antibodies to EB viral capsid antigen. Two animals (#639, #640) with fatal lymphoma died about 30 days after inoculation before antibodies appeared. The other two seronegative animals have been observed for several months. Other animals which received the same inoculum did seroconvert.

Antibodies to viral capsid antigen appeared more rapidly and reached a higher level in marmosets given autologous EBV-converted cells than in animals given cell-free virus. The median time for appearance of detectable antibody was 43 days in eight animals given virus compared with 24 days in four animals given cells. The median maximum antibody titer in those given virus was 1:20 and in those given autologous cells was 1:80. (Fig. 4, 5). Antibody titers remained near the maximum level up to 600 days after inoculation.

Two tumored animals developed antibody titers 4-fold higher than non-tumored animals which received the same inoculum. The anti-VCA titer in marmoset #625 which developed lymphoma after injection of autologous cells was 1:640 220 days after inoculation and in marmoset #667 which developed malignant lymphoma following cell-free virus was 1:80 sixty days after inoculation.

The immunosuppressive regimen did not affect the titers or time of appearance of the antibodies.

Demonstration of Virus: Two general methods were used to detect the presence of EBV in affected lymphoid tissues, namely, direct examination of biopsies for viral particles and antigens and study of continuous lympho-blastoid cell lines derived in vitro.

A survey for particles was made in thin sections of three malignant lymphomas (#625, #642, #667) and in one control node from an animal with a parasitic granuloma (#648). (Table 3). Approximately 150 cell profiles in each specimen were studied by M. Lipman. No virus particles were observed. Viral capsid antigens could not be identified in imprints prepared from lymph nodes of 6 inoculated animals, 3 with hyperplasia and 3 with lymphoma, and from 2 control animals. In one instance (Fig. 6) typical EB nuclear antigen was found in the majority of the cells of an imprint which was a homogeneous collection of tumor cells. Other imprints were studied for EB nuclear antigen after a considerable period of storage and may have been unsatisfactory for this reason.

Cell lines containing viral capsid antigen and viral particles were established from lymphoid organs of 4 animals, 2 with lymphoma and 2 with hyperplasia. The most successful method for deriving lymphoid cell lines was co-cultivation of tissue fragments with placental cells. (Table 4). However cell lines were also derived in each instance without feeder cells.

Once affected nodes had been maintained in vitro for a period of time viral capsid antigen appeared in the cells. The level of antigen was between 5-16% in the es-tablished lines. (Table 3). The one line tested released extracellular herpes virions. Supernatant fluid of this line contained biologically active EBV which immortal-ized human leukocytes. Biologically active EBV from the tumor was partially purified by velocity sedimentation in potassium tartrate gradients. The titer of partially purified virus was reduced 1000-fold by EBV antibody and unaffected by antibody-free human serum. Characterization of the EBV's released from the other cell lines is in progress.

Only once, despite numerous attempts, was a cell line recovered from peripheral blood leukocytes. This line grew from one of six cultures prepared 54 days after inoculation at a time when a biopsy of mesenteric nodes showed hyperplasia. Cell lines with viral capsid antigens have been obtained from the spleen of 2 animals and from the mediastinal lymph nodes and thymus of one animal. We have not demonstrated cytopathic effects or established lymphoid cell lines in cultures of kidney, lung, or liver. EB virus, measurable by the transformation assay, has not been found in the throat, urine or stool of inoculated animals.

DISCUSSION

Comparison between the Experimental Infection and Natural Infection in Man: In experimental infection of marmosets with EBV, as in natural infections of man, there was a spectrum of responses varying from "inapparent" infection, to lymph node hyperplasia to fatal malignant lymphoma. In some animals extensive lymphoid hyperplasia was followed by complete recovery, a finding analogous to infectious mononucleosis. The serologic responses provided another parallel: in two animals with lymphoma which lived long enough to allow assessment of their antibody responses, titers against viral capsid antigen were higher in tumored animals than in those with inapparent infection or hyperplasia. The time of appearance of antibody in the marmosets following inoculation of virus (30-56 days) was in the range known for the incubation period of infectious mononucleosis. The few animals kept for long periods following inoculation maintained antibody titers at the same level, a finding which is comparable to the persistence of EBV antibody after infectious mononucleosis (34).

The cell-virus relationship, too, is similar in the experimental disease and in Burkitt lymphoma. Viral particles or antigens representing viral capsids are not detected in the tumors (35). However, tumor cells explanted in vitro form continuous lines which produce viral capsid antigens and mature virions. EB nuclear antigen is found in cells prepared directly from marmoset and natural tumors (14).

Two respects in which the experimental and natural infections differ must be noted. First, we have not induced a lymphoblastic lymphoma, the usual histologic classification of Burkitt's lymphoma, but a reticulum cell sarcoma. Second, more cells in lines obtained from marmoset tumors exhibit viral capsid antigen than cells in most human lymphoid lines. In the one case studied the marmoset tumor line releases more extracellular biologically active virus than is usual for a Burkitt tumor line. This observation is in accord with our previous findings that EBV-transformed marmoset cells are more productive of EB virus than comparable human cells (36).

Comparison of EBV and H. saimiri and H. ateles
(Table 5): At first glance there are also many similarities between the experimental disease in marmosets induced by EBV and the disease first described by Melendez and coworkers after inoculation of Herpes saimiri and Herpes ateles (37). A malignant lymphoma develops after a short incubation period. Lesions involve the mesenteric lymph node chain and distant lesions are found in many organs especially kidney, liver, lungs and intestine. There are similarities in the serologic responses: marmosets develop detectable antibodies relatively slowly after injection of EBV or HVS (38). There are also similarities in the cell-virus relationship. In neither experimental infection is mature virus detected in vivo, but it can be found once lymphoid cells are explanted in culture. There are even similarities in the epidemiology of the two experimental infections. Both HVS and EBV are transmitted horizontally in their

439

natural hosts but neither appears to be present in the throat of experimentally infected marmosets (39).

Despite these impressive similarities several differences can be described between the behavior of the two viruses in the same host. HVS induces fatal lymphoma with great regularity; 100% of inoculated animals die. EBV is much more variable in its outcome and benign lymphoid hyperplasia is included in the response. For neither virus is the tumorigenic dose known with certainty but it is probably quite low for HVS (40). The tumors following inoculation of HVS have shown histologic variation from reticulum cell sarcome to lymphoblastic lymphoma and leukemia. Thus far EBV induced tumors have only been reticulum cell in type; leukemia has not occurred. According to recent studies HVS transformed marmoset lymphoid cells have "T" cell markers and EBV transformed marmoset leukocytes are "B" cells (41). HVS can be recovered from non-lymphoid organs such as the kidney as well as from lymphoid cells. EBV has only been obtained from lymphoid tissue. The viruses show markedly different properties in cell culture. HVS recovered from experimental tumors induces cytopathic effects in a variety of monolayer cell cultures, whereas no such effect is observed with EBV-recovered from experimental disease. HVS has not yet been shown to transform lymphoid cells in vitro, a property which is characteristic of most EBV strains.

Bearing of the Animal Studies on the Question of the Oncogenicity of EBV in Man: These experiments provide the first direct proof of the oncogenicity of EBV per se in an experimental animal. Furthermore certain features of the experimental infection correspond to EBV infection of man. It is therefore attractive to use these studies as evidence for oncogenicity of EBV in man. However this conclusion does not seem justified. First, the EBV inoculum per se is still poorly characterized and more efforts must be made to prove whether EBV is the only agent in the inoculum. Neutralization of tumor formation with specific antisera is necessary, but first a way must be found for inducing the tumors more consistently. Second, little is known about reasons for the peculiar susceptibility of marmosets to tumorigenesis to a variety of oncogenic viruses including herpes viruses of other New World primates. It is important to emphasize that neither Herpes saimiri or ateles are known to be oncogenic in their natural host. There are now many examples of viruses which are not naturally oncogenic but become so upon transfer to foreign hosts. Finally one must ask the philosophical question whether animal experimentation ever provides evidence of causality of human disease. A more powerful proof of an etiologic association between a micro-organism and a human disease is that removal of the agent leads to a disappearance of the disease.

ACKNOWLEDGEMENT

This work was supported by grants from the American Cancer Society (VC107); U.S. Public Health Service (CA12055) and Damon Runyon Memorial Fund (DRG1147). G.M. is an Investigator of the Howard Hughes Medical Institute.

REFERENCES

1. Henle, G., Henle, W. and Diehl, V. Proc. Nat. Acad. Sci. (Wash.) 59, 94 (1968).
2. Evans, A.S., Niederman, J.C. and McCollum, R.W. New Engl. J. Med. 279, 1121 (1968).
3. Diehl, V., Henle, G., Henle, W. and Kohn, G. J. Virol. 2, 663 (1968).
4. Miller, G., Niederman, J.C. and Andrews, L. New Engl. J. Med. 288, 229 (1973).
5. Epstein, M.A., Henle, G., Achong, B.G. and Barr, Y.M. J. Exp. Med. 121, 761 (1965).
6. Miller, M.H., Stitt, D. and Miller, G. J. Virol. 6, 699 (1970).

7. Walters, M. K. and Pope, J. H. Int. J. Cancer 8, 32 (1971).

8. Reedman, B. M. and Klein, G. Int. J. Cancer 11, 499 (1973).

9. zur Hausen, H. and Schulte-Holthausen, H. Nature (Lond.) 227, 245 (1970).

10. Nonoyama, M. and Pagano, J. S. Nature 233, 103 (1971).

11. Adams, A., Lindahl, T. and Klein, G. Proc. Nat. Acad. Sci. 70, 2888 (1973).

12. Klein, G., Lindahl, T., Jondal, M., Leibold, W. and Ménézes, J. (Manuscript submitted for publication).

13. Pagano, J. S., Huang, C. H. and Levine, P. New Engl. J. Med. 289, 1395 (1973).

14. Reedman, B. M., Klein, G., Pope, J. H., Walters, M. K., Hilgers, J., Singh, S. and Johansson, G. (Manuscript submitted for publication).

15. de-Thé, G., Ambrosioni, J. C., Ho, H. C. and Kwan, H. C. Nature 221, 770 (1969).

16. Nonoyama, M., Huang, C. H., Pagano, J. S., Klein, G., and Singh, S. Proc. Nat. Acad. Sci. 70, 3265 (1973).

17. Wolf, H., zur Hausen, H. and Becker, V. Nature 244, 245 (1973).

18. Rocchi, G., Hewetson, J. and Henle, W. Int. J. Cancer 11, 637 (1973).

19. Henle, W., Henle, G., Gunven, P., Klein, G., Clifford, P. and Singh, S. J. Nat. Cancer Inst. 50, 1163 (1973).

20. Fialkow, P. J., Klein, E., Klein, G., Clifford, P. and Singh, S. J. Exp. Med. 138, 89 (1973).

21. Miller, G. J. Infect. Dis. (To be published August, 1973).

22. Burkitt, D. P. J. Nat. Cancer Inst. 42, 19 (1969).

23. Kufe, D., Magrath, I. T., Ziegler, J. L. and Spiegelman, S. Proc. Nat. Acad. Sci. 70, 737 (1973).

24. Henle, W., Diehl, V., Kohn, G., zur Hausen, H.

and Henle, G. Science 157, 1064 (1967).

25. Pope, J. H., Horne, M. K. and Scott, W. Int. J. Cancer 4, 255 (1969).

26. Gerber, P. and Hoyer, B. H. Nature 231, 46 (1971).

27. Miller, G., Shope, T., Lisco, H., Stitt, D. and Lipman, M. Proc. Nat. Acad. Sci. (USA) 69, 383 (1972).

28. Adams, R. A., Foley, G. E., Farber, S., Flowers, A., Lazarus, H. and Hellerstein, E. Cancer Res. 30, 338 (1970).

29. Shope, T., Dechairo, D. and Miller, G. Proc. Nat. Acad. Sci. 70, 2487 (1973).

30. Werner, J., Pinto, C. A., Haff, R. F., Henle, W., and Henle, G. J. Infect. Dis. 126, 678 (1972).

31. Shope, T. C. and Miller, G. J. Exp. Med. 137, 140 (1973).

32. Epstein, M. A., Hunt, R. D. and Rabin, H. Int. J. Cancer 12, 309 (1973).

33. Miller, G. and Lipman, M. J. Exp. Med. 138, 1398 (1973).

34. Niederman, J. C., Evans, A. S., Subrahmanyan, L. and McCollum, R. W. New Engl. J. Med. 282, 361 (1970).

35. Nadkarni, J. S., Nadkarni, J. J., Klein, G., Henle, W., Henle, G. and Clifford, P. Int. J. Cancer 6, 10 (1970).

36. Miller, G. and Lipman, M. Proc. Nat. Acad. Sci. (USA) 70, 190 (1973).

37. Melendez, L. V., Hunt, R. D., Daniel, M. D., Fraser, C. E. O., Barahona, H. H., Garcia, F. G. and King, V. W. In Biggs, P. M., de-Thé, G., Payne, L. N. (ed.) op cit p. 451-461.

38. Klein, G., Pearson, G., Rabson, A., Ablashi, D. V., Falk, L., Wolfe, L., Deinhardt, F. and Rabin, H. Int. J. Cancer 12, 270 (1973).

39. Wolfe, L. G., Falk, L. A. and Deinhardt, F. J. Nat. Cancer Inst. 47, 1147 (1971).

40. Laufs, R. and Fleckenstein, B. Med. Microbiol. Immunol. 158, 227 (1973).

41. Jondal, M. and Klein, G. J. Exp. Med. 138, 1365 (1973).

TABLE 1

SUMMARY OF INOCULATIONS OF COTTON-TOP MARMOSETS

Expt.	Type of Inoculum	Titer of EBV (TD$_{50}$) in inoculum	No. Animals	No. sacrificed or biopsied	Lymphoma	Hyperplasia	Inapparent Infection	No Infection
EBV Inoculated Animals								
1	Autologous EBV-transformed cells	10^8 cells	4	3	1	0	3	0
2	Cell-Free EBV - B95-8	10$^{4.4}$	4	3	3	0	1	0
3	Throat Washing Virus - Direct	10$^{4.2}$	2	1	0	1	0	1
	- Marmoset adapted	10$^{4.2}$	1	1	0	0	1	0
4	Cell-Free EBV from Cloned Cells	10$^{4.1}$	2	1	0	1	1	0
5	Cell-Free EBV - B95-8 later passage	10$^{5.1}$	4	2	1	1	1	1
	Total EBV inoculated animals		17	11	5	3	7	2
Control Animals								
1	None		2	2				2
2	None		2	0				2^x
3	Medium from Raji cells		2	2				2
4	Medium RPMI 1640		1	0				1
	Total control animals		7	4				7

x These 2 animals were held for 10 months; neither developed antibody or palpable lymph nodes. They were inoculated with virus in experiment #5.

TABLE 2

EFFECT OF IMMUNOSUPPRESSIVE DRUGS ON OUTCOME OF EBV INOCULATIONS

Expt.	Duration of Drugs	Immunosuppressed *				Not Immunosuppressed			
		Lymphoma	Hyperplasia	Inapparent Infection	No Antibody	Lymphoma	Hyperplasia	Inapparent Infection	No Antibody
1	21 days	1		1				2	
2	21 days	2				1		1	
3	3 days		1	1	1				
4	none						1	1	
5	14 days	1	—	1	—	—	1	—	1
	Totals	4	1	3	1	1	2	4	1

* Azathioprine (1 mg/day) prednisilone (0.05 mg/day)

TABLE 3

DEMONSTRATION OF EBV IN MESENTERIC LYMPH NODES AND CELL LINES DERIVED THEREFROM

Expt.	Animal	Diagnosis	Lymph Node			Cell Line			
			EBNA	VCA	Particles	EBNA	VCA	Particles/ml	TD^x_{50}/ml
1	625	Lymphoma	not done	negative	none	no cell line formed			
2	642	Lymphoma	negative	negative	none	100%	5%	10^7	$10^{5.4}$
4	655	Hyperplasia	negative	negative	not done	100%	5%	not done	not done
5	644	Hyperplasia	2%	negative	not done	100%	12%	not done	$10^{3.7}$
	667	Lymphoma	80 - 100%	negative	none	100%	16%	not done	$10^{5.0}$

x TD_{50} = 50% transforming doses
EBNA = EB nuclear antigen
VCA = viral capsid antigen

445

TABLE 4

SUMMARY OF ISOLATION OF LYMPHOBLASTOID CELL LINES
FROM MESENTERIC LYMPH NODES AND OTHER SITES

Expt.	No. animals in the group	No. animals studied	No. successful isolations	Isolation Rate in Successful Attempts from Mesenteric Nodes with different methods			Other Sites of Recovery
				Grids	Fragments plus feeder	Fragments alone	
EBV inoculated animals							
1	4	2	0				
2	4	3	1	3/4	3/5	1/4	spleen
3	3	2	0				
4	2	1	1	4/6	2/2	1/2	spleen
5	4	2	2	0/4 0/2	4/6 8/8	2/6 2/8	leukocytes, thymus mediastinal node
Totals	17	10	4	7/16	17/21	6/20	
Control Animals							
1	2	1	0				
2	2	0	0				
3	2	2	0				
4	1	0	0				
Totals	7	3	0				

TABLE 5

COMPARISON OF THE RESPONSES OF MARMOSETS TO EXPERIMENTAL
TUMORIGENESIS FOLLOWING INOCULATION OF EB VIRUS AND HERPES SAIMIRI VIRUS

	EB Virus	Herpes Saimiri Virus
Biologic Properties of Virus		
Transforms lymphoid cells in vitro	yes	?
Purely productive system	none	several
Clinical Response		
a. Incubation period for tumors	24 – 222 days	18 – 48 days
b. Outcome	variable	invariably fatal
c. Tumor incidence increased by immuno-suppressive drugs	? possibly	not needed
Pathologic Response		
a. histologic type	reticulum cell	reticulum cell; lymphoblastic and lymphocytic lymphoma; leukemia
b. incidence of tumors	~ 30%	100%
c. organs involved	liver, lung, gut, kidney	multiple
d. lymphocyte subtype	B	T
Serologic Response		
a. Time before appearance of ab. to viral capsid antigen after virus	30 – 56 days	28 – 80 days
b. Antibody to early antigen	±	+
Virus Recovery from tumored animals		
a. blood leukocytes	rare	usual
b. tumor	usual	usual
c. non lymphoid tissues	negative to date	kidney
Viral antigens in tumor	EBNA	?
Viral genome in tumor	?	?
Epidemiology		
Horizontal spread by tumored animals	no	no
Horizontal spread by natural host	yes	yes

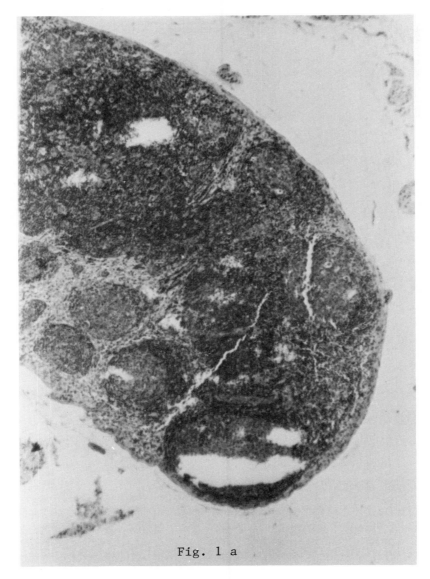

Fig. 1 a

Fig. 1. Normal mesenteric lymph node from uninoculated marmoset No. 628; hematoxylin and eosin stain. a) X 35 b) X 250 original magnification. Note well-preserved architecture and follicular structure.

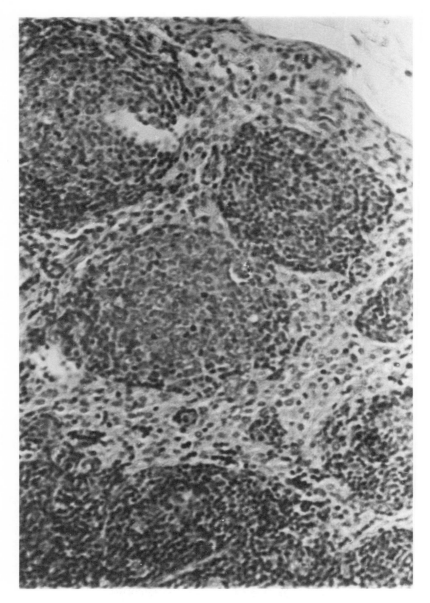

Fig. 1 b

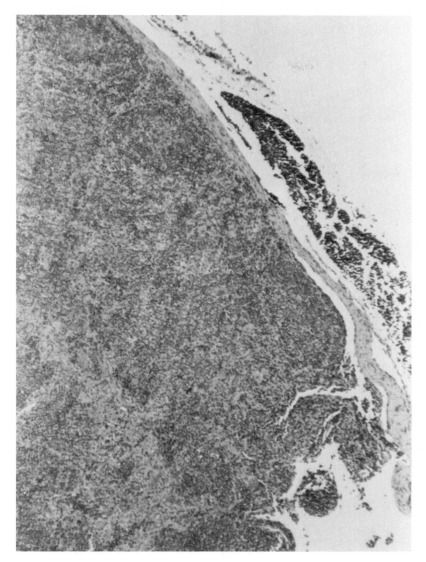

Fig. 2 . Hyperplastic mesenteric lymph node from marmoset No. 644 which received cell-free EBV and no immunosuppressive drugs. Note loss of normal follicles and presence of lymphocytes in perinodal fat. Original magnification X 35.

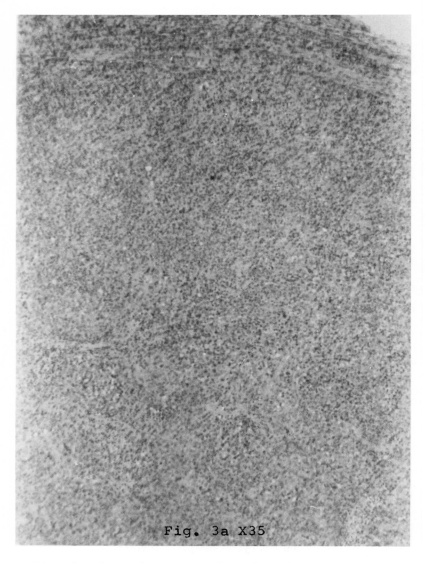

Fig. 3a X35

Fig. 3. Lymphomatous lymph node from marmoset No. 667 which received cell-free EBV and immuno-suppressive drugs. a) X 35 b) X 400. The architecture is totally obscured and the lymph node is replaced by a homogeneous population of reticulum cells.

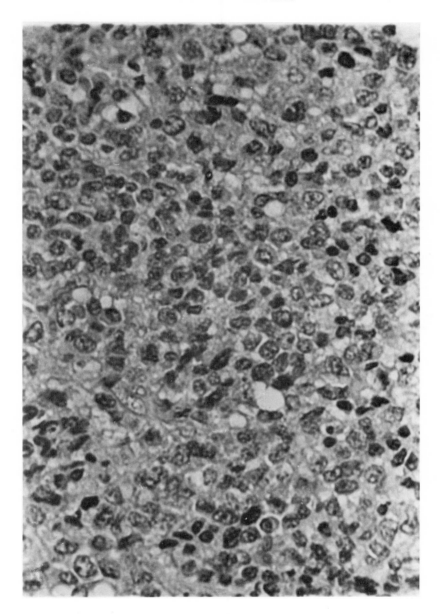

Fig. 3b X400 (see page 450)

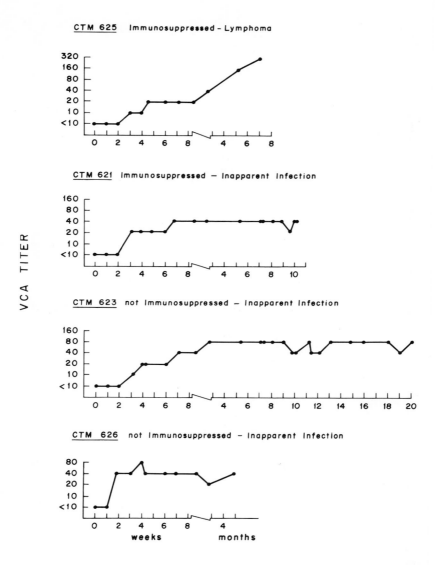

Fig. 4. Time course of development of antibodies to EB viral capsid antigen following administration of autologous EBV-converted cells.

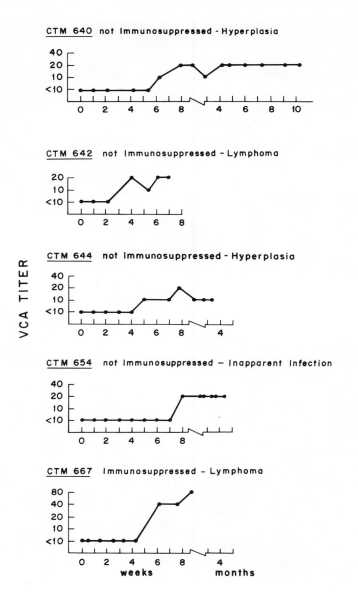

Fig. 5.   Time course of development of antibodies to EB viral capsid antigen following administration of cell-free EBV.

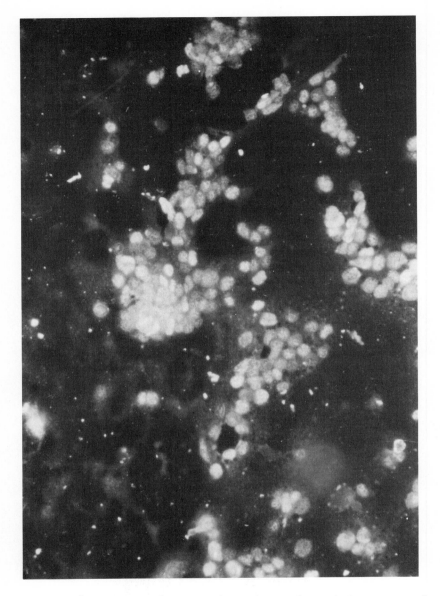

Fig. 6. EB nuclear antigen in an imprint prepared from the tumorous lymph node of marmoset No. 667 illustrated in Fig. 3.

THE REGULATION OF HERPES SIMPLEX VIRUS PROTEIN SYNTHESIS

Robert W. Honess and Bernard Roizman

Departments of Microbiology and Biophysics
University of Chicago
Chicago, Illinois 60637

ABSTRACT. At least 47 virus-specific polypeptides, both
structural and nonstructural, are synthesized as primary
gene products in HEp-2 cells productively infected with
herpes simplex virus. On the basis of the patterns of
their synthesis they form at least 4 temporal classes
(A-D). The polypeptides in B, C and D classes are synthesized at maximum rates early in infection whereas class A
polypeptides are made at progressively increasing rates
until late in infection. Minor virion polypeptides and
nonstructural polypeptides are members of early classes
whereas major structural polypeptides are members of the
late class, A. The temporal regulation of virus specific
polypeptide synthesis appears to result from the sequential
synthesis of 3 coordinately regulated groups of viral polypeptides, designated α, β and γ. Analyses of the transcription of viral DNA and the synthesis of the 3 groups
of polypeptides indicate that, although transcription
appears to be complete in the absence of viral protein synthesis, the only functional messenger accumulating in the
presence of cycloheximide is that for α polypeptides. The
production of β and γ polypeptides requires RNA synthesis
in the presence of α polypeptides. The turning "on" of β
and γ polypeptide synthesis requires the presence of α and
β polypeptides respectively, in order to produce or maintain functional β and γ mRNAs. The turning "off" of the
synthesis of α and β polypeptides appears to be the consequence of post transcriptional events mediated by β and γ
polypeptides, respectively. Properties of both "on" and
"off" controls leading to the sequential production of α,
β and γ polypeptides predict that mRNAs of each coordinately regulated group share cognate signals for their

synthesis and common structural features determining their post-transcriptional processing or functional stability.

INTRODUCTION

Herpes simplex virus has a double-stranded DNA genome with a molecular weight of about 10^8 (1) which is replicated and transcribed as high molecular weight RNA within the nucleus of the infected cell (2). The transcripts are processed to give rise to stable adenylated and non-adenylated RNA species complementary to approximately 50% of viral DNA. The majority of these species are transported from the nucleus and appear on cytoplasmic poly-ribosomes (3,4). This amount of transcribed information is sufficient to specify the sequence of a maximum of 55,000 amino acids. The proteins which the virus is known to produce include virus specific enzymes (5), non-glycosylated components of the virion, some of which accumulate in the nucleus (6), and glycosylated polypeptides which form the envelope of the virus and are incorporated into cytoplasmic and plasma membranes (7,8,9). The virus therefore employs the same basic functional compartmentalization as does the uninfected mammalian cell and produces a qualitatively analogous variety of gene products. Interest in the process of virus replication stems not only from the observation that it mimics many cellular processes but also because a variety of studies have associated the virus with a number of human tumors (10), and with *in vitro* transformation of cells (11). We are therefore interested in the properties of herpes virus gene products and in defining the elements regulating their synthesis and their function in productively infected and in transformed cells.

We currently restrict this account to our studies on the productive infection of human epidermoid carcinoma No. 2 (HEp-2) cells with herpes simplex 1. Our knowledge even of this subject is fragmentary and in beginning this presentation we are reminded of Agatha's reprimand that, "it is because of what we do not understand that we feel a need to declare what we do," and that "There is much more to understand" (Part I, Act I, "The Family Reunion," T. S. Eliot). However although our present declaration is avowedly an interim report we hope that its function will be constructive as well as descriptive.

456

RESULTS

Comparison of the polypeptides synthesized in infected and uninfected cells

A comparison of the polypeptides synthesized by HSV-1 infected and by mock infected HEp-2 cells is shown in Fig. 1. The profile of total infected cell polypeptides obtained by absorbance scanning of Coomassie Brilliant Blue stained gels (Fig. 1) did not differ appreciably from that of uninfected cells. However, the profiles of labeled polypeptides from infected and mock infected cells were readily differentiated (Fig. 1, top and bottom tracings). The profile of labeled polypeptides from mock infected cells reflected the distribution of total cellular proteins, whereas infected cell lysates contained fewer labeled polypeptides and their distribution in the gel did not resemble the distribution of total cellular proteins.

These results indicated that uninfected cells synthesized a very large number of polypeptides and for nearly every infected cell polypeptide (ICP) there existed a component of the uninfected cell characterized by the same or similar electrophoretic mobility. Attempting to differentiate between polypeptides synthesized in infected and uninfected cells solely on the basis of direct comparisons of their electrophoretic mobilities was therefore unprofitable. However, the fact that the profiles of proteins synthesized were different could be used as evidence for selective inhibition or stimulation (induction) to account for these differences.

This type of comparison may be termed the criterion of induction; it provided some evidence for virus specificity of ICP other than those comigrating with prominent components of the uninfected cells ('h,' Fig. 1). These conclusions were reinforced by the results of analyses of the kinetics of synthesis of ICP considered later in the text.

Two additional criteria were applied to determine the specificity of ICP. The first of these criteria required evidence that the properties of ICP were genetically determined by the virus. The second required that they possess immunologic specificities different from those of uninfected cell polypeptides. Operationally, it was shown that (i) the amount and the electrophoretic mobility

457

of some ICP were determined by the virus in that these parameters varied depending on the virus type and intratype variants infecting the cell and (ii) some ICP could be precipitated by the use of antisera specific for viral antigens. The result of an experiment showing that at least some of the ICP possess immunologic specificities different from those of polypeptides of uninfected cells is shown in Fig. 2.

From experiments such as those outlined above we determined that 47 of the polypeptides synthesized in HEp-2 cells after infection with HSV-1 (F1) fulfill one or more criteria for virus specificity (12). The molecular weights of these polypeptides range from more than 250,000 for ICP 1-2 to about 20,000 for ICP 49 (12).

Evidence that HSV-1 ICP identified in short labeling intervals are primary products of translation

In experiments dealing with the kinetics of synthesis of ICP it was important to differentiate between primary products of translation and putative products of rapid post-translational cleavages of newly synthesized polypeptides. The two experiments in this section were designed to determine whether rapid post-translational cleavages of ICP occurred, and to discriminate the precursor from the product.

In the first experiment replicate cultures of cells were exposed to ^{14}C amino acids at 4.5 and 6.5 h postinfection for periods of 10, 30, and 60 min. Additional cultures labeled for 10 min were also incubated for an additional 40 min in medium without labeled precursors. The proteins of the harvested, solubilized cells were then subjected to electrophoresis in parallel on an 8.5% acrylamide gel slab. Comparisons of the autoradiograms (not shown) revealed no significant differences in the mobility or relative quantity of polypeptides accumulating in the cells during 10- to 60-min pulses administered at a given time postinfection. Neither were there any significant differences between the autoradiograms of a 10-min pulse and a 10-min pulse followed by a 40-min chase. As shown in Fig. 3, similar pulse and pulse-chase experiments clearly demonstrated rapid post-translational processing of polypeptides in poliovirus-infected HEp-2 cells.

In the second experiment, we attempted to prevent putative cleavages of newly synthesized polypeptides by adding to the infected cell medium two chloromethyl ketone derivatives which inhibit the proteolytic actions of trypsin (tosyl-lysyl chloromethyl ketone, TLCK) and chymotrypsin (tosyl phenylalanylchloromethyl ketone, TPCK) (see e.g., ref. 15). Other workers have previously shown that these inhibitors can prevent the known post-translational cleavages of poliovirus polypeptides in a number of cell lines (16,17). As a positive control, we included in our test system poliovirus infected cells. The results of this experiment are illustrated in Fig. 3 and showed that the rapid post translational cleavage of poliovirus proteins was readily demonstrated, and that these cleavages were effectively prevented by the inhibitor of chymotrypsin, TPCK. However no rapid post translational cleavages were detected in herpesvirus infected HEp-2 cells. Thus, 10^{-4} M TLCK had no effect on the overall rate of synthesis or on the electrophoretic profiles of ICP from HSV-1 infected cells. Although overall incorporation was reduced in the culture labeled in the presence of 10^{-4} M TPCK, there was no clear difference between the mobilities of ICP made in the presence and absence of the inhibitor. In particular, there was no detectable accumulation of polypeptides of higher molecular weight than those observed in untreated cells.

These experiments suggested that ICP could be regarded as primary products of translation. The aggregate molecular weight of the 47 virus specific ICP can account for 70-80% of the transcribed information content of the viral DNA (12).

The relationship of ICP to virion polypeptides (VP); classification of ICP as structural or nonstructural on the basis of electrophoretic coincidence or non-coincidence with VP

The classification of ICP as either structural or nonstructural constitutes a primary division of the functions of virus specified proteins which is of particular interest in studies on the regulation of viral polypeptide synthesis. The differentiation between structural and nonstructural polypeptides ideally required the demonstration of chemical identity between VP and their putative

459

analogues among ICP. Pending a more complete characterization of these polypeptides, we provisionally designated
ICP as structural or nonstructural solely on the basis of
their electrophoretic coincidence or noncoincidence with
VP. Comparisons of ICP with VP, either by co-electro-
phoresis of ^{3}H-amino acids labeled virions and ^{14}C-labeled
infected cells or by electrophoresis of ^{14}C amino acids
labeled virions and similarly labeled infected cells in
adjacent slots of a polyacrylamide gel slab, led to their
classification into three groups. Thus 23 of the ICP
comigrated with VP and were therefore classified as structural; 16 polypeptides were clearly separated from known
VP and were therefore classified as nonstructural. An
additional 10 polypeptides migrated sufficiently close to
major virion polypeptides to make their designation uncer-
tain and these polypeptides remained unclassified. An
example of a comparison of ICP with VP is shown in Fig. 4.
For our present purposes it is sufficient to note a few
examples of polypeptides classified as structural or nonstructural and to which we shall refer later in the text.
ICP 4, 6 and 8 were all classified as structural since they
comigrated with the minor virion components VP 4, 6, and
VP 6A, respectively. ICP 5, and ICP 21 were also classified as structural polypeptides since they comigrated with
VP 5 and VP 14, respectively. ICP 11, 12 and 29 were
unclassified and ICP 17, 23 and 36 may be cited as examples
of nonstructural polypeptides.

Changes in the synthesis of virus specific polypeptides during the virus growth cycle

The objective of the experiments described in this
section was to outline the time course of synthesis of ICP.
Specifically we wished to determine the temporal patterns
of synthesis of ICP and whether the production of structural and nonstructural polypeptides different systematically in their rates or temporal patterns of synthesis.
These experiments therefore involved labeling infected
cells with ^{14}C amino acids for short periods at different
times throughout the various growth cycle.
    In one such series of experiments samples for
electrophoretic analysis were prepared from infected cells
labeled at 2.5 to 2.9, 3.75 to 4.0, 5.0 to 5.25 and 11.0 to
11.5 h after infection. The labeling intervals were

selected on the basis of the data presented in Fig. 5, which shows the variation in the overall rate of incorporation of labeled amino acids into protein and the time course of accumulation of infectious virus throughout the growth cycle. The interval from 2.5 to 2.9 h coincided with the end of the initial decline in protein synthesis (Fig. 5) and before viral DNA synthesis is normally detected (19). The next two intervals were just before (3.75 to 4.0 h) and at (5.0 to 5.25 h) the time of maximum protein synthesis and high rates of viral DNA synthesis. The last interval (11.0 to 11.5 h) was at a time when the rates of protein and viral DNA synthesis were declining and the rate of accumulation of infectious virus in the cell was near maximal. Fig. 6 shows an autoradiogram of a polyacrylamide gel slab containing electrophoretically separated polypeptides labeled during these intervals. Virual inspection of this figure is sufficient to establish that the synthesis of certain ICP, e.g., ICP 4, 6, 8, increased early in infection and then decreased later in infection, whereas the synthesis of other polypeptides, e.g., ICP 5, 21, increased progressively over the period analyzed. It is also apparent that in general the polypeptides synthesizes at high rates early in infection were largely minor structural polypeptides (e.g., ICP 4, 6, and 8 which comigrated with VP 4, 6, and 6A, respectively (Fig. 4,6), or were nonstructural polypeptides (e.g., ICP 36), whereas those made at increasing rates late in infection comigrated with major structural polypeptides (e.g., ICP 5, 21 which comigrated with VP 5 and VP 14 respectively). Quantitative measurements of the amounts of labeled polypeptides made at different times after infection were obtained by computer-aided planimetry (see Fig. 7) of absorbance tracing from the autoradiogram obtained in this and similar experiments. These quantitative analyses showed that during any one labeling interval the relative molar rates of synthesis (RM--see legend to Fig. 7 for method of computation) of the majority of polypeptides were within an eightfold range and that structural and nonstructural polypeptides were distributed throughout this range. The exceptions were the values of RM for structural polypeptides ICP 1-2 and ICP 31 which differed by 130-fold during the 11.0 to 11.5 h labeling interval (Fig. 6) and formed the extremes of the observed range of values. Analyses of the rates of synthesis of ICP at

461

different times throughout the virus growth cycle permitted their separation into 6 classes (A-F) differing in the temporal patterns of synthesis (Fig. 8). The segregation of ICP among these 6 patterns was independent of the maximum rate of synthesis of the polypeptides. However, the distribution of structural and nonstructural polypeptides among the 6 groups was nonrandom. All but one of the polypeptides presently included in group A are structural. The exception, ICP 17, may be a long-lived precursor since it disappeared on prolonged chase (compare 5.0- to 5.25-h pulse and 5.0- to 5.5-h pulse chased to 9.0 h shown in Fig. 6). Group C contained structural polypeptides only. The structural ICP included in the analysis presented in Fig. 8 had an aggregate molecular weight of 2.3×10^6, and this was distributed in groups A, C, B, F, E, and D in descending order in amounts of 47, 31, 8.1, 8.0, 4.2, and 1.6%, respectively.

The rates of synthesis of polypeptides comprising groups A, B, C, and D show either a gradual increase (A), or an initial increase followed by a leveling off (group B) or a decline (groups C and D). As we noted earlier in the text, the initial stimulation in their rate of synthesis is additional evidence that these polypeptides are virus specific. However, polypeptides of group E could be virus-specific products or host polypeptides with gradually diminishing rates of synthesis. It is noteworthy that several polypeptides which do not fulfill the general criterion of induction, and which are not precipitated by the antiserum (e.g., ICP 34, 35 and ICP 42, 43; see Fig. 1 and Fig. 2) fall into group E. It seems likely that members of group E for which there are criteria for virus specificity (12) are members of group E due to a comigrating host component and not to their own biosynthetic properties (see later).

Patterns F of Fig. 8 were probably consequences of superimpositions of the patterns of synthesis of two or more polypeptides, of which one or more belonged to class E and the others to class A, B, C, or D. This artifactual pattern was observed for polypeptides migrating in gels of a particular strength in multiple, incompletely resolved bands. In the electropherogram illustrating this analysis (Fig. 8, 7.75% gel) the groups of ICP 34 to 36 and 40 to 43 may be cited as examples of poorly resolved species which, in the absence of other data, would be included in category F. Analyses of the same and similar samples on other gel strengths (7 and 9%) permitted classification of ICP 34, 35, 42, and 43 as group E polypeptides.

Controls regulating the temporal sequence of viral protein synthesis

The recognition of multiple temporal classes of virus specific polypeptides clearly implied the existence of controls coordinating the synthesis of these polypeptides. The polypeptides contained in these classes differed in the times at which they attained maximum rates of synthesis. Moreover, the rate of synthesis of polypeptides contained in classes C and D declined late in infection whereas polypeptides in class A were synthesized at progressively higher rates late in infection (Fig. 6,8). Therefore both "on" and "off" controls must be involved in determining the time course of viral protein synthesis. The experiments which follow were designed to demonstrate directly, and to elucidate the nature of these "on" and "off" controls. Operationally, we were concerned with three main questions. The first was whether the synthesis of ICP were interdependent, i.e., whether the synthesis of some ICP required prior synthesis of others. Since this was the case, the second question was whether the synthesis of later or interdependent polypeptides required the presence of early polypeptides only or additional infected cell functions such as new RNA synthesis as well. Thirdly, we wished to know whether the patterns of synthesis of early groups of ICP were influenced by the production of later groups of ICP.

The design of the experiments described in this section was based on the observation that the transcription of viral DNA does not require prior viral protein synthesis. Thus, it has been shown that the amount of DNA transcribed in the presence of inhibitory concentrations of cycloheximide (4, Kozak and Roizman, unpublished data) or puromycin (Silverstein and Roizman, unpublished data) corresponds to at least the amount observed in untreated cells incubated for the same length of time. We therefore examined the polypeptides made after treatment of infected cells with inhibitors of protein synthesis at different intervals during the reproductive cycle.

The effects of inhibition of infected cell protein synthesis on subsequent synthesis of ICP

The effect of inhibiting protein synthesis in infected cells from 1 to 5 h after infection on the polypeptides synthesized during a short interval after the removal of the inhibitor (5 to 5.25 h) is shown in Fig. 9. Also shown in this figure are analyses of polypeptides made in untreated cells from 5 to 5.25 h, and at earlier (2.5 to 2.9 h) and later (11.0 to 11.5 h) times in the virus growth cycle. It is clear from a comparison of these samples that ICP made after the removal of cycloheximide were only a subset of the ICP made in untreated infected cells at the same time, and that the ICP made in largest amounts (e.g., ICP 4, ICP 0 and ICP 27) were those characteristically made at early and not at late times in the virus growth cycle. ICP 0 was not detected in previous analyses of untreated cells (12), probably because it was made in small amounts which were obscured by traces of cellular proteins early in infection and by other viral polypeptides with similar mobility at later times (ICP 8, 9). We found subsequently that ICP 0 was separable from ICP 8,9 in untreated cell lysates by manipulation of the polyacrylamide gel strengths. Resumption of host polypeptide synthesis (e.g., ICP 34, 35) was also observed immediately after the removal of cycloheximide. However, host polypeptides and the subset of viral polypeptides made immediately after the removal of cycloheximide were differentiated in two types of experiment. Thus increasing the multiplicity of infection in the presence of cycloheximide resulted in increased initial rates of synthesis of ICP 4, 0 and 27 and decreasing initial rates of synthesis of host polypeptides. Similarly, increasing the duration of the cycloheximide treatment (beginning at the time of infection) resulted in increasing initial rates of synthesis of viral polypeptides ICP 4, 0 and 27 and in decreasing initial rates of synthesis of host proteins when the inhibitor was withdrawn (see below). The treatment of uninfected cells with cycloheximide for up to 5 h produced a uniform decline in the rate of synthesis of all polypeptides measured subsequent to the withdrawal of the inhibitor.

Control experiments (not illustrated) showed that the selective synthesis of a subset of viral polypeptides was not due to an effect of cycloheximide *per se*, or of the washing procedures required to remove the inhibitor. Thus, the addition and immediate removal of cycloheximide had no effect on the amount or number of polypeptides synthesized by infected or uninfected cells. These experiments indicated that *a period* of inhibition of protein synthesis was required to affect the polypeptides made by infected cells. Moreover puromycin (50 μg/ml) produced results essentially similar to those obtained with cycloheximide.

The relationship between the time of addition of cycloheximide and the rates of synthesis of ICP immediately following removal of the inhibitor

The next series of experiments was designed to determine whether the synthesis of the viral polypeptides which were not made immediately following cycloheximide treatment at or shortly after the time of infection required a *specific* interval of prior protein synthesis in the infected cell and whether virus specific polypeptides could be further differentiated into groups on the basis of such requirements. In these experiments cycloheximide was added to cultures at various times from 0 to 5 h after infection. The inhibitor was removed from all cultures at 7 h post-infection and treated and untreated infected cells were labeled with ^{14}C amino acids from 7 to 7.5 h post-infection. Analyses of the results of such experiments presented in Figs. 10, 11 and 12 show the following:
    (i) The species of polypeptides made immediately after the removal of cycloheximide varied depending upon the time at which cycloheximide was added. The longer the interval between initiation of infection and exposure to the drug, the closer was the resemblance of the electropherograms of polypeptides made immediately upon removal of the drug to those made in untreated infected cells incubated for the same length of time (Fig. 10). Moreover, an equivalent duration of cycloheximide treatment after different intervals of the virus growth cycle did not necessarily produce similar patterns of synthesis of ICP following removal of the inhibitor. This is apparent from comparisons of the polypeptides synthesized after a treatment from 1 to 5.0 h (Fig. 9) with those synthesized after a treatment from 3.17 to 7.0 h (Fig. 10). On the basis of these observations we conclude that an interval of infected

cell protein synthesis prior to the addition of the drug is required for the production of certain virus specific polypeptides immediately after the removal of cyclo-heximide. This interval need not be immediately prior to the amino acid pulse; in fact it may be followed by several hours of exposure to cycloheximide prior to the amino acid pulse.

(ii) Quantitative analyses of the rates of synthe-sis of ICP as a function of the time of addition of cyclo-heximide (Figs. 11 and 12) permitted recognition of three groups of virus specific polypeptides. These groups, designated α, β and γ differed in their requirements for a prior interval of protein synthesis in order for their own synthesis to take place immediately following treatment with cycloheximide.

(iii) Polypeptides of the α group (e.g., ICP 0, ICP 4, ICP 27) were synthesized immediately upon removal of cycloheximide added at the time of infection or a short interval later (Figs. 10, 11, 12). The initial rates of synthesis of α polypeptides, i.e., immediately after removal of the inhibitor, increased with the duration of the drug treatment and with prolonged treatment exceeded the maximum rates observed in untreated infected cells (Fig. 11). Initial rates of synthesis of α polypeptides were progressively reduced by delaying the time of addi-tion of cycloheximide (Figs. 11 and 12). α polypeptides were synthesized in untreated cultures at the highest rates from 3 to 4 h post-infection (Fig. 11). Based on the temporal patterns of their synthesis they were classified as either class C (ICP 4) or were unclassified (ICP 0, 27) (Fig. 6, 8). α polypeptides resembled host polypeptides in two respects. Both α and host polypeptides were made upon removal of cycloheximide added at the time of infec-tion, i.e., their synthesis did not require prior infected cell protein synthesis. In addition, the initial rates of synthesis of both host and α polypeptides were reduced in cultures exposed to cycloheximide at successively later intervals after infection.

(iv) Polypeptides of the second group, β, were not synthesized immediately on removal of cycloheximide added before 1.0 h post-infection (Figs. 10, 11, 12). Additions of cycloheximide later than 1.5 h post-infection resulted in increasing initial rates of synthesis of β polypeptides. In certain instances, for example in cultures treated with cycloheximide beginning between 3.0 and 5.5 h until 7 h post-infection, the initial rates of synthesis exceeded those observed in untreated cells. In untreated cultures β polypeptides were synthesized at highest rates from 5 to 7 h post-infection (Fig. 11). Based on the temporal patterns of their synthesis, they were classified as belonging to class C (e.g., ICP 6 and 8) or D (e.g., ICP 36) (see Fig. 8).

(v) The third group of polypeptides, γ, also required an interval of infected cell protein synthesis before they were synthesized (Figs. 10, 11); they differed from β polypeptides in the duration of this interval and in the initial rates of synthesis following removal of drug. Thus, γ proteins were not made immediately on removal of cycloheximide added before about 2 h post-infection. Between 2 and 5 h post-infection, the later the exposure of infected cells to cycloheximide, the higher were the initial rates of synthesis of γ polypeptides (Figs. 11 and 12). In cells exposed to cycloheximide between 5 h post-infection or later and until 8 h post-infection, the initial rates of synthesis of γ group polypeptides were the same as those in untreated controls. Unlike those of α and β polypeptides, the initial rates of synthesis of γ polypeptides in no instance exceeded those observed in untreated infected cells. On the basis of the kinetics of their synthesis, γ polypeptides (e.g., ICP 5, 17, 21, 31, etc.) were classified (Fig. 8) as belonging to class A, i.e., in untreated infected cells they were made at progressively higher rates until at least 12 h post-infection.

The effect of inhibitors of DNA synthesis on the production of α, β and γ polypeptides

The synthesis of progeny viral DNA is very efficiently prevented by the early inhibition of infected cell protein synthesis (21), probably due to a requirement for the synthesis of the viral DNA polymerase (5) and possibly for other viral proteins which may be essential for viral DNA replication (22). A priori it is therefore possible that the requirement for α polypeptides for subsequent synthesis of β and γ polypeptides reflects a requirement for progeny viral DNA for correct transcription of viral mRNA specifying late classes of polypeptides. Although earlier reports by a number of workers (23,24,25,26) have indicated that herpes virus structural proteins are made in the presence of high concentrations of inhibitors of DNA synthesis, in connection with the present studies, it was necessary to determine whether these inhibitors affected the rates of synthesis of α, β or γ polypeptides. The results of such an experiment are shown in Fig. 13. The inhibitors of DNA synthesis, i.e., cytosine arabinoside or hydroxyurea, did not prevent the synthesis of α, β or γ polypeptides. The inhibitors did selectively reduce the amounts of γ-polypeptide made (e.g., ICP 5, 10, 17; Fig. 13) to 50-60% of the amounts made in untreated cells at the same time. Although we have some reservations about the use of these inhibitors, since low levels of viral DNA synthesis persist even at very high inhibitor concentrations, there is little doubt that the synthesis of β-polypeptides does not require prior DNA synthesis. The relatively small reduction of γ polypeptide synthesis in the presence of these inhibitors likewise indicate that DNA synthesis is not an obligate requirement for the production of these polypeptides. The experiments do suggest, however, that the synthesis of progeny viral DNA may serve to amplify the production of γ-polypeptides.

Effects of actinomycin-D on the synthesis of α, β *and* γ *polypeptides*

In the preceding sections we established that the synthesis of β and γ group virus polypeptides required prior infected cell protein synthesis. The experiments described in this section were designed to determine whether the production of α proteins was the sole requirement for the synthesis of β and γ polypeptides. In one such experiment twelve replicate monolayers of HEp-2 cells were infected at multiplicities of 10 to 20 p.f.u./cell. Cycloheximide was added to six of these cultures at 1.0 h post-infection and removed at 7.0 h. Two treated and two untreated infected cultures were labeled with ^{14}C amino acid from 7.0 to 7.5 h. At the time of removal of cycloheximide, actinomycin-D (10 μg/ml) was added to each of two treated and two untreated cultures and these cultures, together with those not exposed to actinomycin-D, were labeled from 9.5 to 10.0 h post-infection. Labeled polypeptides were separated by electrophoresis on polyacrylamide gel slabs and quantitated as shown in Fig. 7. The results of these analyses for several polypeptides characteristic of α, β and γ groups of virus specific polypeptides and for selected host polypeptides are summarized in Table 1.

The salient features of the data may be summarized as follows: (i) Upon removal of cycloheximide, in the absence of actinomycin-D, the rates of synthesis of α and host polypeptides declined concomitantly with increases in the rates of synthesis of β and γ polypeptides (Table 1, columns 4 and 5). (ii) Addition of actinomycin-D to cultures previously not exposed to cycloheximide resulted in two effects. First, actinomycin-D prevented or reduced the normal decline in the rates of synthesis of α, β and host polypeptides observed in untreated cultures at that time. Second, it caused a rapid decline in the rates of synthesis of γ polypeptides relative to those of untreated cultures. (iii) Actinomycin-D added at the time of removal of cycloheximide reduced the decline in the rate of synthesis of α and host polypeptides and at the same time precluded the synthesis of β and γ polypeptides (column 6). The data indicate that the synthesis of β and γ polypeptides after removal of cycloheximide added at 0 or at 1 h post-infection required RNA synthesis in the presence of α polypeptides. They also show that the decline in the synthesis of α polypeptides in untreated cultures was not due to the action of α polypeptides alone. Also, throughout the period tested the ongoing synthesis of γ polypeptides was more rapidly affected by actinomycin-D than the synthesis of host or of viral α and β polypeptides.

DISCUSSION

In this paper we have presented data showing that, (i) at least 47 polypeptides made in HSV-1 infected cells fulfilled one or more criteria for virus specificity. Included among this number were both structural and non-structural polypeptides with molecular weights from about 15,000 to greater than 250,000. (ii) No evidence was obtained for rapid post-translational cleavages of these polypeptides, suggesting that they were primary products of translation. Based on this conclusion, the size of the viral DNA (1) and the extent of its transcription (4), we estimated that the aggregate molecular weight of the viral

469

polypeptides could account for 70 to 80% of the transcribed information. (iii) The synthesis of viral polypeptides was ordered throughout the virus growth cycle,
some classes of polypeptides were made at high rates early
in infection whereas others were made at increasing rates
late in infection. Structural polypeptides were members
of both early and late classes, whereas most nonstructural
polypeptides were early. (iv) Analysis of the order of
synthesis of viral polypeptides revealed a pattern of cascade regulation of the synthesis of three, sequential,
coordinated groups of polypeptides, designated α, β and γ.
Inherent elements of this cascade regulation are two kinds
of regulatory processes. The first of these turns "on"
the synthesis of polypeptides sequentially. The second
turns "off" or reduces the rates of synthesis, first of α
polypeptides and subsequently of β polypeptides.

In this discussion we would like to focus attention
on both general and specific aspects of cascade regulation
of herpes virus polypeptide synthesis described in this
paper.

Sequential turning "on" of viral polypeptide synthesis

The salient features of the data presented in this
paper are that the onset of synthesis of α, β and γ polypeptides have different requirements. α polypeptides are
synthesized at maximum rates at 3 to 4 h post-infection
in untreated cells. The turning "on" of the synthesis of
α polypeptides does not require prior viral protein synthesis. Rakusanova *et al.* (27) also noted the synthesis
of a selected subset of polypeptides following removal of
cycloheximide from pseudorabies virus infected cells. The
synthesis of β protein does require infected cell protein
synthesis, presumably the synthesis of α polypeptides. In
untreated cells β protein synthesis rises to a maximum at
5 to 7 h post-infection. Production of γ polypeptides is
also dependent on prior virus protein synthesis. However,
the interval required before γ proteins can be synthesized
is longer than that required for β proteins. During this
interval appreciable amounts of both α and β polypeptides
are synthesized. The production of γ proteins may therefore involve either a delayed action of one or more α polypeptides or the participation of one or more β polypeptides by themselves or with α polypeptides.

In the preceding paragraph we have emphasized only requirements for protein synthesis. We should reiterate that although inhibitors of DNA synthesis do not reduce α- and β-polypeptide synthesis, they do reduce the synthesis of γ polypeptides. We conclude that DNA synthesis is not an obligate requirement for the production of any of the three groups of virus polypeptides. However, the synthesis of progeny virus DNA may serve to amplify the production of γ polypeptides.

Functions of α polypeptides and their role in the production of β polypeptides

Of the currently identified α polypeptides only one, ICP 4, is clearly identified as a structural component of the virus by our present criteria. It comigrates with VP 4, a minor virion polypeptide, which is incorporated into virions much less efficiently than major structural components. On the basis of this low efficiency of incorporation we previously suggested it may have a function other than that of a structural polypeptide (12). The remaining polypeptides in the α group have no known electrophoretic counterparts in the virion.

Data obtained from experiments utilizing actinomycin-D indicated that RNA synthesis in the presence of α polypeptides is required for β (and γ) polypeptide synthesis. Since RNA transcribed in the presence of cycloheximide is complementary to the same amount of viral DNA as that transcribed in the absence of the drug, i.e., at least 44% (4), the interpretation of this requirement is not immediately apparent. However, it is clear that mRNAs for α polypeptides are functionally stable, and they either accumulate in the presence of cycloheximide, for as long as 12 h, or their translation is enhanced by the accumulation of a factor whose synthesis is stimulated in the presence of cycloheximide as suggested by Penman et al. (28). By the same considerations functional mRNA for β polypeptides does not accumulate in cells treated with cycloheximide from the time of infection. Therefore, at least one role of α polypeptides involves the production or maintenance of functional β polypeptide mRNA. We cannot exclude the possibility that α polypeptides also function at the level of translation of functional β and γ mRNAs.

In untreated infected cells α protein synthesis declines after about 4 h post-infection. This observation and the data from cycloheximide treated cells (Figs. 10 and 11) show that the continuous synthesis of α polypeptides is not required to sustain their role in subsequent protein synthesis.

Functions of β polypeptides and their role in γ polypeptide synthesis

Polypeptides of the β group are both minor structural components of the virion (e.g., ICP 6) and nonstructural components (e.g., ICP 36). Based on the similarity between the time course of accumulation of β polypeptides (this can be derived from Fig. 11 for ICP 6) and that of a number of herpesvirus specified enzymes (e.g., thymidine kinase, DNA polymerase, DNAse see refs. 5 and 29) our expectation is that these enzymes are members of the β group. In contrast γ polypeptides are typically major structural components of the virus (e.g., ICP 5).

The role of β polypeptides in the production of γ polypeptides is not certain because we cannot at this time entirely dissociate the synthesis of β polypeptides from those of the α group. If β proteins do have such a role, their synthesis is not continuously required to sustain it.

Turning "off" of α and β polypeptide synthesis

In the preceding sections we dealt with requirements for the production of α, β and γ polypeptides. We now wish to draw attention to the finding that, after the synthesis of α and β proteins has begun, the subsequent time course of their synthesis is regulated by the appearance of later groups of viral polypeptides. Specifically, the production of β polypeptides clearly determines the normal decline in α polypeptide synthesis. Thus, when β polypeptide synthesis is prevented either by cycloheximide treatment alone or by cycloheximide followed by actinomycin D the rates of synthesis of α polypeptides exceed those in untreated cultures and the interval of their synthesis is extended. Moreover, the synthesis of α polypeptides is rapidly depressed when β polypeptides are made but before appreciable amounts of γ polypeptides are detected. The data exclude the possibility that α polypeptides directly determine the course of their own biosynthesis.

The mechanism by which β group polypeptides affect the synthesis of α polypeptides is not known. However it is of interest to note that the synthesis of the host polypeptides monitored in this study was also depressed by the synthesis of β polypeptides. This decline was more rapid than that in the presence of α proteins alone.

The rates of synthesis of β polypeptides can also exceed the maximum rates achieved in untreated cells when cycloheximide is added after β polypeptide synthesis has begun but before γ polypeptides are made in large amounts. In this instance the hypothesis that the decline in rates of synthesis in untreated cells is due to the production of γ polypeptides is less compelling and requires further testing.

Implications of coordinate regulation

The observation that viral polypeptides are regulated in a coordinate fashion has a number of implications. First, the different requirement for the production or stability of mRNAs for α, β and γ polypeptides implies either that these groups have differential but coordinate requirements for their transcription or transport or that systematic differences in elements of their structure underlie differences in stability of transcripts not engaged in protein synthesis. In the first instance β mRNAs may be synthesized as a single polycistronic mRNA precursor, which have been reported in herpesvirus infected cells (2), or monocistronic β-polypeptide mRNAs may possess cognate sequences for the initiation of their transcription. Similar considerations would apply to mRNAs for γ polypeptides. The second point is based on the demonstration that the "shut-off" of α and β polypeptides is not due to inhibition of synthesis of their respective mRNAs since actinomycin-D reduces or prevents this "shut-off." It follows that the coordinate depression of α and β polypeptide synthesis is achieved by a post-transcriptional mechanism, also requiring some common elements in the structure of mRNAs within each group to serve as a basis for the discrimination required of this mechanism. The third point is based on the effects of actinomycin-D on ongoing protein synthesis. Although we cannot be certain that measurements of the longevity of protein synthesis in the presence of actinomycin-D are not complicated by indirect effects of the inhibitor, actinomycin-D does discriminate between the synthesis of different groups of polypeptides. The synthesis of γ polypeptides diminishes rapidly in the presence of actinomycin-D whereas that of α and β polypeptides, although not identical in their stability, are in general less sensitive to the inhibitor. These data also suggest differences between mRNAs for α, β and those for γ polypeptides. If the above reasoning is correct, the operation of the coordinate "on" and "off" controls which we have outlined requires that mRNAs for polypeptides within each group share at least one and possibly several common features of their structure which may determine either their synthesis, transport or stability and possibly regulation at the level of their translation or functional half-life.

ACKNOWLEDGMENTS

We thank Chi-Shih Chen for assistance with the computer analyses.

These studies were supported by Public Health Service grant (CA 08494) from the National Cancer Institute, grants from the American Cancer Society (VC 1031), the National Science Foundation (AB 38799), the Whitehall Foundation, and the University of Chicago Cancer Research Center (CA-14599).

R.W.H. is a postfoctoral fellow of the Jane Coffin Childs Memorial fund for Cancer Research.

REFERENCES

1. Kieff, F.D., S.L. Bachenheimer, and B. Roizman, *J. Virol.* **8**, 125 (1971).
2. Wagner, E.K., and B. Roizman, *Proc. Nat. Acad. Sci. U.S.* **64**, 626 (1969).
3. Silverstein, S., S.L. Bachenheimer, N. Frenkel, and B. Roizman, *Proc. Nat. Acad. Sci. U.S.* **70**, 2101 (1973).
4. Frenkel, N., S. Silverstein, E. Cassai, and B. Roizman, *J. Virol.* **11**, 886 (1973).
5. Keir, H.M., In: 18th Symposium of Society for General Microbiology. Cambridge University Press, 1968, p. 67.

6. Spear, P. G. and B. Roizman, *Virology 36*, 545 (1968).
7. Spear, P. G. and B. Roizman, *J. Virol. 9*, 143 (1972).
8. Heine, J. W., P. G. Spear, and B. Roizman, *J. Virol. 9*, 431 (1972).
9. Heine, J. W. and B. Roizman, *J. Virol. 11*, 810 (1973).
10. Nahmias, A. J. and B. Roizman, *New England J. Med. 289*, p. 667, 719, 781 (1973).
11. Duff, R. and F. Rapp, *J. Virol. 12*, 209 (1973).
12. Honess, R. W. and B. Roizman, *J. Virol. 12*, 1347 (1973).
13. Watson, D. H., W. I. H. Shedden, A. Elliot, T. Teksuka, P. Wildy, D. Bourgaux-Ramoisy, and E. Gold, *Immunology 11*, 399 (1966).
14. Honess, R. W. and D. H. Watson, *J. Gen. Virol. 22*, 171 (1974). -
15. Shaw, E., In: Methods in Enzymology. XI, S. P. Colowick and N. O. Kaplan (Eds.); Academic Press, New York, 1967, p. 677.
16. Korant, B. D., *J. Virol. 10*, 751 (1972).
17. Summers, D. F., E. N. Shaw, M. L. Stewart, and J. V. Maizel, Jr., *J. Virol. 10*, 880 (1972).
18. Jacobson, M. F., J. Asso, and D. Baltimore, *J. Mol. Biol. 49*, 667 (1970).
19. Roizman, B., In: Current Topics in Microbiology and Immunology. Vol. 49. B. Benacerraf *et al.* (Eds.), Springer-Verlag, 1969, p. 1.
20. Honess, R. W. and B. Roizman, *J. Virol.*, in press.
21. Roizman, B. and P. R. Roane, Jr., *Virology 22*, 262 (1964).
22. Alberts, B. M., F. J. Amodio, M. Jenkins, E. D. Gutmann, and F. J. Ferris. Cold Spring Harbor Symp. Quant. Biol. *33*, 289 (1968).
23. Levitt, J. and Y. Becker, *Virology 31*, 129 (1967).
24. Nii, S., H. S. Rosencrantz, C. Morgan and H. M. Rose, *J. Virol. 2*, 1163 (1968).
25. Roizman, B., In: Oncogenesis and Herpesvirus. International Agency for Research on Cancer, Lyon, 1972, p. 1.
26. Buchan, A. and S. M. Luff. Personal communication, 1969.
27. Rakusanova, T., T. Ben-Porat, M. Himeno, and A. S. Kaplan, *Virology 46*, 877 (1971).

28. Penman, S., E. Goldstein, M. Reichman, and
    R. Singer, In: 6th Karolinska Symposium on Research
    Methods in Reproductive Endocrinology. Protein
    Synthesis in Reproductive Tissue, 1973, p. 168.
29. Hay, J., P. A. J. Perera, J. M. Morrison,
    G. A. Gentry, and J. H. Subak-Sharpe, In: Strategy
    of the Virus Genome (CIBA Foundation Symposium).
    G. E. W. Wolstenholme and M. O'Connor (Eds.).
    Churchill-Livingstone, 1971, p. 355.

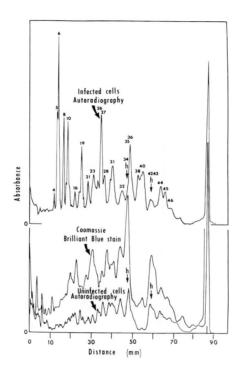

Fig. 1. Absorbance profiles of autoradiographic images of electrophoretically separated polypeptides from infected (top tracing) or mock infected cells (bottom tracing) labeled with ^{14}C-amino acids from 4.5 to 5.0 h after infection or mock infection. The middle tracing shows the profile of electrophoretically separated infected cell proteins obtained by scanning a Coomassie brilliant blue stained gel. Lysates from equal numbers of infected and uninfected cells were separated on 8.5% polyacrylamide gels. The numbers on the upper profile are of selected infected cell polypeptides (ICP) to facilitate comparison with subsequent profiles. The letter "h" identifies proteins in the infected cell (ICP 34, 35 and ICP 42, 43) which were synthesized at rates comparable to proteins of similar mobility in uninfected cells.

Data from Honess and Roizman (12).

477

Fig. 2. The immune precipitation of ICP by antisera specific for viral antigens.
     Photographs of Coomassie brilliant blue stained gels
(right) and the corresponding autoradiograms (left) from
8.5% polyacrylamide gels containing electrophoretically
separated polypeptides from (i) a total cell lysate of
infected cells labeled from 4.25 to 6.5 h post-infection
and harvested immediately after each (total cell), (ii)
the supernatant fluid obtained by sedimentation of the
total cell lysate for 1 h at 35,000 rpm in a Beckman SW40
rotor (Sup. fluid), and (iii) an immune precipitate formed
after incubation of this supernatant fraction with a hyperimmune rabbit antiserum specific for herpes virus antigens
(immune ppt.). Detailed descriptions of the methods used
for the preparation of immune sera and the properties and
use of these sera in immune precipitation of herpes virus
polypeptides were published elsewhere (13,14). Numbers to
the left of the autoradiograms refer to ICP of the total
cell lysate, those at the right indicate the ICP precipitated by the virus specific antiserum. On the right of the
Coomassie brilliant blue stained gels 'heavy' and 'light'
chains of the precipitating immunoglobulin are indicated
together with those stained bands (small solid arrows
annotated with ICP designations) which correspond to prominent labeled components of the immune precipitate.
     Data from Honess and Roizman (12).

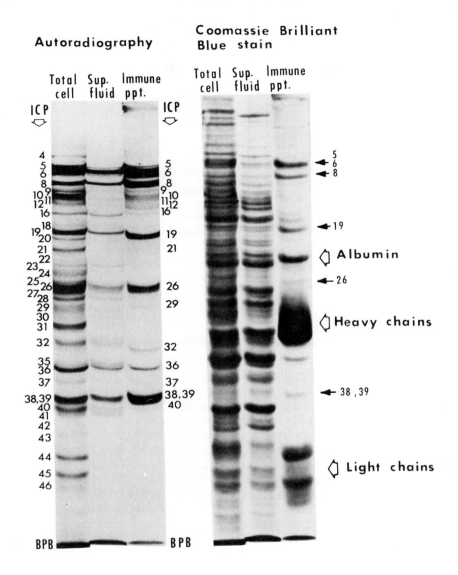

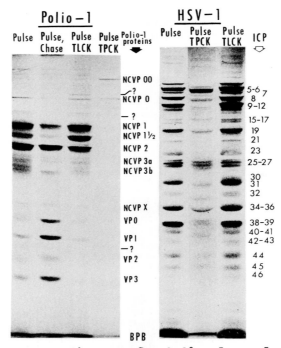

Fig. 3. Autoradiogram of a 9.0% polyacrylamide slab gel containing electrophoretically separated polypeptides synthesized in HSV-1(F) and poliovirus type 1-infected HEp-2 cells labeled with ^{14}C-amino acids in the presence and absence of specific inhibitors of trypsin (TLCK) and chymotrypsin (TPCK) proteases. Left, proteins synthesized in poliovirus-infected cells, pulsed for 15 min from 5 h post-infection in the absence of inhibitors (Pulse), pulsed for 15 min and chased for 30 min in the absence of inhibitors (Pulse, Chase), and pulsed for 15 min in the presence of 10^{-4} M TLCK (Pulse TLCK) and TPCK (Pulse TPCK). Samples on the right are of HSV-1(F) ICP synthesized from 5 to 5.25 h in the absence (Pulse) or presence of inhibitors (TPCK, TLCK). The poliovirus type 1 proteins are designated according to Jacobson, Asso, and Baltimore (18). The numbers to the right of HSV-1(F) samples refer to selected HSV-1(F) ICP. The original autoradiogram was cut for the preparation of this figure, and the exposure interval employed for the printing of the autoradiograms of HSV-1(F)--Pulse TPCK sample was longer than that employed for other samples.

Data from Honess and Roizman (12).

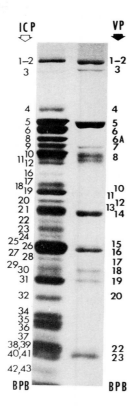

Fig. 4. Comparison of the electrophoretic mobility of ICP and virion polypeptides. Right--autoradiogram of electrophoretically separated ^{14}C-amino acids labeled virion polypeptides. Virions were purified from the cytoplasm of cells labeled from 3 to 20 h post-infection by dextran 10 banding as described by Spear and Roizman (7). Left--autoradiogram of polypeptides of infected cells labeled with ^{14}C-amino acids from 3.5 to 8.7 h post-infection. Solubilized labeled virions and labeled infected cells were subjected to electrophoresis in parallel on a 7.75% slab gel.

Data from Honess and Roizman (12).

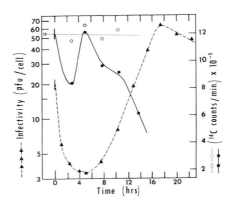

Fig. 5. Accumulation of infectious virus (▲) and rate of amino acid incorporation into acid-insoluble material in infected (●) and mock-infected cells (O). Amino acid incorporation was measured as acid-insoluble radioactivity at the end of 2-h labeling intervals during infection or mock infection and plotted at the midpoint of the interval. Points for infected cultures are the mean of duplicate determinations (2 x 10^6 cells per determination) and those for mock-infected cells are results of a single determination. Accumulation of infectious virus was measured by plaque titrations of duplicate samples of homogenates containing 2 x 10^6 infected cells for each time interval.

Data from Honess and Roizman (12).

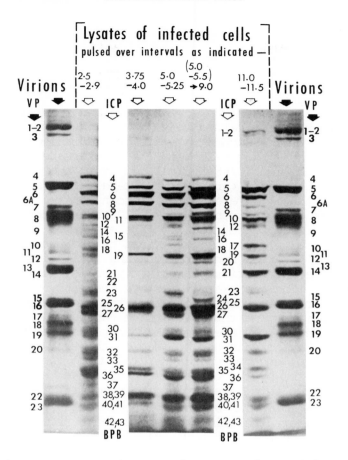

Fig. 6. Autoradiogram of a part of a 7.75% polyacrylamide gel slab containing electrophoretically
separated proteins pulse labeled in HSV-1(F)-infected
cells during intervals shown on top of each sample. The
legend on top of the third gel from the right indicates
that cells were labeled from 5.0 to 5.5 h and then incubated in medium lacking labeled precursors until 9 h post-
infection. Peripheral samples are virion proteins, identified by large numbers to the extreme right and left of
the figure. The autoradiogram was cut in the preparation
of this figure to permit convenient location of numbering
for the ICP (smaller numbers between sample positions 2 and
3 and 5 and 6 of this figure).

Data from Honess and Roizman (12).

Fig. 7. Illustration of the use of computer-aided planimetry to quantitate proteins separated in polyacrylamide gels. The top panel shows the absorbance tracing of an autoradiogram of HSV-1(F) ICP labeled with ^{14}C-amino acids from 3.5 to 8.7 h post-infection and separated on an 8.0% polyacrylamide gel.

The gel was scanned in a Gilford recording spectrophotometer whose photocell output was interfaced with a General Automation 16/45 digital computer, and displayed as a plot of absorbance (arbitrary voltage units) as a function of distance migrated (time of scan) on the oscilloscope screen of a Tektronix Model 4010 control console. The computer was programmed to allow the expansion of regions of the initial profile as determined by the operator and to compute the areas under the tracing for individual bands defined by vertical lines set parallel to the absorbance axis. In this example the regions A, B, C at the top panel indicate those regions of the profile shown in the expanded form in the lower three panels. In each of the lower panels the areas of the bands numbered with the ICP which they contain and bounded by the abscissa, absorbance profile, and broken lines parallel to the ordinate were calculated by the computer and expressed as a percentage of the total area under the complete tracing.

Based on the molecular weights of components in each band, and the estimated relative rate of overall protein synthesis, the amounts of a particular polypeptide can then be expressed as an estimate of either a "relative molar amount synthesized" or, provided the duration of the observation period is sufficiently short, as a "relative molar rate of synthesis," R.M. For example, if K_t is a measure of the overall rate of protein synthesis at the time of the determination, $\Sigma A_i \ldots A_n$ is the total absorbancy of the entire profile, A_i and M_i are the absorbance of band $\underline{i}$ and it molecular weight, respectively, and 10^7 is a constant, then the relative molar amount of protein $\underline{i}$ (RM_i) synthesized is obtained from the relation;

$$RM_i = 10^7 \cdot K_t \cdot \frac{A_i}{M_i (\Sigma A_i \ldots A_n)}$$

Data from Honess and Roizman (12).

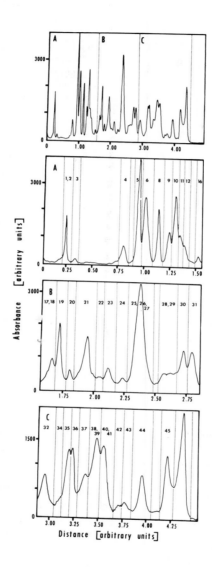

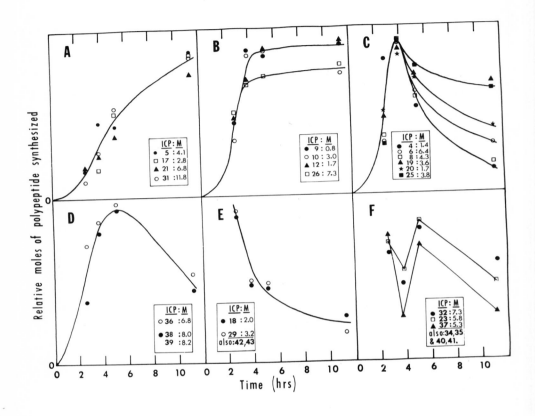

Fig. 8. Patterns of synthesis of ICP in HSV-1(F)-infected cells. The ICP were grouped by the pattern of synthesis designated A to F. Since the RM for the ICP comprising each group are not the same, the plots were normalized. However, the maximum RM observed during the reproductive cycle is shown under column M in the boxed legend next to the number and symbolic representation of the ICP.

Data from Honess and Roizman (12).

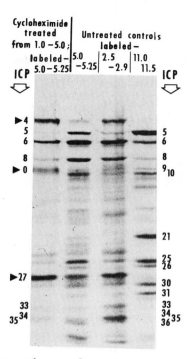

Fig. 9. Comparison of polypeptides made in untreated and in cycloheximide treated infected cells. Replicate cultures of HEp-2 cells were infected with HSV-1(F). Cycloheximide was added to one set of cultures at 1 h post-infection to give a final concentration of 50 µg/ml, a concentration sufficient to produce 98-98% inhibition of overall protein synthesis, and removed followed by thorough washing at 5 h post-infection. Treated and untreated cultures were then labeled with ^{14}C-amino acids from 5 to 5.25 h. Untreated infected cultures were also labeled at earlier (2.5 to 2.9 h) and later (11 to 11.5 h) times in the virus growth cycle. The cells were harvested immediately after the labeling intervals. The figure shows an autoradiogram of a 7.5% polyacrylamide gel slab containing electrophoretically separated polypeptides from lysates of equal numbers of treated and untreated cells. Enumeration of ICP, other than ICP 0, is as in preceding figures. Arrows to the left of the figure identify those viral polypeptides which are synthesized at high rates after the removal of cycloheximide.

Data from Honess and Roizman (20).

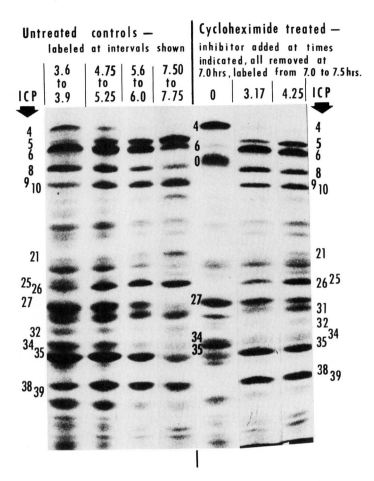

Fig. 10. Autoradiogram of a polyacrylamide gel slab containing electrophoretically separated polypeptides pulse labeled in untreated control cultures with ^{14}C-amino acids at various intervals after infection (four samples on left of figure), and from 7.0 to 7.5 h post-infection immediately following the removal of cycloheximide added at either 0, 3.17 or 4.25 h post-infection, respectively (three samples on right of figure).

Data from Honess and Roizman (20).

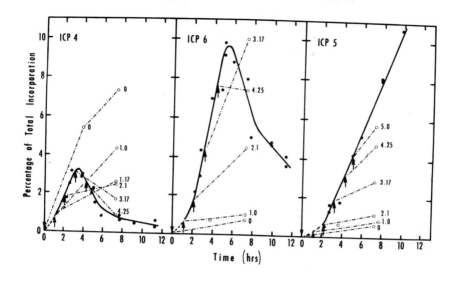

Fig. 11. The synthesis of polypeptides representative of groups α (ICP 4), β (ICP 6) and γ (ICP 5) in cycloheximide treated and in untreated infected cells. The amounts of polypeptide made are expressed in terms of their percentage contribution to the total incorporation of ^{14}C-amino acids into protein during 0.25 to 0.5 h labeling intervals. The filled circles connected by solid lines represent the synthesis of polypeptides at different times after infection in untreated control cultures. The open circles represent the synthesis of polypeptides immediately after the removal of cycloheximide. Cycloheximide was added at the times indicated by arrows to the control curves and the arabic numbers next to the open circles. Corresponding times of addition and removal are interconnected by the dashed lines. The data were derived from planimetry (Fig. 7) of autoradiograms similar to that shown in Fig. 10. Similar data were obtained for other polypeptides of each group, notably for ICP 0 and ICP 8, used as examples of α and β polypeptides and shown in Fig. 12. Data from Honess and Roizman (20).

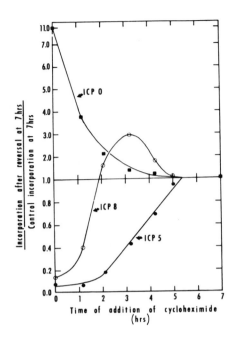

Fig. 12.   Initial rates of synthesis of α (ICP 0,
filled squares), β (ICP 8, open circles) and γ (ICP 5,
filled circles) polypeptides observed on removal of cycloheximide added at different times and removed simultaneously at 7.0 h post-infection. The data are expressed as the
ratio of the percentage of total radioactivity incorporated
in the polypeptide immediately after removal of cycloheximide (cycloheximide was removed at 7.0 h and cultures
labeled from 7.0 to 7.5 h) to the percentage of incorporation into the same polypeptide in untreated cultures
labeled from 7.5 to 7.75 h.   Data points were plotted as a
function of the time of addition of the inhibitor and are
based on analyses of autoradiograms similar to that shown
in Fig. 10. Almost identical plots were obtained for other
polypeptides of each group, notably for ICP 4 and ICP 6
used as examples of α and β polypeptides and shown in
Fig. 11.
    Data from Honess and Roizman (20).

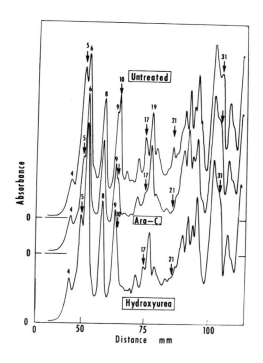

Fig. 13. Absorbance tracings of autoradiograms of electrophoretically separated polypeptides from infected cells labeled with ^{14}C-amino acids from 5.5 to 6.0 h after infection in untreated cells (top tracings) and in cells treated from 0 to 5.5 h with 50 µg/ml of cytosine arabinoside (Ara-C, middle tracing) or 50 µg/ml of hydroxyurea (bottom tracing). Selected ICP are identified by their numbers, those annotated with arrows directed downward were reduced in treated cultures. Absorbance scales for the three tracings are directly comparable. The zero absorbance values for middle and top tracings are indicated by short lines to the ordinate.

Data from Honess and Roizman (20).

TABLE 1

Effects of actinomycin D on synthesis of polypeptides in untreated infected cells and after removal of cycloheximide

Group	Polypeptide	Amounts of polypeptide synthesized[a]					
		(1)	(2)	(3)	(4)	(5)	(6)
					Cycloheximide treated from 1.0 to 7.0 h		
		Untreated cells		Actinomycin D from 7.0 to 9.5			Actinomycin D from 7.0 to 9.5 h
		Pulse 7.0 to 7.5	Pulse 9.5 to 10.0	Pulse 9.5 to 10.0	Pulse 7.0 to 7.5 h	Pulse 9.5 to 10.0 h	Pulse 9.5 to 10.0 h
α	ICP 4	2.2	1.3[c]	1.6	7.4	2.9	6.8
	ICP 0	-	-	1.6	13.9	1.5	5.1
β	ICP 6	13.7	7.1	10.6	3.0	5.4	2.5
	ICP 8	9.8	5.1	5.8	1.7[c]	3.7	1.7[c]
γ	ICP 5	12.5	13.6	6.7	1.5[c]	2.8	1.1[c]
Host	ICP 34,35	9.5	4.2	9.7	14.9	7.7	10.1
Relative incorporation of ^{14}C amino acids into total protein in sample[b]		1.54	1.27	1.16	1.68	1.00	1.38

Footnotes to Table 1[d]

[a] Data were obtained by analysis of absorbance tracings of autoradiograms of electrophoretically separated polypeptides. The percentage of total incorporation in each polypeptide was determined by computer-aided planimetry of the absorbance tracing of the autoradiogram (12). These percentages were then corrected for differences in the total incorporation of labeled amino acids so that amounts of polypeptide synthesized in different samples could be compared.

[b] Relative incorporation of ^{14}C-amino acids into total protein in various samples, expressed as the ratios of the total integrated absorbance of autoradiograms from electrophoretically separated samples. Note that the amount of polypeptide synthesized is the product of the relative incorporation into the sample and the percentage of total integrated absorbance due to a given polypeptide. These data are shown to indicate the extent of variation in total amino acid incorporation observed in these samples.

[c] Values are maximum estimates for amounts of these minor components.

[d] Data from Honess and Roizman (20).

THE LUCKÉ TUMOR VIRUS SYSTEM

Allan Granoff and Robert F. Naegele

Laboratories of Virology and Immunology
St. Jude Children's Research Hospital
Memphis, Tennessee 38101

ABSTRACT. The renal adenocarcinoma (Lucké tumor) of the common leopard frog, *Rana pipiens*, occurs spontaneously with high frequency. The etiologic agent has been shown to be the herpesvirus associated with this tumor. An important recent advance is the successful *in vitro* propagation of the virus. This virus-tumor system provides the only available model for study of a naturally occurring cancer of herpesvirus etiology unconfused by the presence of C type virus.

> *What a wonderful bird the frog are—*
> *When he stand he sit almost;*
> *When he hop he fly almost.*
> *He ain't got no sense hardly;*
> *He ain't got no tail hardly either.*
> *When he sit, he sit on what he ain't got almost.*[1]
>
> — *Anonymous*

INTRODUCTION

The renal adenocarcinoma (Lucké tumor) of the common leopard frog, *Rana pipiens,* was one of the earliest tumors of suspected virus etiology (1,2). This supposition was based on the presence of acidophilic intranuclear inclusion bodies in tumor cells and on cell-free transmission experiments (2,3). Fawcett (4) and

---

[1] Cited in "The Frog Book" by Richard Shaw. Kaye and Ward, Publisher.

Lunger (5) established that a herpesvirus was present in tumor cells but corroborative transmission experiments until recently were equivocal (6). With the demonstration by Tweedell (7) that herpesvirus-containing tumor extracts induced tvpical renal tumors in developing frog embryos, the stage wa set for study of herpesvirus oncogenesis in a naturally occurr ɪg tumor. A number of comprehensive reviews have been written on the Lucke tumor and the reader should refer to them for more detailed and illustrative presentations (6, 8-11). Here we will present a minireview of facts presently available and provide evidence suggesting that the Lucke tumor-virus system may be the most relevant model for studying the natural history of oncogenesis by herpesvirus.

THE TUMOR: GEOGRAPHIC DISTRIBUTION, INCIDENCE, AND PATHOLOGY

The north central and northeastern parts of the United States, and adjacent southern Canada are the major areas where Lucke tumor-bearing frogs are found (3,12,13). The frequency of tumor-bearing frogs taken directly from individual collection sites in nature may vary from less than 1% to 9% (14), a range comparable to that obtained from data on commercially purchased frogs. When large adult frogs are held in the laboratory at 25°C for about 8 months, either isolated or under crowded conditions, 25-50% of them may develop tumors (15,16).

The Lucke tumor can range in size from small, single or multicentric, early tumors to large masses that have replaced most of the kidney and which may comprise half the body weight of the animal. Simultaneous development of several foci is a likely occurrence. Involvement of kidneys can be unilateral or bilateral, with the liver and lung the most frequent sites of metastases.

Histologically, tumors are usually well-differentiated adenocarcinomas consisting of rather large basophilic cells. Frequently such growths are cystic with pronounced papillary ingrowths. In some tumors the component cells are less atypical and are arranged in a more orderly fashion, resembling adenomas rather than adenocarcinomas. Thus, all gradations are found: from the malignant adenocarcinoma to the structurally benign adenoma, cystadenoma and papillary cystadenoma. It is generally agreed that the tumor cells arise in proximal tubules (6), although cells other than those of the proximal tubule (*e.g.* Wolffian ducts, collecting ducts) may also be sites of malignant transformation (17). The frog tumor fulfills all the criteria by which a tumor is recognized as a

494

malignant neoplasm, whether in man or other vertebrates; that is, it invades and destroys the tissue of its origin and it can metastasize.

An important feature of the Lucké tumor, already alluded to in the Introduction, is the frequent presence of acidophilic intranuclear inclusions. The presence of these inclusions is invariably correlated with the presence of virus as determined by electron microscopy. Although Lucké (3) in his early studies recognized that the presence or absence of inclusions had a seasonal variation (more frequent in winter and spring than in summer or autumn), this phenomenon has only recently been firmly established (see below). Tumors from frogs captured in the warm summer months or held in the laboratory at 20-25°C do not contain nuclear inclusions and have a high mitotic index. However, cells of tumors in frogs collected while in hibernation or held cold (4-9°C) in the laboratory have inclusions. The number of inclusion-bearing cells in the neoplastic tissue varies greatly: sometimes relatively few are present, sometimes nearly every cell in some portion of the tumor is affected and such cells appear degenerated.

Fawcett (4) was the first to describe the presence of "virus particles" similar to herpes simplex virus in cells bearing inclusions, an observation subsequently corroborated (12,18,19). Lunger (5) was able to extract virus particles from inclusion-bearing tumors and showed that their ultrastructure was compatible with known herpesviruses (162 capsomeres). The cells containing virus are degenerating cells, indicating that the presence of virions is incompatible with cell survival.

TEMPERATURE AND ITS RELATIONSHIP TO THE PRESENCE OF VIRUS

As noted earlier, the presence of intranuclear inclusions and the presence of herpesvirus are invariably correlated. The first well-documented study on the temperature dependence of inclusion-body formation was made by Roberts (20), who found that renal tumors of frogs held at 20-25°C never had intranuclear inclusions whereas those of frogs held at 5°C did. Rafferty (21), by biopsy, demonstrated the development of intranuclear inclusions in tumor cells of frogs after 5-7 months at 4°C. Mizell et al. (22) and Skinner and Mizell (23) placed inclusion-free tumor fragments in the anterior eye chambers of R. pipiens as well as other species and followed the development of inclusions (light microscopy) and virus (electron microscopy) in the tumor transplants at various times after the frogs were placed at temperatures ranging from 4-26°C. There was a direct correlation between the presence of virus and the time and the temperature of incubation. Replication of herpesvirus was induced up to 11.5°C with 7.5-9.5°C the optimal range; above 11.5°C the tumor cells remained virus-free. Under optimal conditions about 30% of cells examined were virus-positive by 3 months.

Urine from tumor-bearing frogs held at 4°C frequently contains large amounts of herpesvirus while urine from tumor-bearing frogs held at 25°C does not (24). Moreover, ascitic fluid from tumor-bearing frogs held at low temperature may also contain herpesvirus (25).

Breidenbach *et al.* (26) demonstrated that the intact host is not required for induction of virus replication at low temperature. Tissue culture explants of virus-free tumors maintained *in vitro* at 7.5°C produced virus after 3 months.

The opposite effect can also be demonstrated: virus-containing tumor cells degenerate and are replaced by virus-free cells at temperatures from 15-26°C. When frogs bearing virus-positive tumors are moved from 4°C to 20-22°C, cellular debris and virus are observed in the lumina and no virus-containing inclusions are present by 7 days (27). Transplantation of fragments of inclusion-positive tumors to the frog anterior eye chamber also results in disappearance of virus within 2-6 weeks at 15-26°C (18, 23).

Evidence for transcription of viral information in virus-free tumors has been obtained (28). Tumor-bearing frogs held at 20-25°C were given [^{3}H] uridine and [^{3}H] RNA extracted from tumors hybridized with Lucké tumor herpesvirus obtained from herpesvirus isolated and purified from tumors. Normal frog kidney RNA did not bind to viral DNA and purified virus-specific RNA from tumors did not hybridize to cellular DNA. Thus, virus-free tumors contain herpesvirus genetic information, providing additional evidence for an etiological role of the virus in tumor formation.

From the evidence thus far accumulated it is clear that replication of the herpesvirus associated with the Lucké tumor is dependent on temperature both *in vivo* and *in vitro*. Neither the mechanism of this dependence nor the significance of the role of temperature in virus replication and Lucké tumor formation is known. Although it is possible that the cell and not the virus is the main temperature-dependent factor, there is no reason to believe that virus and cell are mutually exclusive contributors to the observed temperature effect. Worthy of note are the similarities between induction of the Lucké tumor-associated herpesvirus by cold treatment and induction of other herpesviruses of suspected oncogenicity, such as Epstein-Barr virus by 5-bromodeoxyuridine (29).

PHYSICAL, CHEMICAL, AND BIOLOGICAL PROPERTIES OF THE LUCKÉ TUMOR-ASSOCIATED HERPESVIRUS

Little information is available on the physical and chemical properties of the herpesvirus obtained from the Lucké tumor. There appears to be nothing distinctive in virus ultrastructure (5,30) or in development of the virus in tumor cells as reconstructed from electron micrographs (12,31). Viral DNA is a linear double-stranded molecule with a base composition of 45-47% guanine plus cytosine (32,33).

Although Lucké's (2,3) early transmission experiments with cell-free preparations of tumors suggested a viral etiology, the results of subsequent experiements, as indicated in the Introduction, were generally equivocal (6). Tweedell (7) made the first significant advance in firmly establishing a virus etiology of the Lucké tumor by showing that as high as 90% of R. pipiens embryos or larvae receiving injections of cytoplasmic fractions of inclusion-containing Lucké tumors and held at 20°C developed typical renal tumors as they reached metamorphosis. The material injected contained herpesvirus as determined by electron microscopy, and filtrates of this material retained activity although it was somewhat diminished. Comparable fractions of normal adult frog kidneys or inclusion-free tumors failed to induce tumors. Tweedell (34) also demonstrated that exposure of oocytes to herpesvirus extracted from a Lucké tumor led to tumor development only when oocytes were exposed during ovulation and not when exposed after they had left the animal.

Tumor-inducing activity is destroyed by ether (Naegele and Granoff, unpublished observation) and by protease or by lyophilization, but it is stable to sonication (35). Rate zonal centrifugation of cytoplasmic fractions of virus-containing tumors yields oncogenic preparations rich in enveloped herpesvirus (36). Lucké tumors have been induced in embryos of R. clamitans and R. palustris, and in interspecific hybrids between R. palustris and R. pipiens (37). Transmission of the tumor also has been demonstrated with herpesvirus-containing ascitic fluid obtained from a tumor-bearing frog (25).

It is clear that the cell-free induction of Lucké tumors by herpesvirus-containing fractions of tumors or ascitic fluid has been conclusively demonstrated in the laboratory. However, the association of other viruses with the Lucké tumor (9) indicated a need to more firmly establish the relationship of the Lucké herpesvirus (LHV) to tumor formation. An experiment was therefore designed (38) to as nearly as possible fulfill the classical

497

Koch-Henle postulates (39) for identifying the causal agent of the Lucké tumor.

LHV was extracted from a naturally occurring "cold" tumor and 63% of frog embryos inoculated with the virus developed typical virus-free tumors; these animals were raised at 20-22°C. None of the surviving sham-infected control embryos developed tumors.

To determine whether the LHV genome was present in induced tumors and could be made to replicate *in vitro* by low temperature treatment, fragments of a tumor were placed in culture. The cultures were divided into 2 groups; one group was incubated at 22°C and the other at 7.5°C. Tissue samples were taken periodically and examined by light and electron microscopy for the presence of intranuclear inclusions and herpesvirus.

Typical intranuclear inclusions and herpesvirus were detected in the cells of tumor fragments maintained at 7.5°C. By day 50 the frequency of cells containing herpesvirus was 4.5%, in good agreement with the frequency of cells containing inclusions (4.8%). By day 70 at 7.5°C the percentage of inclusion-bearing tumor cells reached 30% and those containing virus 39.4%. Neither intranuclear inclusions nor virus was seen in tumor fragments incubated at 22°C, confirming the low temperature dependence of virus replication.

These results clearly demonstrated the full expression of the LHV genome in induced tumors under *in vitro* conditions in the absence of possible host-contributing factors. However, Koch-Henle's third postulate requires that the recovered microorganism must be shown to be the same as that inoculated. The criterion we used to satisfy this requirement was the demonstration that the virus recovered from the tumor fragments was oncogenic. For this purpose a group of tailbud embryos were inoculated with virus extracted from tumor fragments maintained at 7.5°C.

A second group of embryos were inoculated with an identically prepared extract obtained from tumor fragments maintained at 22°C. Additionally, a group of embryos were inoculated with diluent alone. All animals were reared at 22°C.

Tumors were first detected at 4 months; after 5 1/2 months all surviving animals were sacrificed and examined for tumors. Typical Lucké tumors were found at high frequency (65%) in the animals receiving the LHV-containing extract of 7.5°C tumor fragments; none occurred in animals receiving extracts of tissue incubated at 22°C or diluent alone. The tumors were free of intranuclear inclusions. Thus, the herpesvirus present in induced tumors retained its oncogenic activity and was with little doubt the same agent as originally isolated from the wild tumor.

Figure 1 schematically illustrates the entire experiment starting with the original tumor-bearing frog.

VIRUS ISOLATION STUDIES

Attempts to grow tumor-inducing herpesvirus from Lucké tumors in cultured cells have until now been unsuccessful (9). Several viruses have been isolated from Lucké tumors and have been propagated *in vitro*; *they do not induce tumors.* The properties of these viruses have been the subject of several reviews (8,9,40) and will not be dealt with further. However, it is important to emphasize that one of these isolates, FV 4 (21), is a herpesvirus distinct from the one physically separable from the tumor (33,41). These differences include base composition, base sequence homology, and antigenic composition. It is equally important to point out that none of the isolates is a C type virus and that we have failed to obtain evidence for the presence of C type virus in warm and cold tumors and in Lucké tumor cells cultured *in vitro* (Naegele and Granoff, unpublished observation). Likewise, we have not been able to induce C type particles by chemicals such as BrdU.

One of the major obstacles in the study of the Lucké virus tumor system has been the lack of *in vitro*-cultured host cells susceptible to infection by LHV. Recently, a frog pronephric cell line has been established (42) which supports the replication of LHV (43). These cells were infected at 25°C with LHV obtained from a "cold" Lucké tumor. A cytopathic effect, which included the development of typical intranuclear inclusions in about five percent of the cells, could be serially passaged. Infected cells in the third passage contained typical herpesvirus particles as determined by electron microscopy. When inoculated into frog embryos, herpesvirus-containing extracts of the cells induced renal tumors in these animals. Thus it appears that the etiologic agent of the Lucké tumor has now been successfully cultured *in vitro*. This achievement makes possible a comprehensive study of the natural history of the tumor and of molecular mechanisms operative in a herpesvirus-induced tumor in a natural host. The finding that LHV can replicate at 25°C in monolayer cultures, in contrast to its low-temperature dependence in *in vivo* or *in vitro* fragment cultures, requires further elucidation.

DISCUSSION

Evidence for a herpesvirus etiology of human malignancy is circumstantial. Seroepidemiological studies have been used to implicate herpes simplex viruses types 1 and 2 and Epstein-Barr virus (EBV) in a number of human malignancies (44-47). The fact that HSV inactivated by ultraviolet light can transform hamster embryo cells *in vitro* (48,49) has supported the idea that these agents have oncogenic potential. The ability of EBV to produce lymphomas in simians (50-52) also reinforces the notion that these viruses may cause cancer in humans. We would like to point out, however, that evidence for virally-produced cancer in an unnatural host is not unique and cannot be taken to indicate a similar role for the virus in a natural host. The only herpesvirus which causes a malignant disease in its natural host is Marek's disease virus (53). Here the picture becomes cloudy because of the possible participation of C type particles (54). Similarly, indirect evidence for the presence of C type particles has been suggested for Burkitt lymphomas (55).

Thus, as we view it — and contrary to the belief expressed by Albert B. Sabin at a recent meeting[1] that it has no relevancy to human cancer — the Lucke' tumor is the only system to date in which a naturally occurring tumor is caused by a herpesvirus in the absence of detectable C type particle participation. Thus, one of the oldest virus-tumor systems may now be used as a model for learning about herpesvirus oncogenesis in higher vertebrates. Cancer is cancer — be it in frog or man. The history of science tells us that model systems do provide relevant information to understanding human disease; the Lucké herpesvirus system is one such example.

ACKNOWLEDGMENTS

This work was supported by Research Grant CA-07055, Contract 71-2134 of the Virus Cancer Program, and Childhood Cancer Research Center Grant CA-08480 from the National Cancer Institute, Grant 1073 from the Damon Runyon Memorial Fund for Cancer Research, and by ALSAC.

REFERENCES

1. B. Lucke', *Amer. J. Cancer* 20, 352 (1934).
2. B. Lucke', *J. Exp. Med.* 68, 457 (1938).

---

[1] Eighth Annual Joint Working Conference of the Virus Cancer Program, National Cancer Institute, Hershey, PA, Nov. 4-7, 1973.

3.   B. Lucke′, *Ann. N.Y. Acad. Sci. 54*, 1093 (1952).
4.   D.W. Fawcett, *J. Biophys. Biochem. Cytol. 2*, 725 (1956).
5.   P.D. Lunger, *Virology 24*, 138 (1964).
6.   K.A. Rafferty, Jr., *Cancer Res. 24*, 169 (1964).
7.   K.S. Tweedell, *Cancer Res. 27*, 2042 (1967).
8.   A. Granoff, M. Gravell and R.W. Darlington, *In* Recent Results in Cancer Research, Springer-Verlag, Berlin-Heidelberg-New York, 1969, p. 279.
9.   A. Granoff, *Fed. Proc. 31*, 1626 (1972).
10. A. Granoff, *In* The Herpesviruses, A. Kaplan (Ed.), Academic Press, New York, 1973, p. 93.
11. R.G. McKinnell, *Amer. Zool. 13*, 97 (1973).
12. P.D. Lunger, R.W. Darlington and A. Granoff, *Ann. N.Y. Acad. Sci. 126*, 289 (1965).
13. R.G. McKinnell, *Ann. N.Y. Acad. Sci. 126*, 85 (1965).
14. R.G. McKinnell and B.K. McKinnell, *Cancer Res. 28*, 440 (1968).
15. K.A. Rafferty, Jr. and N.S. Rafferty, *Science 133*, 702 (1961).
16. K.A. Rafferty, Jr., *Science 141*, 720 (1963).
17. K.A. Rafferty, Jr., *In* Oncogenesis and Herpesviruses, P.M. Biggs, G. deThé and L.N. Payne (Eds.), IARC, Lyon, 1972, p. 159.
18. J. Zambernard and M. Mizell, *Ann. N.Y. Acad. Sci. 126*, 127 (1965).
19. J. Zambernard, A.E. Vatter and R.G. McKinnell, *Cancer Res. 26*, 1688 (1966).
20. M.E. Roberts, *Cancer Res. 23*, 1709 (1963).
21. K.A. Rafferty, Jr., *Ann. N.Y. Acad. Sci. 126*, 3 (1965).
22. M. Mizell, C.W. Stackpole and S. Halperen, *Proc. Soc. Exp. Biol. Med. 127*, 808 (1968).
23. M.S. Skinner and M. Mizell, *Lab. Invest. 26*, 671 (1972).
24. A. Granoff and R.W. Darlington, *Virology 38*, 197 (1969).
25. R.F. Naegele and A. Granoff, *J. Nat. Cancer Inst. 49*, 299 (1972).
26. G.P. Breidenbach, M.S. Skinner, J.H. Wallace and M. Mizell, *J. Virol. 7*, 679 (1971).
27. J. Zambernard and A.E. Vatter, *Cancer Res. 26*, 2148 (1966).
28. W. Collard, H. Thornton, M. Mizell and M. Green, *Science 181*, 448 (1973).
29. P. Gerber, *Proc. Nat. Acad. Sci. U.S.A. 69*, 83 (1972).
30. I. Toplin, M. Mizell, P. Sottong and J. Monroe, *Appl. Microbiol. 21*, 132 (1971).
31. C.W. Stackpole, *J. Virol. 4*, 75 (1969).
32. E.K. Wagner, B. Roizman, T. Savage, P.G. Spear, M. Mizell, F.E. Durr and D. Sypowicz, *Virology 42*, 257 (1970).

33. M. Gravell, *Virology 43*, 730 (1971).
34. K.S. Tweedell, *In* Recent Results in Cancer Research, M. Mizell (Ed.), Springer-Verlag, New York, 1969, p. 229.
35. K.S. Tweedell, *Proc. Soc. Exp. Biol. Med. 140*, 1246 (1972).
36. M. Mizell, I. Toplin and J.J. Isaacs, *Science 165*, 1134 (1969).
37. D.J. Mulcare, *In* Recent Results in Cancer Research, M. Mizell (Ed.), Springer-Verlag, New York, 1969, p. 240.
38. R.F. Naegele, A. Granoff and R.W. Darlington, *Proc. Nat. Acad. Sci. U.S.A.* (In press, 1974).
39. T.M. Rivers, *J. Bacteriol. 33*, 1 (1936).
40. A. Granoff, *In* Current Topics in Microbiology and Immunology, *50*, Springer-Verlag, Berlin-Heidelberg-New York, 1969, p. 107.
41. M. Gravell, A. Granoff and R.W. Darlington, *Virology 36*, 467 (1968).
42. W.Y. Wong and K.S. Tweedell, *Proc. Soc. Exp. Biol. Med.* (In press, 1974).
43. K.S. Tweedell and W.Y. Wong, *J. Nat. Cancer Inst.* (In press, 1974).
44. M.A. Epstein, *In* Oncogenesis and Herpesviruses, P.M. Biggs, G. deThé and L.N. Payne (Eds.), IARC, Lyon, 1972, p. 261.
45. G. deThé, *In* Oncogenesis and Herpesviruses, P.M. Biggs, G. deThé and L.N. Payne (Eds.), IARC, Lyon, 1972, p. 275.
46. W. Henle and G. Henle, *Cancer Res. 33*, 1419 (1973).
47. A.B. Sabin and G. Tarro, *Proc. Nat. Acad. Sci. U.S.A. 70*, 3225 (1973).
48. R. Duff and F. Rapp, *Nature New Biol. 233*, 48 (1971).
49. R. Duff and F. Rapp, *J. Virol. 12*, 209 (1973).
50. T. Shope, D. Dechairo and G. Miller, *Proc. Nat. Acad. Sci. U.S.A. 70*, 2487 (1973).
51. M.A. Epstein, R.D. Hunt and H. Rabin, *Int. J. Cancer 12*, 309 (1973).
52. M.A. Epstein, H. Rabin, G. Ball, A.B. Rickinson, J. Jarvis and L.V. Melendez, *Int. J. Cancer 12*, 319 (1973).
53. H.G. Purchase, *Fed. Proc. 31*, 1634 (1972).
54. W.P. Peters, D. Kufe, J. Schlom, J.W. Frankel, C.O. Prickett, V. Groupé and S. Spiegelman, *Proc. Nat. Acad. Sci. U.S.A. 70*, 3175 (1973).
55. D.W. Kufe, W.P. Peters and S. Spiegelman, *Proc. Nat. Acad. Sci. U.S.A. 70*, 3810 (1973).

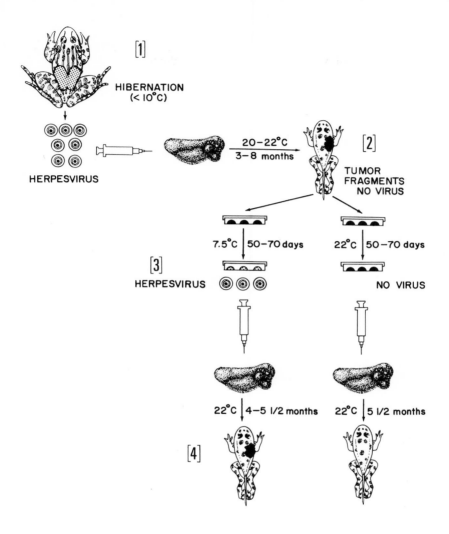

Fig. 1. Schematic representation of the Lucke' tumor experiment fulfilling Koch-Henle postulates (38). [1] Association of the agent with the disease. [2] The agent must induce the same disease in a susceptible host. [3] The agent must be isolated from the induced disease. [4] The isolated agent must be identified as the same agent originally associated with the disease.

LATENT GENOMES OF EPSTEIN-BARR VIRUS

Meihan Nonoyama and Akiko Tanaka

Departments of Microbiology
Rush-Presbyterian-St. Luke's
and University of Illinois Medical Centers
Chicago, Illinois 60612

Berge Hampar

National Cancer Institute
Bethesda, Maryland 20014

Jeffery G. Derge
Flow Laboratories Inc.
Rockville, Maryland 20852

ABSTRACT. EBV DNA becomes latent in human leukocytes as well as in tumor tissues. The majority of such DNA does not seem to be covalently integrated into large chromosomal DNA although it is located in chromosomes. This DNA replicates in the early S phase before or at the time of onset of cell DNA replication. Whether the majority of EBV-DNA attaches to a small piece of cell DNA and whether very small amounts of EBV genomes are integrated into large cell DNA has not been determined yet.

INTRODUCTION

Epstein-Barr virus (EBV) was first discovered in human leukocyte cells established from a Burkitt's lymphoma patient (1). The association of this virus with various diseases has been studied immunologically (2,3,4). African Burkitt's lymphoma patients have generally high titers of serum antibody against EBV and nasopharyngeal carcinoma patients also show such a tendency. In addition EBV is strongly associated with infectious mononucleosis.

Nucleic acid hybridization methods have been developed to detect EBV DNA in tumor cells or tissues and confirm the immunological association of the virus with the tumors. The methods used for the hybridization studies were DNA-DNA (5) or complementary RNA (C-RNA) hybridization on a nitrocellulose filter (6) and DNA-DNA reassociation kinetics (7). C-RNA hybridization can only detect more than 2 viral genome equivalents per cell whereas DNA-DNA reassociation kinetics can detect one complete viral genome in 10 to 50 cells (7,8). Although an association of EBV DNA with African Burkitt's lymphoma and nasopharyngeal carcinoma was found (5,9), it was rather surprising that some of other African tumors (8 of 24) also contained EBV DNA (9). These included adenocarcinoma, carcinoma, melanoma, sarcoma and leukemia. In contrast, American tumor biopsies did not contain such significant amounts of EBV genomes (10,11). Thus the association of EBV with tumors seems to be restricted geographically to a certain area even though the virus is present universally.

Not only tumor tissues but all human B type lymphocytes established as cell lines *in vitro* carry the viral DNA (6,12,13,14). Raji cells which were established from a Burkitt's lymphoma, for example, contained 50 genomes of EBV per cell. How the viral genomes are persisting in these cells is an interesting question. Are the viral genomes covalently integrated into chromosomal DNA just as DNA of other tumor viruses (15) or do they exist as plasmid DNA? The discussion will focus on this question.

RESULTS AND DISCUSSION

Separation of EBV DNA from large molecular weight cell DNA by velocity sedimentation. EBV DNA has a molecular weight of 10^8 daltons. Since cell DNA should be larger than the viral DNA, the viral DNA should be separated from cell DNA by velocity sedimentation if it is not covalently integrated. If it is linearly integrated through phosphodiester bonds the viral DNA and cell DNA should be cosedimented even in an alkaline condition.

As reported previously (16), Raji cells were gently lysed by 0.5 N NaOH and sarkosyl-97 (1%) and large molecular weight DNA was sedimented through a 10 to 30% alkaline glycerol gradient. Hela cells (viral genome

free) were mixed with EBV and treated in the same way. The
location of EBV DNA in the gradients was determined by EBV
specific C-RNA hybridization. As seen in Figures 1a and
1b, EBV DNA did not sediment with cell DNA and was
completely separated. Although the fastest sedimenting
peak of hybridized fractions was 68S which corresponds
5x10^7 daltons (full length of single stranded EBV DNA),
the hybridized fractions were rather broad from 68S to
30S. This indicates that EBV DNA both in Raji cells and
in purified virus particles had single stranded nicks in
the molecules.

The presence of nicks in EBV DNA made interpretation
of the above experiment rather complicated and all the
following possibilities should be considered.

1.   EBV DNA in Raji cells is covalently integrated into
cell DNA with the same pattern of nicks in the molecules
as in the virus particles.

2.   EBV DNA is linearly integrated into cell DNA through
alkaline labile bonding, such as RNA (17) or hydrogen
bonding (18).

3.   EBV DNA is not integrated into cell DNA in linear
form.

Since full size EBV DNA was recovered in velocity
sedimentation from Raji cells and the pattern of strand
nicks were very similar to that of virus particles,
integration of fragmented EBV DNA may not be likely.

To distinguish the third possibility from the first
and the second, any denaturing conditions should be
avoided. Thus large molecular weight DNA was isolated by
lysing cells by pronase and sarkosyl or by sarkosyl alone
and sedimented through a neutral glycerol gradient.
Under this condition EBV DNA which now has 53S should be
separated from cell DNA only if the third possibility is
correct.

Raji cells were lysed by sarkosyl alone and the
viscous materials were poured on top of a gradient containing 5 to 10% glycerol with a bottom cushion of 20%
glycerol. Figure 2a shows that the majority of hybridization was seen in the region of cell DNA which had sedimented onto the 20% glycerol cushion. However there was a

small peak which appeared in the viral DNA region.
Addition of pronase to sarkosyl lysate of Raji cells
enlarged the hybridized peak in the viral DNA region
(Figure 2b); 70 to 80% of the total hybridizable amounts
appeared in the viral DNA region and only 20 to 30%
sedimented with the large cell DNA. A mixture of EBV
genome free human leukocytes (simpson cells) (8) and EBV
particles were treated with pronase and sarkosyl and
sedimented through the same type of the glycerol gradient
(Figure 2c). Again 70 to 80% of the viral DNA appeared
in the viral DNA region and the rest were aggregated with
cell DNA. The large cell DNA fraction was isolated from
the gradient of the pronase-sarkosyl lysate of Raji cells
and recentrifuged through a 5 to 10% glycerol gradient
with a 20% glycerol cushion (Figure 3). About 40% of the
viral DNA was released from the cell DNA fraction. From
these experiments about 80 to 90% of EBV DNA in Raji cells
which contained 50 to 60 genomes per cell seems to exist
as nonintegrated DNA. These viral genomes were located
in chromosomes (6) and the EBV DNA was isolated tightly
bound to cell DNA through proteins as shown by lysing
cells with sarkosyl alone. Since all the viral genomes
in Raji cells were located in chromosomes and *in situ*
hybridization showed about equal numbers of grains in each
Raji cell (16), the cell suspensions should not contain
spontaneously induced cells. Therefore the experiments
reported here clearly showed that the latent EBV DNA
present in Raji cells can be separated from cell DNA
without fragmentation. However whether the isolated
viral DNA is covalently linked to a small piece of cell
DNA and whether a few genomes are covalently integrated
into cell DNA remain to be determined.

Control of latent EBV DNA replication in Raji cells.
It has been discussed in the previous section that the
majority of EBV genomes in Raji cells may not be linearly
integrated into cell DNA. Throughout passages Raji cells
contained the same amount of EBV genomes, which indicates
that replication of the latent viral genomes is well
controlled by cellular mechanisms of DNA replication even
though the viral genomes exist as plasmid DNA. Then a
question to be answered (19) is whether the viral DNA
replicates together with cell DNA throughout the S phase
or if viral DNA replication only occurs at a certain

point of the cell growth cycle.

Raji cells were synchronized by double thymidine block (20) and total cell DNA replication was followed by thymidine-H^3 uptake. The viral DNA replication was determined by C-RNA hybridization after extraction of whole DNA from cells. If the viral DNA replicated before cell DNA replication, the number of EBV genomes per cell should become doubled at the end of the viral DNA replication and should decrease with cell DNA replication, reaching 50 genomes per cell again at the end of cell DNA replication. If the viral DNA replicated after cell DNA replication, the number of EBV genomes should decrease to one half at the end of cell DNA replication and should come back to 50 genomes per cell at the end of the viral DNA replication. If the viral DNA replicates together with total cell DNA synthesis, the number of EBV genomes per cell should not be changed. After release of the double thymidine block, S phase started immediately and maximum DNA synthesis occurred between 2 and 4 hours. It was completed in 4 to 5 hours. C-RNA hybridization was conducted for each time period and the number of EBV genomes were calculated. As seen in Figure 4a the number of EBV genomes per cell doubled in 60 to 90 minutes after thymidine release and gradually decreased to 50 genomes per cell. The result indicates that the latent EBV genomes replicated at the specific time just before or at the time of onset of cell DNA replication, Figure 4b showed that EBV DNA replicated also in the second early S phase indicating that the result obtained here should not be the immediate artifact of thymidine block.

ACKNOWLEDGMENTS

This work was supported in part by contracts NOI-CP-33219 and NOI-CP-3-3247 from the Virus Cancer Program, National Cancer Institute, National Institutes of Health, Bethesda, Maryland, and by grants from the American Cancer Society, Illinois Division (No. 73-23) and the National Institutes of Health (No. CA-15281-01).

REFERENCES

1. M.A. Epatein, B.G. Achong and Y.M. Barr, *Lancet 1*, 702 (1964).

2. P. Gunven, G. Klein, G. Henle, W. Henle and P. Clifford, *Nature 228,* 1053 (1970).
3. W. Henle, G. Henle, H. Ho, P. Burtiss, Y. Cachin, P. Clifford, A. Deschryrer, G. DeThe, V. Diehl and G. Klein, *J. Nat. Cancer Inst. 44,* 225, (1970).
4. G. Henle, W. Henle and W. Diehl, *Proc. Nat. Acad. Sci. U.S. 59,* 94 (1968).
5. H. Zurhausen, H. Schulte-Holthausen, G. Klein, W. Henle, G. Henle, P. Clifford and L. Santessen, *Nature 228,* 1056 (1970).
6. M. Nonoyama and J.S. Pagano, *Nature New Biol. 233,* 103 (1971).
7. M. Nonoyama and J.S. Pagano, *Nature 242,* 44 (1973).
8. Y. Kawai, M. Nonoyama and J.S. Pagano, *J. Virol. 12,* 1006 (1973).
9. M. Nonoyama, C.H. Huang, J.S. Pagano, G. Klein and S. Singh, *Proc. Nat. Acad. Sci. U.S. 70,* 3265 (1973).
10. J.S. Pagano, C.H. Huang and P. Levine, *New England J. Med. 289,* 1395 (1973).
11. M. Nonoyama, Y. Kawai, C.H. Huang, J.S. Pagano, Y. Hirshaut and P.H. Levine, *Cancer Resch. in press.*
12. H. Zurhausen and H. Schulte-Holthausen, *Nature 227,* 245 (1970).
13. H. Zurhausen, V. Diehl, H. Wolfe, H. Schulte-Holthausen and U. Schneider, *Nature New Biol. 237,* 189 (1972).
14. J. Minowada, M. Nonoyama, G.E. Moore, A.M. Rauch and J.S. Pagano, *Cancer Resch. in press.*
15. J. Sambrook, H. Westphal, P.R. Srinivasan and R. Dulbecco, *Proc. Nat. Acad. Sci. U.S. 60,* 1280 (1968).
16. M. Nonoyama and J.S. Pagano, *Nature New Biol. 238,* 169 (1972).
17. A. Adams, T. Lindahl and G. Klein, *Proc. Nat. Acad. Sci. U.S. 70,* 2888 (1973).
18. J. Tomizawa and N. Anraku, *J. Mol. Biol. 8,* 516 (1964).
19. B. Hampar, A. Tanaka, M. Nonoyama and J.G. Derge, *Proc. Nat. Acad. Sci. U.S. in press.*
20. B. Hampar, J.G. Derge, L.M. Martos, M.A. Tagamets, S-Y. Chang and M. Chakrabarty, *Nature New Biol. 244,* 214 (1973).

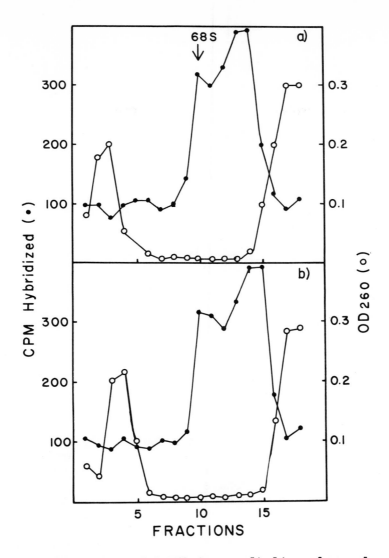

Fig. 1.   Latent EBV DNA in an alkaline glycerol
gradient (16) 5x10⁶ or Raji cells (a) or Hela Cells with
EBV (b) were treated with 0.5 N NaOH, 1% sarkosyl and
0.1M EDTA overnight at 4°C on top of a 10 to 30% alkaline
glycerol gradient containing 0.1 M NaOH and 0.9 M NaCl in
a SW 27 tube.   Centrifugation was at 25,000 rpm for 5
hours at 4°.   The gradients were fractionated from the top
of the tubes and C-RNA hybridizations were carried out for
each fraction after measurement of OD260.   C-RNA
hybridization specific to EBV DNA was described previously
(6).   ●-● c-RNA hybridization, o-o OD260.

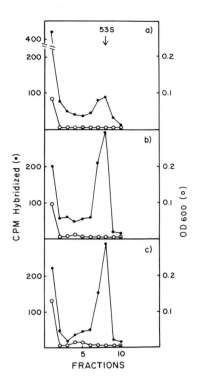

Fig. 2.   Latent EBV DNA in a neutral glycerol gradient 10^6 Raji cells were treated with 1% sarkosyl and 0.025 M EDTA pH 7.4 (a) or with 1% sarkosyl, 0.025 M EDTA pH 7.4 and 1 mg/ml of pronase (**b**) for 12 hours at 37°. Simpson cells mixed with EBV were treated with sarkosyl-EDTA-pronase (c) for 12 hours at 37°. The lysates were poured onto 5 to 10% glycerol gradient cushioned with 20% glycerol, all containing tris 0.01 M and EDTA 0.001 M, pH 7.4 in Corex 30 ml centrifuge tubes. The centrifugations were at 12,500 rpm for 12 hours at 4°C in a JS-13 rotor in a Beckman J-21 centrifuge. The gradients were fractionated from the bottom of the tubes through an inserted glass tubing by suction. Each fraction (3 ml) was treated with 1.0 N NaOH for 5 hours at 37° and DNA was fixed onto a nitrocellulose filter after neutralization. C-RNA hybridization was carried out for each fraction and DNA concentration on the filters was determined by diphenylamine test. ●-● C-RNA hybridization, o-o OD600 for diphenylamine reaction.

512

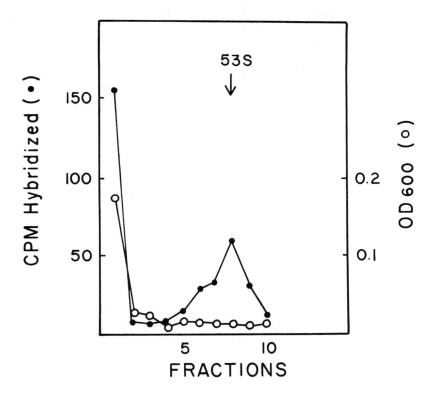

Fig. 3. Recentrifugation of large molecular weight cell DNA fraction. Large molecular weight cell DNA fraction (bottom tube) as in Figure 2b was diluted with tris, 0.01 M, 0.001 M EDTA pH 7.4 and recentrifuged through the same type of the gradient as in Figure 2. Each fraction was hybridized with EBV specific C-RNA. DNA concentration was determined on the filters by diphenylamine after the hybridization. ●-● C-RNA hybridization, o-o OD600 for diphenylamine reaction.

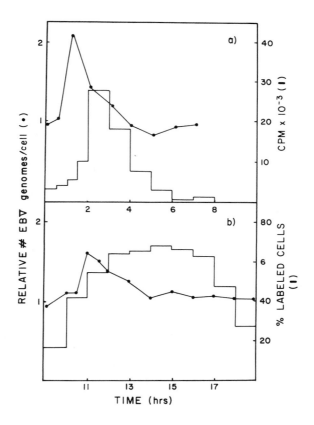

Fig. 4. Replication of latent EBV DNA in synchronized Raji cells. Raji cells were synchronized by double
thymidine block as previously described (20) and
thymidine-H^3 uptake determination and c-RNA hybridization
were carried out for each period. C-RNA hybridization
values were expressed in relative numbers; 50 genomes per
cell obtained for a random culture of Raji cells (6) was
taken as an unit of relative number. a) first S phase,
b) second S phase.

514

THE ONCOGENIC POTENTIAL OF HUMAN HERPESVIRUS

Ronald Duff and Fred Rapp

Department of Microbiology
The Milton S. Hershey Medical Center
The Pennsylvania State University
Hershey, Pennsylvania 17033

ABSTRACT. The in vitro transformation of normal cells
into oncogenic cells by human herpesvirus is dependent
upon inhibition of the lytic potential of the virus. This
inhibition can be accomplished by inactivation of the
virus genome (UV-irradiation or photodynamic inactivation)
or selection of a cell type which is only partially permissive for the replicative cycle of the infectious
herpesvirus. These techniques have been used to demonstrate that herpes simplex virus type 1 (HSV-1), herpes
simplex virus type 2 (HSV-2) and human cytomegalovirus
have the potential to transform normal hamster embryo
fibroblast (HEF) cells into cells with oncogenic potential.
HSV-1 and HSV-2 have transformed normal HEF into cells with
either a fibroblastic morphology or an epithelial
morphology. Fibroblastic cells induced fibrosarcomas
and epithelial cells induced adenocarcinomas when injected
into newborn Syrian hamsters. Both cell types contained
HSV-specific antigens before injection into the host
hamster and the antigens were conserved after animal
passage of the tumor cells. The results directly implicate
human herpesviruses in the oncogenic transformation of
normal cells and provide a model system with which to
study the characteristics of an oncogenic virus utilizing
the in vitro transformed cells in an experimental animal.

INTRODUCTION

Human herpesviruses have been implicated in cancer by
a variety of experimental methods. An extensively studied
herpesvirus of human origin is the Epstein-Barr (EB) virus
which was originally identified in and isolated from
Burkitt's lymphoma cells (1,2). Further studies have
demonstrated that a correlation exists between the presence and levels of circulating antibody directed against

the EB virus and the prognosis of the disease in patients
with Burkitt's lymphoma (3,4,5). EB virus has been
implicated as the causative agent of infectious mononucleosis (6) and has also been found to transform primate leukocytes in tissue culture (7,8,9,10). The injection of EB
virus into marmosets induces a lymphoma in the experimental
animal and further implicates this virus in the induction
of the human tumor (11). However, the question of why
EB virus induces a malignant lymphoma in some humans
within a geographically defined area and the non-mali-
gnant infectious mononucleosis in a second geographical
area has not yet been determined. It is likely that some
co-factor is necessary, either to inhibit or enhance the
oncogenic potential of the virus.

A second group of human herpesviruses which has been
associated with cancer are the herpes simplex viruses. Two
distinct types of herpes simplex viruses can be identified
based upon the site of isolation within the host (12,13).
Herpes simplex virus type 1 (HSV-1) has been isolated most
frequently from the oral region and has been implicated
in several cancers of the oral region. Herpes simplex
virus type 2 (HSV-2) has been isolated most frequently
from the genital region and as a result has been most
strongly associated with carcinoma of the cervix.

The initial evidence which associated HSV and cancer
was the casual observation by physicians that tumors often
appeared at sites which were previously occupied by a
herpetic lesion (14). The next step was the epidemiolog-
ical demonstration that patients with cervical cancer had
a higher history of herpetic lesions of the genital area
than did individuals without cervical cancer (15,16,17).
Additional experiments enhanced the relationship of HSV to
cervical cancer by demonstrating that cervical carcinoma
patients had a significally increased incidence of antibody directed against HSV-2 than did matched controls (18,
19,20). This correlation has been confirmed by several
investigators in independent laboratories among most populations studied.

The relationship of HSV-2 to cervical cancer was
strengthened by additional studies that identified herpesvirus antigens in exfoliated cervical carcinoma cells and

isolated the virus from similar cells (21,22). Subsequently, it was demonstrated that HSV-2-specific DNA could be identified in a cervical tumor by DNA hybridization techniques (23). However, the results described above have not yet been independently confirmed in other laboratories and the possibility of a prior nonrelated infection in the host or an accidental laboratory contamination can not be excluded.

Recently, several laboratories have reported the identification of antibodies directed against a non-virion or early herpesvirus antigen in the sera of patients with several types of cancer including cancer of the lip, mouth, oropharynx, nasopharynx, bladder, vulva, cervix, kidney and prostate (24,25,26,27,28). Control sera from individuals with high neutralizing antibody titers did not contain detectable antibodies against the early antigens. These observations demonstrated that the prolonged exposure of the individual to the tumor resulted in the stimulation of a humoral immune response specifically directed against a herpes simplex virus induced antigen and as a result strongly associates herpes simplex virus with a variety of human cancers.

The final method which has been used to link herpesviruses and cancer is the transformation of cells in tissue culture by herpesviruses, followed by the demonstration of the oncogenicity of transformed cells in compatible experimental animals. This approach, which has been repeated in several laboratories using hamster, mouse, human and rat cells (29,30,31,32,33,34), will be the subject of the remainder of this paper.

METHODS OF TRANSFORMATION BY HERPESVIRUSES

Herpes simplex virus is extremely lytic in most cell systems. Therefore, the rapid cell death induced by the virus infection must be inhibited to enable the detection of cellular transforming potential. Three methods have been used in this laboratory designed to inhibit the lytic cycle of HSV. These methods (UV-irradiation, photodynamic inactivation and cell mediated resistance) are outlined in Figure 1. The inactivation of HSV by UV-irradiation has been studied most extensively (29,30,31,32,35) and is a simple but efficient way to partially inactivate the virus genome, removing lytic activity without removing transforming activity. In addition to the demonstration of the transforming potential of HSV using this method, human cytomegalovirus has been found to induce the transformation of hamster cells after UV-irradiation of the virus (36).

The growth of HSV-1 and HSV-2 in the presence of neutral red followed by the exposure of the virus to fluorescent light also resulted in the partial inactivation of the virus. Treatment of hamster embryo fibroblast (HEF) cells with this photodynamically inactivated virus induced the oncogenic transformation of these cells (37). Recently, this technique of virus inactivation has been used as a therapeutic treatment for recurrent herpes simplex infections (38). However the observation that such treatment can render the inactivated virus potentially oncogenic necessitates a re-evaluation of the usefulness of photodynamic inactivation as a therapeutic measure.

The two methods previously mentioned are dependent upon the physical inactivation of the virus genome before infection of the host cell. Without virus inactivation the cell would be destroyed and obviously no transformation detectable. This type of system is of necessity somewhat artificial. Therefore, a system utilizing non-inactivated herpesvirus was developed. A hamster cell line (2-cT-1a) previously transformed by the PARA (defective SV40)-adenovirus 7 hybrid was found to be highly resistant to infection with HSV-2. However, HSV-2 specific antigens could be detected by immunofluorescence techniques in 2-cT-1a cells soon after virus infection. The cells infected by HSV-2 remained viable and were passaged several times without release of detectable virus. At that time the HSV-2 infected cells were found to be morphology distinct from the parental 2-cT-1a cells indicating that these cells were transformed by HSV-2 in addition to the initial transformation by the PARA-adenovirus 7 hybrid. Similar results using rat cells doubly transformed by an oncornavirus and HSV have also been recently described by other investigators (34).

MORPHOLOGY OF CELLS TRANSFORMED BY HERPESVIRUS

The majority of virus-transformation systems have been concerned exclusively with cells of a fibroblastic morphology. Initially most hamster cells isolated after transformation with inactivated herpesviruses were predominantly fibroblastic (29,30,35). However, hamster cells with a definite epithelial morphology have been described after transformation by HSV-1 (31). Recently a similar epithelial morphology has been observed in some hamster cells transformed by UV-irradiated HSV-2. The comparative morphological features of cells transformed by HSV-1 and HSV-2 are shown in Figure 2 and Figure 3.

Whether the morphologically distinct type of cell after transformation by HSV is a result of different target cells within the heterologous HEF cell population or is a result of a multi-potential of the genome of the transforming virus has not been determined with certainty. However, the 2-cT-1a cell line was derived from a single cell isolate which was originally fibroblastic. Following transformation with HSV-2 the resultant cells were primarily epithelial in morphology (Figure 4). More recently, results using a clonal line of the mouse 3T3 cells have also indicated a multi-potential for transformed cell morphology within the transforming HSV genome. Transformed 3T3 cells can be identified and isolated after HSV-2 injection with either an epithelial or fibroblastic morphology (Duff, unpublished observations). Therefore, preliminary evidence supports the hypothesis that HSV-2 has the potential to induce epithelial or fibroblastic transformation in a homologous cell population.

ONCOGENIC CHARACTERISTICS OF

HERPESVIRUS TRANSFORMED HAMSTER CELLS

The morphological transformation of HEF cells by inactivated HSV-1 or HSV-2 does not mean that all transformed cells acquire oncogenic potential (11). When tested in HEF cells 11 out of 21 HSV-2 strains, or 52%, induced transformation. However, only 3 of 21 HSV-2 strains (14%) induced oncogenic conversion of the HEF cells. Similar results have been obtained with HSV-1 with the exception

that both transforming potential (4 of 22 or 18%) and
oncogenic conversion potential (1 of 22 or 5%) are reduced
when HSV-1 is compared to HSV-2 (39). Furthermore, the
potential of oncogenic conversion is not randomly distributed among all virus strains but is concentrated to a
limited number of HSV strains which can consistently transform normal cells into cells which have oncogenic potential.

The type of tumor induced by an oncogenic cell line of
HSV transformed cells depends upon the morphology of the
in vitro cell. Fibroblastic cells induced fibrosarcomas
after the injection of 2 X 10^5 cells into a newborn hamster (Figure 5). Under the same conditions, in vitro transformed cells with an epithelial morphology induced adenocarcinomas (Figure 5). At the present time both types of
tumors have been obtained using HSV-2 transformed cells.
Only epithelial tumors have been obtained using HSV-1 transformed cells. Whether this difference represents a real
difference or an artificial difference due to the limited
number of cell lines tested is not known at present; however, experiments are now in progress designed to answer
this question.

Cell lines transformed with either HSV-1 or HSV-2 contained virus-specific antigens in the cytoplasm of the
transformed cells. These antigens were detectable by
immunofluorescence techniques (Figure 6). Similar antigens
were detected in tissue culture grown cells obtained from
tumors induced by the injection of HSV transformed cells
and the antigens persisted in the transformed cells through
at least 5 passages in weanling hamsters.

Tumor-bearing hamsters also developed HSV-specific
neutralizing antibodies in their sera. These antibodies
could be detected in the sera of hamsters with tumors
induced by HSV transformed cells that had been previously
passed 5 times in a weanling hamster (Figure 7). The
specificity of the neutralizing antibodies induced in the
tumor bearing hamsters is dependent upon the type of virus
used to initially transform the HEF cells in vitro (30,31).
Antibodies resulting from tumors induced by cells transformed by HSV-2 were specific for the neutralization of
HSV-2. However, antibodies induced in tumors induced

520

after the induction of tumors with HSV-1 transformed
cells neutralized HSV-1 and HSV-2 with a nearly equal
efficiency (Figure 8).

An additional characteristic of tumors induced by HSV
transformed cells is the ability of these tumors to rapidly invade surrounding tissue in the host animal and to
metastasize to distal organs. Both fibrosarcomas and
adenocarcinomas rapidly invaded surrounding tissue (Figure
9) and metastasized to the lungs and kidneys (Figure
10). However, only cells from an adenocarcinoma have
been observed to metastasize through the lymphatic system
of the host hamster.

DISCUSSION

The conversion of normal cells into transformed cells
by human herpesviruses is a technique which has been repeated in several laboratories by several independent investigators using several cell types (29,30,31,32,33,34).
The success of this technique depends upon the inhibition
of the lytic potential of the virus. Such inhibition can
be accomplished either by direct inactivation of the virus
genome or the use of a partially susceptible cell type.
Whether either type of mechanism plays a role in the
natural induction of human neoplasia is a matter for spec-
ulation and further research.

In addition to the demonstration of oncogenic potential
by human herpesviruses one major contribution of the in
vitro transformation system has been the development of
model systems with which to study carcinomas.
Most viral induced transformation and/or the resulting
tumor do not closely resemble natural neoplasms. After
injection into the host animal oncogenic HSV transformed
cells behave very much like a naturally occurring tumor.
The cells are extremely invasive, and as many as 70%
metastasize under reproducible conditions (40). Such
systems should prove invaluable for the study and characterization of tumor growth using a defined system in an
experimental animal.

ACKNOWLEDGEMENTS

This study was conducted under Contract No. 70-2024 within the Virus Cancer Program of the National Cancer Institute, National Institutes of Health, U.S. Public Health Service.

REFERENCES

1. Epstein, M.A., Achong, B.G. and Barr, Y.M., Lancet 1, 702 (1964).
2. Epstein, M.A., Barr, Y.M. and Achong, B.G., Pathol. Biol. (Paris) 12, 1233 (1964).
3. Henle, G. and Henle, W., J. Bacteriol. 91, 1248 (1966).
4. Henle, G., Henle, W., Klein, G., Gunven, P., Clifford, P., Morrow, R.H. and Ziegler, J.L., J. Nat. Cancer Inst. 46, 861 (1971).
5. Henle, W. and Henle, G., Cancer Res. 33, 1419 (1973).
6. Henle, W. and Henle, G., In Oncogenesis and Herpes- viruses, Lyon, France: International Agency for Research Cancer, WHD (P.M., Biggs, G. De-The and L.N. Payne, eds) 269 (1971).
7. Pope, J.H., Hoine, M.K. and Scott, W., Int. J. Cancer 3, 857 (1968).
8. Chang, R.S., Hsieh, M. and Blankenship, W.J., Nat. Cancer Inst. 47, 479 (1971).
9. Miller, G., Lisco, H., Kohn, H.I. and Stitt, D., Proc. Soc. Exp. Biol. Med. 137, 1459 (1971).
10. Miller, G., Shope, T., Lisco, H., Stitt, D. and Lipman, M., Proc. Nat. Acad. Sci. 69, 383 (1972).
11. Shope, T., Dechairo, D. and Miller, G., Proc. Nat. Acad. Sci. 70, 2487 (1973).
12. Dowdle, W.R., Nahmias, A.J., Harwell, R.W. and Pauls, F.P., J. Immunol. 99, 974 (1967).
13. Pauls, F.P. and Dowdle, W.R., J. Immunol. 98, 941 (1967).
14. Wyburn-Mason, R., British Med. Journal 2, 615 (1957).
15. Naib, Z., Nahmias, A. and Josey, W., Cancer 19, 1026 (1966).
16. Naib, Z., Nahmias, A., Josey, W. and Krawer, J., Cancer 23, 940 (1969).
17. Rawls, W.E., Tompkins, W.A.F., Figueroa, M. and

Melnick, J.L., Science <u>161</u>, 1255 (1968).

18. Nahmias, A.J., Josey, W.E., Naib, Z.M., Luce, C.F. and Guest, B.A., Amer. J. Epidemiol. <u>91</u>, 547 (1970).

19. Rawls, W.E., Tompkins, W.A.F. and Melnick, J.L., Amer. J. Epidemiol. <u>89</u>, 547 (1969).

20. Royston, I. and Aurelian, L., Amer. J. Epidemiol. <u>91</u>, 531 (1970).

21. Royston, I. and Aurelian, L., Proc. Nat. Acad. Sci. <u>67</u>, 204 (1972).

22. Aurelian, L., Strandberg, J.D., Melendez, L.V. and Johnson, L.A., Science <u>174</u>, 704 (1971).

23. Frenkel, N., Roizman, B., Cassai, E. and Nahmias, A.J., Proc. Nat. Acad. Sci. <u>69</u>, 3784 (1972).

24. Aurelian, L., Schumann, B., Marcus, R.L. and Davis, H.J., Science <u>181</u>, 161 (1973).

25. Hollinshead, A.C., Lee, O., Chretien, P.B., Tarpley, J.L., Rawls, W.E. and Adam, E., Science <u>182</u>, 713 (1973).

26. Tarro, G. and Sabin, A.B., Proc. Nat. Acad. Sci. <u>65</u>, 753 (1970).

27. Tarro, G. and Sabin, A.B., Proc. Nat. Acad. Sci. <u>70</u>, 1032 (1973).

28. Sabin, A.B. and Tarro, G., Proc. Nat. Acad. Sci. <u>70</u>, 3225 (1973).

29. Duff, R. and Rapp, F., Nature (New Biol.) <u>233</u>, 48 (1971).

30. Duff, R. and Rapp, F., J. Virol. <u>8</u>, 469 (1971).

31. Duff, R. and Rapp, F., J. Virol. <u>12</u>, 209 (1973).

32. Munyon, W., Kraiselburd, E., Davis, D. and Mann, J., J. Virol. <u>7</u>, 813 (1971).

33. Darai, B. and Munk, K., Nature (New Biol.) <u>241</u>, 265 (1973).

34. Garfinkle, B. and McAuslan, B.R., Proc. Nat. Acad. Sci. <u>71</u>, 220 (1974).

35. Duff, R. and Rapp, F., Gustav Stern. Symp. <u>Perspectives</u> Virol. VIII, <u>189</u> (1973).

36. Albrecht, T. and Rapp, F., Virology <u>55</u>, 53 (1973).

37. Rapp, F., Li, J.H. and Jerkofsky, M., Virology <u>55</u>, 339 (1973).

38. Moore, C., Wallis, C., Melnick, J.L. and Kuns, M.D., Infect. Immunol. <u>5</u>, 169 (1972).

39. Rapp, F. and Duff, R., Cancer, in press.

40. Duff, R., Doller, E. and Rapp, F., Science <u>180</u>, 79 (1973).

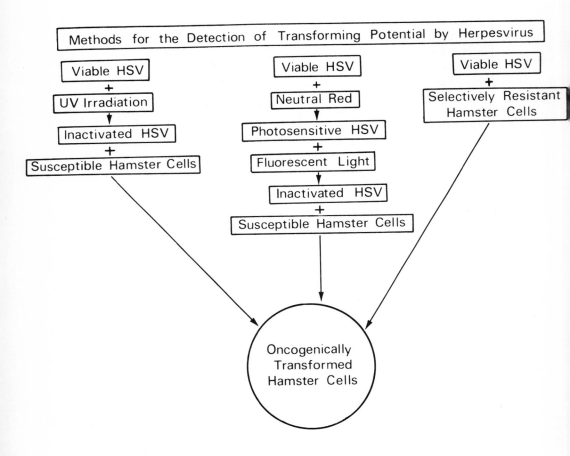

Fig. 1.

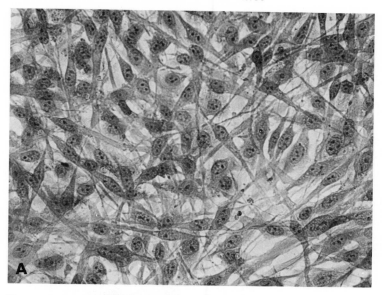

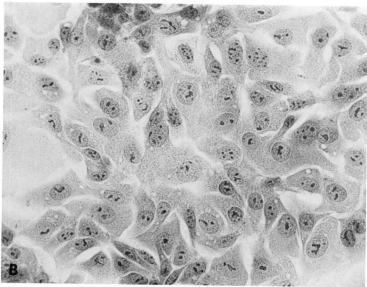

Fig. 2. Photomicrograph of hamster embryo cells transformed after infection by HSV-1. Cells with a fibroblastic morphology (A) and cells with an epithelial morphology (B) were stained with hematoxylin and eosin. X300.

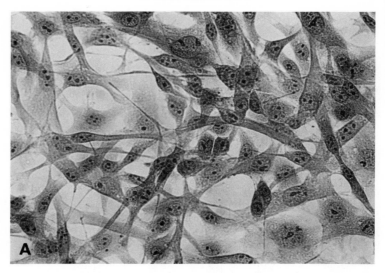

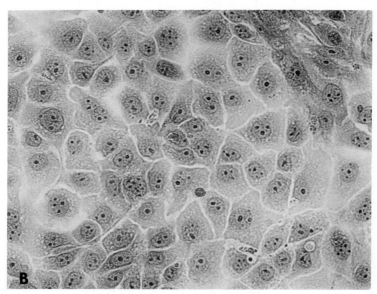

Fig. 3.   Photomicrograph of hamster embryo cells transformed after infection by HSV-2.   Cells with a fibroblastic morphology (A) and cells with an epithelial morphology (B) were stained with hematoxylin and eosin.   X300.

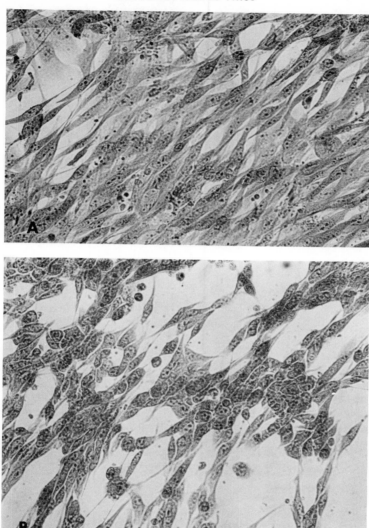

Fig. 4. Photomicrograph of transformed hamster embryo cells. Cells transformed by the PARA (defective SV40)-adenovirus 7 hybrid (A) and cells transformed initially by the PARA-adenovirus 7 hybrid, followed by transformation with HSV-2 (B) were stained with hematoxylin and eosin. X300.

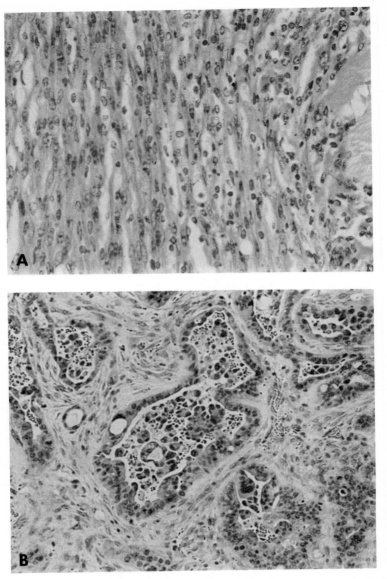

Fig. 5. Photomicrograph of cells from a tumor induced in a newborn hamster after the injection of HSV-1 or HSV-2 transformed cells. Cells transformed by HSV-2 induced tumors identified as fibrosarcomas (A). Cells transformed by HSV-1 induced tumors identified as adenocarcinomas (B). Cells were stained with hematoxylin and eosin. X300.

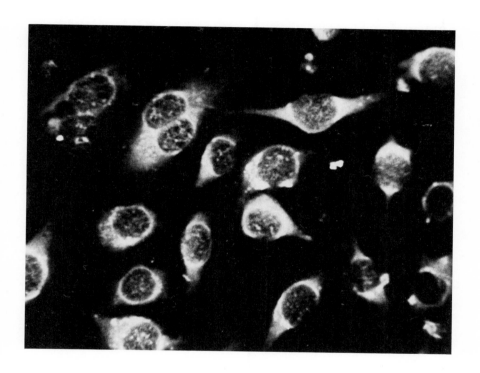

Fig. 6. Immunofluorescent photomicrograph of HSV specific antigens in the cytoplasm of cells transformed by UV-irradiated HSV-2. X450.

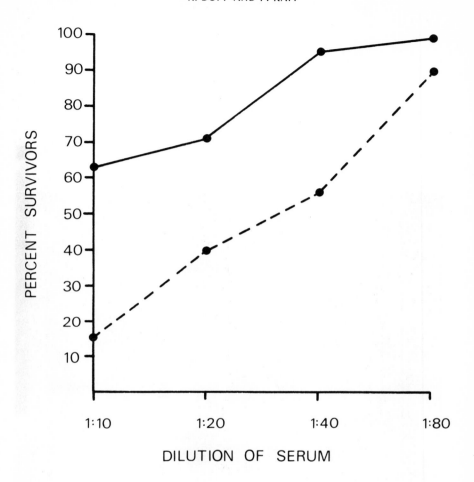

Fig. 7. Neutralization of HSV-1 (——) and HSV-2 (---) by sera from tumor bearing hamsters. Tumors were induced after the injection of HSV-2 transformed hamster cells. The cells that were used to induce the tumors in weanling hamsters had been previously passed 5 times in weanling hamsters. The results are expressed as the percent of 1000 infectious HSV particles which survived incubation with the antiserum for 40 min at 37°C.

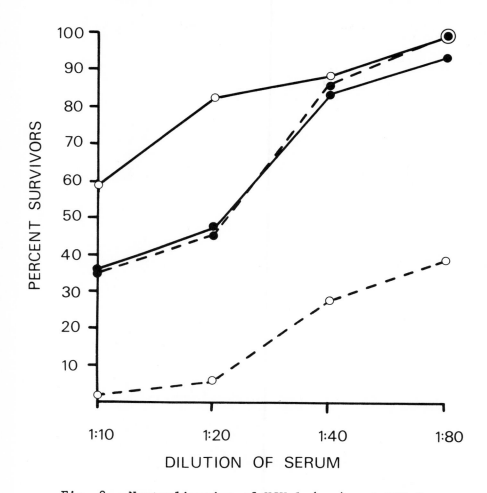

Fig. 8. Neutralization of HSV-1 (——) and HSV-2 (---) by sera from hamsters with tumors induced by the injection of HSV transformed cells. The tumors were induced by HSV-1 transformed hamster cells (●) or HSV-2 transformed hamster cells (○). The results are expressed as the percent of 1000 infectious HSV particles which survived incubation with the antiserum for 40 min at 37°C.

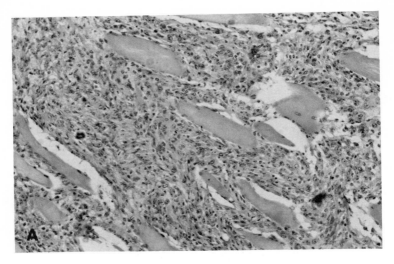

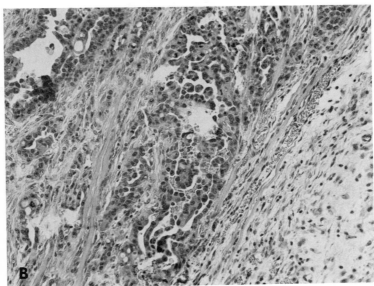

Fig. 9.   Photomicrograph of cells from tumors
induced by HSV transformed cells.   Fig. 9A illustrates the invasion of normal muscle fibers by
fibrosarcoma cells originally transformed by HSV-2.
Fig. 9B illustrates the invasion of muscle fibers
by adenocarcinoma cells originally transformed by
HSV-1.   The primary tumor in both animals was induced by a dorsal subcutaneous injection of a
weanling hamster with 10^5 viable cells.   Stained
with hematoxylin and eosin.   X120.

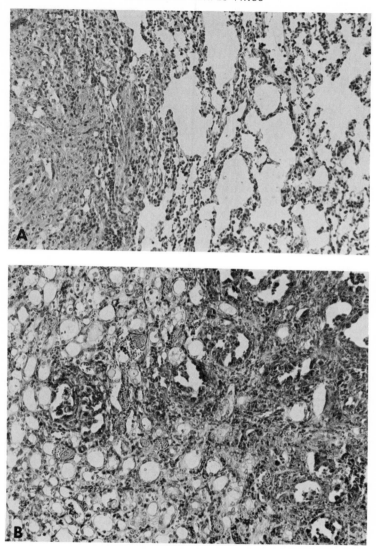

Fig. 10.   Photomicrograph of cells from metastatic tumors initially induced by the injection of HSV transformed cells.   Fig. 10A illustrates a lung metastasis from cells transformed by HSV-2.   Fig. 10B illustrates a kidney metastasis of cells transformed by HSV-1. The primary tumor in both animals was induced by a dorsal subcutaneous injection of a weanling hamster with 10^5 viable cells.   Stained with hematoxylin and eosin.   X120.

SUBJECT INDEX

Genetically controlled
    resistance, 147
Genomes,
    latent, 505
    polyploid, 287
    virus, 515
Group B arbovirus, 147
Growth, serum requirement,
    262
Growth control, 261
H-2 type, 41
HA polypeptide, 347
HB$_{core}$Ag, 245
HEp-2 cells, 455
HSV-specific antigens, 515
Halogenated pyrimidines, 49
Hamsters, 203
Hamster embryo fibroblast
    (HEF) cell, 515
Heat-dissociated 60-70s
    RNA, 288
"Helper effect" of SV40 for
    adenovirus growth,
    259
Helper phage, 385
Hemagglutination inhibiting
    antibody, 191
Hemagglutinin, particle-
    associated, 191
Hemagglutinin polypeptide,
    347
Hemophilus influenzae re-
    striction endonu-
    clease preparations,
    190
Hepatitis B
    antigen, 215
    virus, 243
    virus candidate, 225
Hepatocytes, 245, 247
Herpes saimiri, 439
Herpes simplex 1, 456, 515
Herpes simplex 2, 515
Herpes simplex virus, 455,
    515

Herpes simplex virus growth
    cycle, 460
Herpesvirus, frog renal
    tumor, 493
Heterotypic interference,
    107
Hexose transport, 327
Hodgkin's disease, compli-
    cation of, 188
Host genes, 69
Host range marker (leuko-
    sis virus), 287, 288
    289
Host restriction, 69
Human
    amnion cells, 280
    cytomegalovirus, 515
    fetal brain cells, 191
    fetal glial cells, 193
    herpesvirus, 515
    papovirus, 190
    S+L- cells, 273, 280
Hydrocephalus, 161
Hydroxyurea, 468
Immortalization, 432
Immune complexes, 19
Immune precipitation, 478
Immune response,
    cell mediated, 25, 189
    disease producing, 19
Immunity, 134
    to superinfection, 386
Immunofluorescence, 245
Immunology, 25
Immunosuppression, 187, 203,
    427, 435
Immunosuppressive drugs,
    187
In vitro latent infection,
    200
In vitro transformation,
    515
Inability to assemble outer
    coat peptides, 161
Inclusion bodies, 87

538